DooH005.

Nursing Research

DATE DUE			

Nursing Research

Principles, Process and Issues

SECOND EDITION

Kader Parahoo

palgrave
macmillan

First edition 1997
Second edition 2006 published

First published 1997 by
PALGRAVE MACMILLAN

Palgrave Macmillan in the UK is an imprint of Macmillan Publishers Limited,
registered in England, company number 785998, of Houndmills, Basingstoke,
Hampshire RG21 6XS.

Palgrave Macmillan in the US is a division of St Martin's Press LLC,
175 Fifth Avenue, New York, NY 10010.

Palgrave Macmillan is the global academic imprint of the above companies
and has companies and representatives throughout the world.

Palgrave® and Macmillan® are registered trademarks in the United States,
the United Kingdom, Europe and other countries

ISBN-13: 978–0–333–98727–8
ISBN 10: 0–333–98727–6

This book is printed on paper suitable for recycling and made from fully
managed and sustained forest sources. Logging, pulping and manufacturing
processes are expected to conform to the environmental regulations of the
country of origin

A catalogue record for this book is available from the British Library.

10   9   8   7
15   14   13   12   11   10   09

Printed in China

Contents

List of Research Examples

List of Figures and Tables

Figures

Tables

Preface to the Second Edition

Writing a second edition is like making improvements to a house built many years ago. While recognising the need for change, one must be careful not to alter the character and purpose of the original building. So it is with this book.

Almost nine years on, nursing research has developed rapidly. There are more journals, books, conferences, workshops and courses on research. There is now greater emphasis on evidence-based practice, systematic reviews, research governance, the dissemination and utilisation of research, multi-disciplinary collaboration and the combination of different methods in the same study. There is more evidence of research on methodology and of a higher level of methodological discussions in nursing and other journals. On-line access to databases, electronic journals and other information have brought research nearer to the workplace and to the home! All these changes needed to be reflected in this new edition to keep readers up to date.

While the structure of the book has been maintained, three new chapters have been added (Chapter 4: 'Qualitative Research', Chapter 5: 'Combining Quantitative and Qualitative Methods', and Chapter 19: 'Evidence-based Practice').

A number of other chapters have been substantially enhanced. These include Chapter 3 on quantitative research, Chapter 6 which now includes an expanded section on ethical issues and research governance, Chapter 7 on systematic reviews, and Chapter 18 where more discussion has been devoted to strategies for translating research into practice. The rest of the book has been updated, in particular the research examples. It is hoped that the expanded glossary and a more extensive index will facilitate readers to navigate their way and increase their understanding of research.

I was encouraged by, and grateful for, the feedback I received from readers of the first edition, in particular, from students in different parts of the United Kingdom and beyond. The positive response was unexpected and overwhelming. To them I dedicate this book.

As usual there are a number of people to whom I owe a debt of gratitude. They are Julie Cummins, Kate Thompson, Jerome Marley and Sharon McCaffrey. I am grateful to, and appreciate the contribution of, the anonymous reviewers whose comments have helped to enhance the quality of the final product. I am deeply indebted to Eilís whose unflinching support and love made the load a lot lighter. My children Roisín, Yasmin and Ciarán (the last two are additions since the first edition) have been remarkably tolerant when I have been lost in thought or simply 'busy' in the study. I hope the effort is worthwhile.

K.P.

Introduction

The International Council of Nurses (2005) provides the following definition of Nursing:

> **Nursing** encompasses autonomous and collaborative care of individuals of all ages, families, groups and communities, sick or well and in all settings. Nursing includes the promotion of health, prevention of illness, and the care of ill, disabled and dying people. Advocacy, promotion of a safe environment, research, participation in shaping health policy and in patient and health systems management, and education are also key nursing roles.

There is significant scope and potential for research to inform all these areas of policy, practice and education. The extent to which this is achieved depends on how nurses perceive their role in research. This is likely to vary according to the levels at which they practise. First-level (qualified) nurses are expected to be able to search for and evaluate the relevant evidence to inform their decisions and actions.

By questioning their practice, they should be able to identify problems and issues which require research investigation. Nurses need to understand the ethical implications of different methodologies in order to be in a better position to protect patients from potential harm when participating in research and to safeguard their rights.

To do this, they must first acquire the necessary skills and knowledge. There is sometimes a naïve view that they can start critiquing research articles without a prior knowledge of the basics of research. One student, when asked to critique a research article after a two-hour introduction to research, remarked that 'the cart was being put in front of the horse'. No one would dare attempt a sociological analysis without first learning concepts such as class, socialisation and social structure.

This book is written mainly for those who have little or no prior knowledge of research. It is intended to equip them with a comprehensive understanding of the concepts and principles of nursing research so that they can begin to read research critically. Postgraduate students will also find sections of the book useful.

The code of professional conduct of the Nursing and Midwifery Council (NMC) of the United Kingdom states that professional nurses, midwives and health visitors have 'a responsibility to deliver care based on current evidence, best practice, and where applicable, validated research when it is available' (NMC, 2004).

Of necessity, this book provides only a basic introduction to the principles, process and issues in nursing research, as it is intended for beginners. Each chapter could be expanded into one or more books and their topics can be discussed from a number of different perspectives to illustrate how they vary. The challenge in writing this book was to keep things simple enough to attract the interest of those who want or need to gain a basic understanding of research. No doubt readers will want to know more. For this, there are whole books written on, for example, interviewing, randomised controlled trials or grounded theory. One of the key features in this book is the list of references at the end of each chapter which provide examples of 'real' research and discussions of key issues.

Content and layout

This book opens with a discussion of the relationship between research and practice. It puts research in the context of other ways of knowing, such as intuition, tradition and experience, as well as the potential contribution of research to clinical effectiveness and to the development of nursing as a profession. Chapter 2 offers an exploration of the philosophical roots of research approaches. It puts research in perspective (in relation to other belief systems). It helps to explain how research has become a dominant form of knowledge production, and how our perception of reality or truth and the means to study them can influence our choice of approaches and methods. Unavoidably, a large number of concepts and issues are introduced at this stage. They are, however, dealt with further throughout the book. For example, concepts such as induction, deduction, validity and reliability are fully integrated in the text.

What constitutes nursing research and research evidence is itself problematic. There are different perspectives on research, on how it should be carried out and on its actual and potential benefits. The debate about the value of quantitative and qualitative approaches to nursing has been going on for the last 30 years. Although such discussions are considered to be outdated, these terms continue to be used in the nursing and health research literature. This book deals with many of the issues raised in this debate. The potential contribution of both approaches is compared and contrasted, and the benefits and drawbacks of mixing them are explored. The strengths and weaknesses of a range of methodologies, in particular research methods, are also discussed. These issues are dealt with in Chapters 3, 4 and 5.

The rest of the chapters follow closely the stages of the research process. Chapter 6 gives an insight into the process of different types of research as well as the main ethical implications of doing research with humans. These issues are further raised at relevant points in the book. Chapters 7 and 8 explore the meaning and processes of literature reviews and the relationship between theory and research in quantitative and qualitative studies, while Chapter 9 deals with the formulation of questions and operational definitions.

Although a range of research designs is discussed in Chapter 10, experimental and quasi-experimental designs are given a separate and lengthy treatment in Chapter 11. The current emphasis on the evaluation of, and comparisons between, treatment programmes have focused attention on a lesser-used design in nursing research – that of the randomised controlled trial (RCT). The strengths and weaknesses of the RCT, as well as its appropriateness for the study of nursing phenomena, are also considered.

Data collection methods, samples and sampling techniques are described and discussed in Chapters 12, 13, 14 and 15, while Chapters 16 and 17 are designed to help readers make sense of research findings.

The utilisation of research in practice warrants a chapter on its own. Chapter 18 examines the evidence relating to factors which facilitate or impede research utilisation. It also discusses the strategies and theories for addressing the complexity of change in clinical practice. The book ends with a critical look at the concept of evidence-based practice, and its relevance to nursing.

One of the main features of the book is the use of examples to explain abstract concepts. In these Research Examples (boxed), the relevant parts of the articles are described or quoted, and are followed by comments designed to illustrate concepts or issues raised in the text. Therefore they should be treated as part of the text. These excerpts stand on their own, but readers who may wish to read the original articles will not find them difficult to access. The rationale for using real examples is that one useful way to learn about research is to find out how research studies are carried out.

Finally, in an attempt to avoid the clumsy and inelegant form 'she/he', the female gender is used in this book to refer to researchers. The flipping of a coin was the 'scientific' strategy used to select the pronoun. It is, of course, acknowledged that researchers are both men and women.

To conclude, this book is not designed to teach how to do research but to help readers to acquire a thorough and comprehensive understanding of research principles, concepts, processes and issues in order to be able to read research critically. The view taken here is that both qualitative and quantitative approaches have a contribution to make towards advancing knowledge. Research is put in the context of other ways of knowing. Throughout this book, both the potential benefits of research and the danger of blind faith in research findings are emphasised.

References

International Council of Nurses (2005) http://www.icn.ch/definition.htm, accessed 1 February 2005.

Nursing and Midwifery Council (2004) *The NMC Code of Professional Conduct: Standards for Conduct, Performance and Ethics* (London: Nursing and Midwifery Council).

1 Research and Nursing Practice

▶ Research without practice is like building castles in the air. Practice without research is building castles on slippery grounds.

Introduction

This introductory chapter will examine the sources of knowledge for practice, and the meaning of, and rationale for nursing research. The role of nurses in research and the relationship between research and practice will be explored. Finally a brief overview of the development of nursing research worldwide will be offered.

Sources of knowledge for nursing practice

Much has been written about the variety of sources of knowledge from which practitioners draw. Of these the main ones are tradition, intuition, experience and research.

Traditional knowledge

The bulk of our knowledge has been accumulated over centuries and passed down to us through literature, art, music, oral history and other such media. Traditional nursing knowledge is learnt mainly from books and journals, by word of mouth and by observing the practice of others. Much traditional practice takes the form of rituals. For example, it may be tradition in some hospitals that patients are routinely shaved before an operation. This ritual is performed consistently with little thought to the rationale behind it. Walsh and Ford (1990) explain:

> Ritual action implies carrying out a task without thinking it through in a prob-
> lem-solving, logical way. The nurse does something because this is the way it
> has always been done. Perhaps actions have become enshrined in the holy

tablets of stone known as the procedure book, or just: 'This is the way Sister likes it done'. Either way, the nurse does not have to think about the problem and work out an individual solution; the action is ritual.

O'Brien and Davison (1994), referring to the routine taking of blood pressure 'at fixed and pre-determined times unrelated to the clinical status of the individual patients', suggest what such practices mean to practitioners:

> Once established, such rituals readily became part of the nursing culture and provided comfort and certainty to nurses in their daily work. It is not surprising that nurses are reluctant to challenge cherished and established approaches to practice, especially when the alternatives demand individualised considerations, notions of appropriate clinical decision making and professional accountability.

Traditions are important not only in passing down knowledge, but also in giving groups in society a sense of identity, belonging and pride. Through socialisation, we learn the culture of those who have gone before us. Similarly, traditional nursing knowledge and practice are learnt by novice nurses through the process of socialisation in educational institutions and clinical areas. Much of this traditional knowledge and many ritual practices are the outcomes of sound reasoning. Today's new knowledge and practices will likewise eventually become traditional. The term 'traditional' is sometimes used in a negative sense, meaning backward, outdated or unprogressive. Knowledge in itself is harmless; it is the use people make of it which can be harmful or beneficial. It should neither be rejected too quickly nor clung to rigidly if we are to benefit from the experiences of our predecessors and continue to make progress.

Biley and Wright (1997) argue that there is much to be said in defence of routine and rituals in nursing and health care. In particular they suggest that rituals are 'in some way a part of healing, that they have some positive action, ritualistic symbolism, latent function and meaning for the patient and the nurse'. The danger with rituals, however, is when the rationale for their practice is long forgotten and never questioned.

Intuition

Intuition by its very nature is not easy to define. Intuition is a form of knowing and behaving not apparently based on rational reasoning. The use of intuition in nursing is only beginning to attract nurse researchers, so not much is known about 'how' nurses come to know there is something 'wrong' or whether they have a 'sixth' sense that tells them what to do. According to Kenny (1994), nurses use empathetic intuition in their daily practice:

> This type of intuitive thinking often occurs within the context of a nursing situation, and feeling, rather than conscious thinking, seems to predominate. Nurses know that there is something wrong but cannot explain what it is.

Intuition involves the use of all human senses such as touch, smell, hearing, sight and even taste as well as previous experience (in the form of tacit knowledge) to assess, and react to, a situation. It happens in ways which seem to be beyond comprehension. McCutcheon and Pincombe (2001) studied nurses' understanding of intuition, their perceptions of their use of intuition, and assessed the impact of intuition on nursing practice. They found that intuition is the result of complex interaction between a number of factors including knowledge, experience, expertise, personality and environment.

Despite the recognition that intuition is an important 'tool' in the human repertoire of knowing, concern has been raised regarding the 'process of apprehension and action without apparent reason' (Aggleton and Chalmers, 1986). Even the strongest intuition is sometimes proved false when put to an empirical test (Polgar and Thomas, 1991). In scientific terms, that which cannot be researched seems to be less reliable than that which can be empirically observed.

Experience and reflective practice

Nurses and midwives base their practice on their own experience and on the experience of others. A study by Luker and Kenrick (1992) of 47 community nurses from four district health authorities in Britain showed that:

> The effects of past experience and situational variables were identified by all the nurses as having an important impact on the decision-making process, and both these influences were deemed to be practice-based knowledge, with experience having 82% (n = 39) agreement and the situational context having 76% (n = 36) agreement. Another factor which all nurses identified as being an important source of influence was discussions with nurse colleagues, described as experiential knowledge by 82% (n = 39) of respondents.

Mander (1992) interviewed 40 midwives and found that 'knowledge derived from their occupational experience was of overwhelming significance' to them. In a recent study by Thompson et al. (2001) on 'the accessibility of research-based knowledge for nurses in the United Kingdom acute care settings', it was reported that the most common source of information for reducing clinical uncertainty was their colleagues' experience.

Experience is a useful way of learning. There is a wealth of untapped knowledge embedded in the practice and 'know-how' of expert nurse clinicians (Benner, 1984). It is also reckoned that what we learn by experience is more enduring than what we are taught. However, our experience is in itself rather narrow. For example, in treating depression, a nurse may use one or two approaches. While the experience obtained is invaluable, she will be unfamiliar with other treatments and may either be reluctant to try them or may reject them out of hand.

There is also a degree of trial and error when learning by experience. While this may be inevitable in a few cases, there is, by and large, a risk of reinventing the wheel and a greater risk of unsafe practice. Experience is therefore an important source of nursing knowledge, but relying solely on it and overstating its importance can be detrimental to nursing practice.

One way to use one's experience to improve practice is through 'reflective practice'. There is confusion as to what reflective practice is and how it can be implemented (Mackintosh, 1998) although much has been written about it. Reflective practice requires practitioners to think though the process of decision making which leads to particular actions. The two types of reflective practice which are generally referred to are 'reflection-on-action' and 'reflection-in-action' (Schon, 1987). The former is a retrospective 'analysis' of an action which has already taken place, while the latter involves reflecting while the action is taking place.

Reflective practice is a learning process designed to gain insight into one's own practice with the intention of improving it. Now and then we must stop and consider what we do, why and how we do it and to what effect, otherwise we turn what we do into thoughtless routines. For progress to take place, we must ask if we are doing the right things and if there are alternative ways to make things better. Stuart (1998), referring to midwifery practice, explains that routinisation 'leads to unthinking, unhelpful care-giving, with little possibility of the midwife learning from experience'. According to Rolfe (2001), in order to become 'knowledge generators', practitioners can use reflective practice 'to uncover the rich store of experiential knowledge that lies buried within their own practice'.

Reflective practice is not without its problems and limitations. Mackintosh (1998) divides the problems into three main categories: the process by which reflection takes place (Burnard, 1995), the ability of individuals to reflect in a meaningful way (Aitkens and Murphy, 1993; Richardson and Maltby, 1995; Waterworth, 1995); and the benefits that the process of reflection may have for nursing practice (Burnard, 1995).

Reflective practice assumes that the practitioner is capable of reflecting in a meaningful way on his or her decisions leading to a particular action, despite the acknowledgement that the rationale for action can be intuitive and difficult to verbalise. It is also believed that we can examine our prejudices which can underpin our practice. Yet people are generally reluctant to admit their prejudices, many of which they may not be conscious of. The process of group reflection can be a daunting and threatening experience with ethical and political implications. The use of diaries and journals for reflective purposes has been criticised by Mackintosh (1998) as giving rise to issues of confidentiality. Journals and diaries also have the potential to identify bad practices which the reflective practitioner may not be in a position to address, thereby leading to frustration and low morale.

There is a lack of empirical evidence into the outcomes of reflective practice (Paget, 2001). Hannigan (2001) calls for research to generate answers to questions such, as 'How does reflection assist in the development of more effective practice?'

Reflection as a concept to learn about our actions and about ourselves has much to commend. Despite its problems and limitations, it should not be rejected 'out of hand', nor should it be the only strategy for developing practice. It must be recognised that all methods of generating knowledge have limitations and closing our minds to other methods can be unproductive and often dangerous.

Reflective practice has the potential to raise questions which can thereafter be explored by other means, including research. In Paget's (2001) study of practitioners' views of how reflective practice has influenced their clinical practice, some of the respondents reported that reflective practice encouraged the use of research findings in their practice.

Research

Research, in contrast to tradition, intuition and reflective practice, is a systematic way of knowing and lays bare its methods for all to see. Researchers collect and analyse data systematically and rigorously, and this process is described to others by means of oral and/or written presentation. Research findings by themselves are not solutions to problems. They provide new insight into phenomena or add to, confirm or reject what is already known. Decisions still have to be taken about whether they should be used or not, and how.

One may argue that, by using common sense, nurses can take the right decisions. However, they still need relevant and valid information in order to do so. What may seem simple and straightforward is not necessarily so. For example, in many developing countries babies suffering from diarrhoea are not given fluids because it is believed that this will aggravate the situation. To the parents, it makes sense that in order to stop the baby from passing 'watery' faeces, they must stop the administration of fluids. In doing this, the baby is put at risk of dying from dehydration. Jackson (1994) recalls that in midwifery practice, 'it used to be common sense to give an enema to prevent soiling during delivery until Romney and Gordon (1981) published their research which showed that this procedure was not necessary'.

One of the important factors in decision making is the availability of relevant and up-to-date information. Traditional knowledge, although an important source of information, needs to be updated. What was relevant a decade ago may not be so now, as illustrated by Jackson (1994):

> Many of the observations that we make on pregnant women today were probably implemented when the health of the pregnant population was much less robust than it is today. In many instances, the pregnant woman would have been less than well and this probably influenced the way she was cared for.

Research has the potential to provide up-to-date information that may facilitate decision making. The perception of research data as superior to other forms of knowledge is not purely a matter of personal preference, but is dependent on the quality of the research itself. Traditional knowledge may have suited a world in which 'authority' was not questioned, people did what they were told and things were right because someone 'important' said so. We now live in an age when most clients are no longer passive recipients of services and those who hold the purse strings require business plans for the allocation and use of funds. The need to justify one's practice is greater now than it has ever been.

Using more than one source of knowledge

By separating the sources of knowledge for the sake of explanation, the impression may be given that practitioners use one source at the exclusion of others. In practice, nurses and other practitioners use a combination of these, consciously and unconsciously, depending on what their interventions consist of. Referring to the lack of consensus about what kind of knowledge is at work in the actions of social workers, Nygren and Blom (2001) ask:

> What is the role of theoretical knowledge in the moment of action, when a child is separated from its parents, when a dialogue is opened with a drug abuser, or when the client is told how much money she or he will get? To what extent is it a question of personal talent, creativity or charisma that is crucial to what will happen? Is knowledge applied in a prescriptive or instrumental way, or does it take the shape of a 'mass' or a matrix of knowledge – a more or less conscious background against which social workers reflect their sensory impressions.

Berragan (1998) echoes the same thoughts in pointing out that the knowledge from a variety of sources which nurses draw upon has 'something to offer to holistic nursing practice'. However, it must be acknowledged that there can be potential conflict when knowledge drawn from various sources is different and contradictory.

The meaning of nursing research

Nursing research is a broad term for all research into nursing practice and issues. It aims to provide insights into, and understanding of, nursing practice, its effects on patients and their carers and on the use of resources. Other areas of nursing research include the education and training of nurses, the organisation and delivery of services, the conditions in which nurses work, their influence on the work environment as well as the effects of work on themselves.

Definitions of nursing research are difficult to find mainly because of the lack of consensus in the definition of nursing and because nurses' roles are constantly evolving and expanding in order to meet new demands. Often the definition of nursing research is implicit in the goals of nursing organisations. For example, the National Institute of Nursing Research (NINR) in the United States describes the type of research it supports as 'the care of individuals across the life span – from management of patients during illness and recovery to the reduction of risks for disease and disability, the promotion of healthy lifestyles, promoting quality of life in those with chronic illness, and care for individuals at the end of life' (National Institute of Nursing Research, 2004). The NINR goes on to explain that nursing research includes families within a context and involves clinical care in a variety of settings including community and home in addition to more traditional health care sites.

Health care is delivered not by nurses only but by multi-professional teams whose aim is to provide the best possible care for patients and their families. It follows then that multi-disciplinary research should be an approach of choice. Yet there are boundaries around the areas that each professional group deals with, and although these areas can overlap, health professionals generally are aware of what constitutes their domain of practice. There are aspects of care which are entirely or mostly delivered by nurses, and it is legitimate that nurses seek to develop their practice with the use of research. Both multi-disciplinary and uni-disciplinary research are important and one should not be developed at the expense of the other.

One can ask if nursing research should be carried out by nurses only. In theory it may not seem important that research is 'produced by members of the professions to whose practice it is directly or indirectly relevant' (Higher Education Funding Council for England [HEFCE], 2001). In practice it would be odd if members of these professions did not engage in researching their practice. Clinically relevant questions can be developed mainly by clinicians themselves.

Practitioners are also well placed to decide on priority areas for research. According to the Department of Health (DoH) (2000), there are 'two principal dimensions to influencing the research and development agenda: ensuring that important areas of research about nursing receive appropriate priority; and ensuring that general priority setting benefits from a nursing perspective'. The HEFCE (2001) explains that because it 'recognised the importance of maintaining healthy links between research, practice and teaching, it would be concerned if entire sub-fields became dominated by researchers from outside the professions'.

Nursing research uses designs and methods mainly from the natural and the social sciences, since nursing is concerned with the physical, psychological, social, environmental and spiritual aspects of patients and their carers. In return, nursing also provides fertile grounds for testing the theories and methods of these sciences. Nursing research is eclectic (uses a variety of methods and approaches) and sometimes modifies these methods to suit its own ends. In doing so nursing research further develops these approaches and methods, and often gives them particular 'slants' or interpretations more suited to the context and the reality of nursing practice. Thus nursing research makes a unique contribution to the development of approaches and methods for the study of its core issues.

Rationale for nursing research

Nurses are the largest professional group among health care workers worldwide. In the UK alone nurses, midwives and health visitors represent the largest workforce within the National Health Service (NHS), consuming 70 per cent of the NHS wage bill and 40 per cent of the NHS budget (Rafferty et al., 2000). How such a workforce fulfils the health service agenda and what use they make of such a sizeable budget should be of concern to those responsible for the health of the population, to nurses and to society itself. Nurses are the health professionals who have most person-to-person contact with patients. They carry out thousands of interventions with patients and their carers, and their decisions and actions affect the lives of whole populations. It makes sense, therefore, that nursing practice should be based on sound evidence. According to the American Nurses Association (2003), research-based practice is essential if the nursing profession is to meet its mandate to society.

If what nurses do is important, then it needs to be done well. To ensure that nursing practice is efficient and effective both from patients' and nurses' perspectives, it has to be questioned and, where necessary, improved. Research is one of the main tools available to question practice and seek answers. Aristotle differentiated between two types of knowledge: 'know-how' and 'know-why' (Laudan, 1996). Put simply, 'know-how' is the knowledge which the craftsman possesses as, for example, when a shipbuilder knows that wood, when properly sealed, floats (Laudan, 1996). 'Know-why' would require him to know the principle by which wood floats over water (buoyancy). 'Know-why' knowledge is mainly generated by research, both basic and applied. Basic research involves answering general questions such as, for example, why, and in which circumstances, do people conform? This type of knowledge can be used to understand why patients conform. Applied research focuses on a specific question in an area of practice: for example, why do patients with diabetes comply (or not) with professional advice?

'Know-how' knowledge is necessary but not enough for progress. This type of knowledge involves learning by 'trial and error', which can be costly and time-consuming. If practitioners are reasonably satisfied with their work it could lead to a tendency to leave things as they are, thus maintaining the status quo. 'Know-why' knowledge, on the other hand, can be divorced from practice. This is why this type of knowledge needs to be generated in collaboration with practitioners, otherwise it could remain in 'ivory towers'. Together, 'know-how' and 'know-why' knowledge can provide the knowledge for the enhancement of nursing practice.

Another reason for using research to generate knowledge for nursing practice is to contribute towards the development of nursing as a profession. The accumulation of knowledge on different aspects of nursing constitutes a 'body of knowledge' that nurses and others can draw upon and contribute to. This body of knowledge is the sum total of nursing knowledge (theories, research findings, reflections on practice, and so forth) contained mainly in books, journals, reports, theses and other audiovisual forms. The progress made in the creation of nursing's body of knowledge can be gauged by the availability of books on different aspects of nursing and the number of nursing journals currently on the market compared with the early 1970s, when the number of books on nursing in the UK probably amounted to only a handful. The creation of a body of knowledge distinct to nursing is an important step in establishing nursing as a profession. One of the hallmarks of a profession is the possession of a body of knowledge based on research, and in the progress of nursing towards true professional status, the acquisition of a research basis for practice is essential (Royal College of Nursing) [RCN, 1982]. Nursing relies heavily on knowledge from other disciplines, such as biology, chemistry, sociology and psychology. While nursing will continue to draw upon, and contribute to, knowledge from these other disciplines, it is imperative that it continues to create a body of knowledge to inform its own practice.

The status of nursing as a profession will be enhanced when other professions recognise that nursing is not just common sense but is based on knowledge derived from research and organised in the form of concepts and theories.

The contribution of research towards the status of a profession is also recognised by the allied health professions (AHPs). Sackley (1994) reported that 'physiotherapists in the UK have recognised the trend towards becoming research-based practitioners, ready to justify their techniques and procedures'.

The creation of a body of knowledge is the means by which parity with other professions can be achieved, and research is the process by which this knowledge can be developed and validated.

The role of nurses in research

As explained above, nurses have an important role in creating a body of knowledge and using it to inform their practice. This is what is meant by nursing being a research-based profession (Briggs, 1972). Yet it is not always clear to nurses what exactly they are expected to do. With competing demands on their time and the need to acquire a range of skills, they may wonder whether they are expected to be researchers as well as nurses. This perception may be based on the fact that research is relatively new to nursing.

Nurses' primary duty is to give the best possible care to patients. This involves creating and maintaining a safe, caring environment and using interventions which, to the best of their knowledge, are the most appropriate and effective in bringing about the desired effects. To do so they should question the knowledge and rationale on which they base their practice and seek to develop new ways to improve what they do. The answers to some of these questions can be obtained in various ways, including research. An important step in integrating research and practice is for nurses to be research-minded.

To be research-minded involves an attitude and an ability to ask questions of one's practice which can be answered through the process of research. While the next step involves finding the answers to those questions, it does not mean that practitioners are expected to carry out research studies, although some do. The answers may already be available in the form of published research. In this case a literature search and review would be undertaken. In cases where there is no research, the role of nurses is to identify and work with those who have research experience and who are in a position to carry out a new study. To complete the process, the findings of the literature review or the research study should be critically appraised, and where appropriate, they should be disseminated and implemented.

Nurses' role in research extends beyond asking questions, and seeking and implementing evidence. It includes protecting patients' rights by ensuring that patients are fully informed of the implications of participating in research, that informed consent is sought, that no pressure is exerted – directly or indirectly – on them to participate, and that their right to withdraw at any time is respected. This advocacy role applies throughout the duration of the project and beyond. (See Chapter 6 for more discussion of these issues.)

The methods and skills used by researchers can also be of use to nurses in their daily practice. Kirkham (1994) states that 'the basic skills of research, i.e. listening and observation, are also the basic skills of midwifery'. Nurses and midwives engage in problem solving. They consistently collect and analyse data in the assessment of patients and in the evaluation of outcomes. The skills of interviewing and observing in clinical practice can be sharpened though learning some of the research method skills. Hayes (2002) explains how her research experience prior to starting nurse training was useful to her as a nurse:

> My research background has helped me develop an enquiring mind and the ability to see the broader picture. It helps me question my practice and its impact on patients. The skills I developed while working as a researcher are relevant to everyday practice on the wards. For example, they give me the confidence to tackle new information and communicate with people. Interview skills help me to sensitively obtain information for patient assessments and analytical skills help me develop care plans.

Although it is rare that a student nurse would have research experience before undertaking nurse training, this example shows how learning research skills can benefit practice.

To maximise the potential contribution of research to practice requires knowledge of what research means, its strengths and limitations, knowledge of the research process (including the main research designs) and an appreciation of the ethical and political implications of research. Knowledge of support systems and available resources is often very important. The skills required include the ability to identify aspects of practice which would benefit from research, to formulate research questions, to differentiate between questions which can be answered by research and those which can be answered by other means such as audit and reflection on practice (or by a combination of these).

Another fundamental skill for research-based practice is the ability to search and critically appraise research studies. Information technology has greatly facilitated access to research and other literature. To fully reap the benefits nurses need the skills to search, obtain and critically read appropriate and relevant literature. Critical appraisal skills are likely to be more useful to most nurses than the skills to carry out research. Finally, the skills to implement findings and to manage and evaluate change are crucial if research is to have any impact on practice.

How nurses should acquire these fundamental skills remains a subject for discussion. Anecdotal evidence in the UK suggests that this has been interpreted differently by different institutions, with the result that some courses require students to carry out a literature review on a topic related to practice, while others expect students to formulate a research proposal or even carry out a small-scale project. The consensus in the nursing profession seems to be that qualified nurses should be able to read and use research critically and have a sense of the need for research to underpin their practice. The task of conducting research should rest with those who have acquired further education and training, especially in research methodology.

The role of nurses in research-based practice as described above applies to all nurses, since they all should identify researchable questions and seek and implement evidence. However, depending on the nature of their jobs, positions or responsibilities, some nurses may put more emphasis on certain aspects of these roles than others. For example, nurse managers may have more of a leadership role in encouraging and facilitating others to enhance their practice through research and by supporting them with the necessary resources. Specialist nurses may be required to have a greater awareness of research in their own area of specialism, and to act as a useful resource for other less specialised nurses.

There are a number of triggers and reasons which can make you question your practice. These include:

1. When you carry out a task, even though you have doubts about whether it is effective, harmful or even necessary, as shown in Research Example 1.

RESEARCH EXAMPLE 1

So much for common sense   *Jackson (1994)*

'It is current practice to note a woman's temperature, pulse and blood pressure when she is admitted in labour and to record the foetal heart rate. Normally these readings are then recorded at regular intervals throughout labour . . .

There is no research base to support the need for some of these observations in the first instance or to use as a basis for determining the frequency of others. Yet I, like many others, would be reluctant to abandon them. There does seem to be a logical explanation for performing the observations and I could, like all midwives, explain why they are thought to be necessary. On the other hand, I cannot recall ever finding a woman's temperature to be raised at the beginning of labour except in circumstances where pyrexia would have been expected or anticipated. So why have I continued to take and record it? If I am honest, it's because I've never really thought about it before writing this piece.' (Jackson, 1994).

2. When you want to know more about something which arouses your curiosity (Research Example 2).
3. When you wonder whether there is a better way to care for patients (Research Example 3).

RESEARCH EXAMPLE 2

Choosing a research topic that has personal and professional significance helps with motivation

Duffy (2002)

Duffy shows how her experience influenced her motivation and interest in exploring a particular topic.

'As a staff nurse I had been involved in failing a student on a clinical placement, an experience that I will never forget. Then as a lecturer I was involved in supporting mentors who were trying to decide whether or not to fail students. So issues around failing students in clinical practice was something that held my interest for some time.'

She explains that the professional significance of exploring this topic came when she read research findings which suggested that students whose performance was unsatisfactory were allowed to pass their clinical assessments. Her concern about patient care and safety were also prime reasons for choosing this topic for a Ph.D. study.

Under the skin of any nurse researcher you will find a colleague quite like yourself
Laight (2002)

Laight (2002) explains how, prior to becoming a nurse researcher, she used research to improve her practice.

'My introduction to research occurred in response to a patient I can still picture now, ten years later. He was critically ill and receiving intensive care for multi-system failure. His eyes became bloodshot, oedematous and ulcerated. I wondered if better eye care could prevent this.

I embarked on a project to investigate and standardise the eye care we delivered on the intensive therapy unit and ultimately compared the effectiveness of two forms of eye care.'

Laight (2002) went on to explain the difficulties she experienced in doing her study but concluded that it increased her understanding of the factors that contributed to the eye conditions shown by her original patient.

4. When you want to introduce a new policy or practice (Research Example 4).

RESEARCH EXAMPLE 4

Research at a local level not only helps improve care, but also brings dividends for staff
Cole (2002)

Cole (2002) explains how he wanted to review the policy on visits to patients by friends and relatives.

'The staff felt this was an important issue that was often overlooked. They wanted to revise the current policy, and rather than merely changing it to what the staff thought was best, they decided to use research to find out what the patients, visitors and staff actually thought about the whole topic.'

Cole (2002) expected that the research project would lead to improvement in clinical care and to an increase in the awareness of the research process and issues for all those involved.

These are examples where nurses decided, for good reasons, to collect data to answer their questions. However, before engaging in a project it is wise to search and review the literature as the answers may already be available. One must also be careful when using research findings that are not conclusive.

It is important in any profession that some of its members focus their attention on research. In the UK, Briggs (1972) proposed that the 'active pursuit of serious research must be limited to a minority within the nursing profession'. To carry out serious research, nurses need a degree of knowledge and skills, not usually attainable in basic training. The research training of undergraduate nurses varies in the UK, as explained earlier. Anecdotal evidence, as well as a perusal of the nursing literature, shows that more and more staff nurses in the UK conduct research, albeit small-scale projects, mainly as part of their courses. Some take part in projects led by doctors and other health care professionals.

Practising nurses are frequently asked to collect data for other researchers, be they nurse researchers, doctors, psychologists or others. Their clinical nursing experience can be valuable to the research enterprise. Nurses are in a position to identify problems that need investigation through research. On the other hand, the researcher can also bring her detached perspective to bear on the problem being researched. This is illustrated by the following example. A researcher was called upon to help to improve care in a ward of older people through research. She had a hunch that constipation might be a problem in this group of patients. The ward sister did not think so until they both examined the Kardex and found that 11 out of 19 patients were prescribed laxatives, some three times daily. While discussing each patient individually, the ward sister also observed that those who were not prescribed laxatives were also the most confused patients on the ward and would probably not have been able to ask for medication. Without clinical insight, the researcher would have missed this important observation. This highlights the important and unique contribution that nurses can make to the research enterprise in nursing. The research–practitioner collaboration is further discussed in Chapter 18.

The American Nurses Association's (ANA) (2003) position statement on education for participation in nursing research states that at undergraduate level, 'an attitude of enquiry, as well as an introduction to the research process should be initiated'. They should also learn about how to look for, critique and utilise, research in their practice. According to the ANA (2003) the responsibility for the conduct of research begins at master's level, when they are prepared to be active members of research teams. At doctoral level, nurses should be able to contribute to knowledge through 'the conduct of research aimed at theory generation or theory testing' (American Nurses Association, 2003).

The danger of leaving the conduct of research to a minority of nurses within the profession is that practitioners may not see research as integral to their practice. While there is some evidence from nursing journals of staff nurses conducting research, it is too much to expect first-level nurses to do so, even though many are very capable of doing so. Whether they conduct research or not will depend on their research training, their interests and their skills, and on available opportunities. Although nurses should collaborate with others, they must seek to become full members of the research team. The opportunities to register for a higher degree must also be considered. Nurses have grown in confidence from the early days when they were mostly handmaidens to medical and other researchers, collecting data with little to show for it.

Research and clinical effectiveness

The primary goal of nursing research is to improve the quality of care given to patients and clients. The drive towards clinical and cost effectiveness has been at the heart of health policies in the UK in the last two decades. The aim is to strive 'continuously to improve the overall standard of clinical care, to reduce unacceptable variations in practice and ensure care is based on the most up-to-date evidence of what is known to be effective' (Department of Health, 1999). Clinical effectiveness is defined as:

> The extent to which specific clinical interventions, when deployed in the field for a particular patient or population, do what they are intended to do, i.e., maintain and improve health and secure the greatest possible gain from the available resources.   (NHS Executive, 1996)

To coordinate and maximise individual nurses' and other health professionals' contribution to clinical effectiveness, a number of policies and measures have been introduced in the UK. They are designed to:

● set clear national quality standards through National Service Frameworks and the National Institute for Clinical Excellence (NICE);

● ensure local delivery of high-quality clinical services through clinical governance;

● monitor delivery of quality standards in the form of a statutory Commission for Health Improvement (CHI) and the National Performance Frameworks and national patient and users survey. (Department of Health, 1999)

Since then the CHI has been replaced by the Healthcare Commission (http://www.healthcarecommission.org.uk).

In effect, these national measures set the standards by which quality is to be measured, provide a framework to facilitate and coordinate the implementation of these standards and create structures to monitor and evaluate the extent to which they are achieved.

Research plays a key role in providing evidence on the value and limitations of clinical interventions and on their cost effectiveness. This was recognised by the UK government when it launched its NHS Research and Development Strategy in 1992, at the heart of which is evidence-based health care (Department of Health, 1992). However, it must be emphasised that clinical effectiveness is not achieved through research only. Other strategies used by health professionals to develop and enhance their practice include the development and use of clinical guidelines (see Chapter 18), client pathways, clinical audit, patient feedback and reflection on practice.

In the health service audit is carried out to monitor if and how the standards and objectives set by a particular service are achieved. Thus audit is an activity which monitors, through the collection of data, the targets and standards set. The findings of audit are primarily designed to measure how these targets are achieved. In doing so it can identify gaps in practice; then new standards and goals are set, and the audit cycle can start again. It is, therefore, a continuous monitoring of targets and performance.

Research, on the other hand, seeks answers to particular questions and uses a range of designs and rigorous methods of data collection and analysis. Research is expected to enhance our understanding of phenomena or test particular theories. Audit, on the other hand, is a monitoring function using limited (often already available) data to inform practitioners of the extent to which they are achieving their objectives. Balogh (1996) and Closs and Cheater (1996) have provided useful discussions of audit and its relationship with research.

Finally, the role of professional organisations in promoting clinical effectiveness is vital in providing guidance and support for their members. In 1996, the RCN launched its Clinical Effectiveness Initiative, which aimed to provide nurses with information, support and advice (Royal College of Nursing, 1996). Other relevant publications include *Guidance for Nurses on Clinical Governance* (Royal College of Nursing, 1998) and *Doing the Right Thing – Clinical Effectiveness for Nurses* (Royal College of Nursing, 1999).

Development of nursing research

The origins of nursing research can be traced back to the time of the Crimean War when Florence Nightingale collected statistical data on mortality rates in the hospital where she worked. However, it was not until the beginning of the twentieth century in the USA, and in the 1950s in the UK, that nursing research began to develop.

Although the pace and extent of the development of nursing research worldwide vary from country to country, there are remarkable similarities in the way nursing research began and progressed thereafter. This is mainly due to some of the similar issues faced by nurses everywhere, namely the low status of nursing relative to other health professions, the education and training of nurses at the margins of higher education and the lack of resources to carry out research.

Tierney (1997) offered an insightful analysis of the development of nursing research in some European countries. She described the 1960s as the emerging years in which 'lone pioneers' played a great part. The 1970s are credited with the 'beginnings of collective activity', both internationally and nationally, throughout Europe. Tierney (1997) explained that collaboration among pioneer nurse researchers across Europe led to the formation of the Workgroup of European Nurse Researchers (WENR) in 1978. The 1980s are described as the period of 'growth of activity and infrastructure', underpinned by the nursing profession's expanding association with universities. Finally, the 1990s was an era in which 'the development of research in nursing in Europe' was steered 'strategically and with a greater sense of political acumen'.

Tierney (1997) also recognised that the advancement of nursing research has occurred more rapidly in countries with strong and stable economies. Not unsurprisingly, therefore, the development of nursing research in less developed countries has lagged behind; not much is written about nursing research in these places. The lack of funding and the low status of nursing in many of these countries have been factors contributing to the slow development of nursing research. Mangay-Maglacas pointed out in 1992 that nursing research in the developing and least developed countries was 'in its infancy', although 'much development had taken place in improved educational patterns and increased recognition of nursing as an important element of health care systems'. More recently Uys (1998) observed that 'nursing research in most developing countries is still in an early developmental stage', while Lee (2003) believes that the majority of nurses in developing countries have been data collectors rather than researchers, although things are beginning to improve.

While research carried out in developed counties can be useful to nurses and midwives in developing countries, there are many areas – such as 'nursing care of endemic diseases, approaches to health education with illiterate/oral groups, inclusion of traditional healers in health terms' – which remain unresearched because they are not priority areas for nurse researchers in Europe or the USA (Uys, 1998).

It is not wise to generalise about developing countries as they vary according to their stages of economic development. In some of those countries nursing research is more developed than others. There are also examples of joint projects in education and research between richer and poorer countries. This is seen as beneficial as well as a hindrance. Joint ventures involve transfer of skills and useful learning opportunities. However, they can lead to developments in the image of Western societies. Mancia and Gastaldo (2004), referring to the relationship between Brazil and the USA, point out that:

> So far, the dominance of the scientific model of American nursing has prevented fruitful exchanges between Brazilian (Portuguese-speaking) and English-speaking nurses. In this model, which mirrors the commercial relationships between first world countries and third world countries, English-speaking nurses are producers of knowledge, while non-English speaking nurses are its supposed consumers. When Brazilian, Portuguese-speaking nurses try to resist this dominant model and establish equal relationships, a series of subtle but effective barriers comes into play.

It is difficult to know what the current situation regarding nursing research in developing countries is since there is a dearth of publications on this issue, and some are in languages other than English. The impression is that nurses in these non-Western countries are rising to the challenge of developing a research culture and acquiring funding for training and projects. There is ample evidence, for example, from South Africa (Brink, 1992), Taiwan (Tsai, 2000), Brazil (Collet et al., 2000) and Iran (Valizadeh and Zamanzadeh, 2003) of nurses engaging in research development and research utilisation.

To understand further how nursing research developed, and the contributing factors, we need to look at the following areas: the role of professional organisations, the focus of nursing research, the trend in approaches used in nursing studies, research capacity building and research funding.

The role of nursing organisations

Nursing organisations have played a vital role in promoting the need for research, in providing support, as well as in advocating state recognition and funding for nursing research. Tierney (1997) acknowledges the significant contribution of national nurses' associations:

> There is no doubt that the developments of nursing research in Europe has been greatly strengthened by the active support of national nurses' associations (NNAs) and, indeed, in many countries, they have done more than any other single organisation to advance the cause of research in nursing.

She gave the example of the Royal College of Nursing's contribution to nursing research in the UK by pointing out how it supported researchers as early as 1959, through the establishment of a nursing research discussion group. The RCN Nursing Research Conference, organised by the Nursing Research Society, is an annual fixture for nurse researchers in the UK and beyond. In 2003, the RCN published its position statement, *Promoting Excellence in Care through Research and Development* (Royal College of Nursing, 2003). This document outlines the role of the individual nurse, the health care provider and the higher education institution in research and development of nursing practice.

Other examples of NNAs' role in nursing research include the founding of the Irish Nurses Research Interest Group (INRIG) in the mid-1970s. The Department of Health and Children in Ireland (2003) recognised the contribution of INRIG, who 'pioneered research appreciation, research thinking, and research utilisation and ensured research was included on the nursing and midwifery agenda in Ireland'. For other examples see the special edition of the *International Journal of Nursing Studies* in 1990 (vol. 27, no. 2), which focused on the development of nursing research in the UK, Canada, Norway, Sweden, Denmark and Finland.

The focus of nursing research

The early phase of nursing research development was characterised by a focus on nurses rather than on clinical practice, although there are still signs that the situation has not quite reversed. In the USA, 'studies about nurses outnumbered clinical studies by 10 to 1, in the early years' (Henderson, 1994). In New Zealand, 'prior to 1973 the history of nursing research is scant and very much a history of research on nurses, conducted mostly by non-nurses and always from the perspective of another discipline' (Chick, 1987). Borbasi et al. (2002) analysed topics in Australian nursing research publications between 1995 and 2000. They found more research on 'education of nurses' than on 'practice issues', and that data were collected more often from nurses (40.7 per cent) than from patients (25.5 per cent). Traynor et al. (2001) found 'research concerned with problems and issues to do with nursing as a profession' (endogenous) more than doubled between 1988–1991 and 1992–5, in the UK. At the same time research concerned with the nursing of patients (exogenous) had a 'lower rate of growth in output'.

Early research studies in nursing were invariably carried out by non-nurses. Macleod-Clark and Hockey (1986) remarked that up to the mid-1960s nurses in the UK had been dependent on members of other disciplines, especially the social scientists, for the study of their own profession. This is supported by Traynor et al. (2001), who pointed out that early studies of nurses and nursing tended to be undertaken by sociologists or industrial psychologists. According to Flaherty (1990), 'although Canadian nurses have been involved in research for more than half a century, in the beginning the research activity consisted largely of co-operation with and/or assistance to members of other disciplines'.

Traynor et al. (2001) suggest that research studies which focused on nurses and were carried out by outsiders provided nurses with a 'medium for consciousness raising and self-definition for the profession'; resulting in the 'expulsion' of those who 'lurk in the margins' of the nursing profession.

Nursing research was also dominated, in its early phase, by quantitative approaches. This may be because these studies were carried out by social scientists trained in these methods. Early nurse researchers would also have been trained mostly by researchers in other disciplines which were steeped in quantitative methods, at a time when qualitative research was in its early phase of development. In the last two decades, the number of published qualitative studies have increased significantly. There are signs that they may have overtaken quantitative ones. According to Curzio (1998), much of nursing research is qualitative in nature. Borbasi et al.'s (2002) analysis of Australian nursing research publications found that 41 per cent used quantitative and 47 per cent qualitative approaches. Using a combination of these approaches has become popular recently (see Chapter 5).

Research training and education

One of the main barriers to the development of nursing research is the lack of resources and training opportunities for nurses. Although the situation has improved in some countries, it still remains problematic in others. Doctoral programmes in many countries are recent, and in some countries like Spain there are no Ph.D. programmes, although nurses can earn doctorates in other fields (Moreno-Casba and de Frutos-Sánchez, 2002). In Canada the first doctoral programmes in nursing date back to the early 1990s. In the UK, which has a longer history of doctoral programmes, there were 3,700 postgraduate students in 1998–9 (Traynor and Rafferty, 2001). However, as Hale (2002) points out, once nurses have obtained their Ph.D.s, there are few opportunities for them to consolidate their experience.

One of the reasons for the lack of a research tradition in nursing is that nurse education in many countries took place outside the university sector. Wright et al. (1995) explain that the move of nurse education into universities brought a whole new meaning to nurse education in Australia and, in particular, nursing research. The integration of nurse education into higher education in the UK seems to have acted as a catalyst for the education of nurses to doctoral level. Although much progress has been made there is a shortfall of capable researchers in nursing to meet the demands of evidence-based practice (Rafferty et al., 2003). This was recognised by the Higher Education Funding Council for England (HEFCE) who, in partnership with the Department of Health (DoH) set up a task group to report on research capacity building in nursing and the allied health professions (AHPs). The Report (HEFCE, 2001) recognised the underfunding of nursing and AHPs' research relative to comparable professions such as education. It also found that funding was 'skewed towards short-term projects'. One of its main recommendations was the establishment of a fund to develop and expand the capacity for high-quality research in nursing and AHPs over a period of seven years. Without meaningful investment in the training of nurse researchers, it is difficult for nurses to deliver the evidence-based practice agenda.

Funding nursing research

Funding research training is only a symptom of the general lack of funding for nursing research. The amount of funding available for nursing research varies according to individual countries. In Europe, some countries like the UK have been able to attract considerable funding for research, while others, especially in Eastern Europe, have virtually no access to research funds (Tierney, 1997). From their 'mapping exercise' of 50 nursing and midwifery departments in UK universities, Traynor and Rafferty (2001) showed that research income increased from £3 million in 1996–7 to £9.7 million in 1999–2000. Nonetheless, funding provision in the UK remains patchy, fragmented and uncoordinated

(Rafferty et al., 2000). A task force to report on the Strategy for Research in Nursing, Midwifery and Health Visiting (Department of Health, 1992) recognised the need for 'ring-fenced' funding but rejected the call for a research council. The reasons put forward by the task force was that 'separate development would lead to marginalisation' and constrain the contribution of nurses, midwives and health visitors to the National Health Service Research and Development Strategy (NHS R&D) (Rafferty et al., 2000).

In the USA, nursing research has fared better. The National Institute of Nursing Research, which began life as a 'Center' in 1986, was established in 1993. Its annual budget, which rose from $6 million in 1986 to $90 million in 2004, is spent on grants for clinical and basic research (74 per cent) on pre- and postdoctoral training and career development (12 per cent) and other aspects such as research management and support (National Institute of Nursing Research, 2004). Such a model of research structure and funding ensures a co-ordinated and holistic approach to the development, support and promotion of nursing research. A nursing research council in the UK would similarly ensure that the profession sets its own agenda within the national R&D framework and allocate funds as appropriate to research programmes and training. Such a council could balance the need for nursing research to address clinical and related issues directly with the need to invest in basic research designed to produce new knowledge. It could take a strategic role by facilitating, coordinating and monitoring research activities in the profession.

The Research Assessment Exercise (RAE) carried out periodically in the UK is an audit of the volume and quality of research and related activities in universities and other academic institutions. Nursing was ranked last in the 1996 and the 2001 RAE among all disciplines which took part in the exercise. It seems that as well as being marginalised, nursing continues to 'hang at the coat tails' of other professions and disciplines.

Other countries, such as Canada, have different support systems and funding sources. According to Wood (2001), nurses in Canada in the early 1980s struggled for recognition of their research efforts, and the Canadian Nurses Association and the Canadian Association at University Schools lobbied extensively for dedicated funding to support nursing research. More than 20 years later the funding situation had improved greatly. Three main sources of funding for nursing research and research capacity building are the Canada Foundation for Innovation, the Canadian Health Services Research Foundation (under its auspices, funds dedicated to nursing research are administered) and the Canadian Institutes of Health Research (Wood, 2001). In other countries nurses continue to struggle in their efforts to secure funding for their research. Wright et al. (1995) point out that nursing research in Australia 'has received low priority in funding, especially from prestigious academic funding bodies, such as the Australian Research Council and the National Health and Medical Research Council'. In Ireland funding for nursing research has remained 'ad hoc' over the years (Department of Health and Children, 2003). Recently some funding has been made available by the Health Research Board and An Board Altranais for research capacity building and for research projects (ibid.). The Research Strategy for Nursing and Midwifery in Ireland recommended that 'additional funding should be provided to finance a variety of nursing and midwifery research activities through the Health Research Board and that finance for postgraduate, doctoral and postdoctoral research should be enhanced' (ibid.).

The overall picture of funding for nursing research worldwide is that the USA remains the envy of nurse researchers elsewhere. In some countries of Europe funding has increased over the years but this is less than for comparable professions. Finally, some countries have little, if any, access to funds for nurses to engage in research.

Putting the development of nursing research in perspective

Although the development of nursing research has been slow in many of the countries mentioned above, there are real signs of progress in terms of research activities and research infrastructure and support. There is also growing recognition by the state of the importance and benefits of nursing research. In contrast, nursing research in poorer countries remains undeveloped and poorly supported.

Progress is reflected in the growing number of nursing journals and in the number of research papers published. According to Dawson et al. (1998) nursing research, in terms of publications, is one of the six most rapidly expanding sub-fields of biomedicine in the UK. However, this needs to be put in context. As Rafferty et al. (2003) point out, 73 per cent of (published) research in nursing remain unfunded despite the fact that the UK invests almost £3.5 billion in medical research.

Research is now well integrated in nursing curriculae in most developed countries. The number of nurses trained to doctoral level has also increased and continues to rise. More support in terms of studentships and fellowships are available to nurses. Yet apart from the USA and a few other countries most research projects remain small with little potential impact on practice. With few exceptions, research programmes supported by significant funding remain outside the grip of nurse researchers. Giving the tools of research to nurses by training them at postgraduate level and not providing funding for nursing research thereafter prevents them from fulfilling their potential and from making their contribution to evidence-based practice.

There is growing recognition by governments of the potential for nursing research to contribute towards the clinical and cost effectiveness of nursing care. In the UK the DoH (1999) published the document *Making a Difference: Strengthening the Nursing, Midwifery and Health Visiting Contribution to Health and Healthcare* in which it pointed out that for practice to be evidence-based nurses, midwives and health visitors 'need better appraisal skills to translate research findings into practice'. If research findings relevant to nurses' work do not exist, nurses have little to implement. This document also recommended the development of a strategy to influence the research and development agenda. In 2000 *Towards a Strategy for Nursing Research and Development* (Department of Health, 2000) was published and it made a number of recommendations including the need 'to explore options for pump-priming a handful of designated centres with thematic research and development programmes to help build capacity through partnerships and collaboration, focusing on links with the NHS and service delivery'. This strategy did not seem to address the issue of 'ring-fenced' or dedicated funds for research projects in its recommendations. Rafferty et al. (2003) believe that without 'targeted investment the service will fail to deliver the benefits of evidence-based practice'.

In Ireland, the Department of Health and Children (2003) published the first ever *Research Strategy for Nursing and Midwifery in Ireland*. It recognised the 'considerable importance' of research in providing a solid base for nursing and midwifery practice. It also made a number of recommendations including the provision of additional funding through the Health Research Board.

There is a growing recognition of the importance and value of nursing research worldwide. This is reflected in nursing curriculae, in the increase in studies, journals, books, conferences and workshops, and in the thirst for research training and development. More remains to be achieved, in particular in countries where nurses and midwives still face an uphill battle in making their voices heard.

SUMMARY

Summary and conclusion

The role of research-based knowledge in decision making is crucial for effective practice, and the need to have a sound rationale for one's practice has increased over the last decade. It is not incumbent on every nurse to carry out research, but all should be research-minded enough to value the contribution of research to practice, identify problems that can be explored through research, be aware of research findings, collaborate with others in research activities and protect the rights of patients with regard to their involvement in research projects.

While nursing research must be carried out by nurses in order to create a nursing body of knowledge, a multi-disciplinary approach is also required as nurses work with other health professionals and share the same goal.

Nursing research has come of age in some countries, while in others it is still in its infancy. The momentum created by nursing research must be maintained and increased if it is to contribute positively to patient care and achieve the recognition it deserves.

References

Aggleton P and Chalmers H (1986) Nursing research, nursing theory and the nursing process. *Journal of Advanced Nursing*, 11:197–202.

Aitkens S and Murphy K (1993) Reflection: a review of the literature. *Journal of Clinical Nursing*, 18:1188–192.

American Nurses Association (2003) Education for participation in nursing research. http://nursingworld.org/readroom/position/research/rseducat.htm; accessed 18 April 2003.

Balogh R (1996) Exploring links between audit and the research process. *Nurse Researcher*, 3, 3:5–16.

Benner R (1984) *From Novice to Expert – Excellence and Power in Clinical Nursing Practice.* (Menlo Park, CA: Addison-Wesley).

Berragan L (1998) Nursing practice draws upon several different ways of knowing. *Journal of Clinical Nursing*, 7:209–17.

Biley F C and Wright S G (1997) Towards a defence of nursing routine and ritual. *Journal of Clinical Nursing*, 6:115–19.

Borbasi S, Hawes C, Wilkes L, Stewart M and May D (2002) Measuring the outputs of Australian nursing research published 1995–2000. *Journal of Advanced Nursing*, 38, 5:489–97.

Briggs A (1972) *Report on the Committee on Nursing* (Briggs Report). Cmnd 5115 (London: HMSO).

Brink H (1992) The status of nursing research in the Republic of South Africa: past and present perspectives. *Curationis*, 15, 4:28–31.

Burnard P (1995) Nurse educators' perceptions of reflection and reflective practice: a report of a descriptive study. *Journal of Advanced Nursing*, 21:1167–174.

Chick N P (1987) Nursing research in New Zealand. *Western Journal of Nursing Research*, 9, 3:317–33.

Closs S J and Cheater F M (1996) Audit or research – what is the difference? *Journal of Clinical Nursing*, 5, 4:249–56.

Cole N (2002) Research at a local level not only helps improve care, but also brings dividends for staff. *Nursing Standard*, 16, 30:19.

Collet N, Schneider J F and Correa A K (2000) Nursing research: advances and challenges. *Revista Brasileira de Enfermagem*, 53, 1:75–80.

Curzio J (1998) Funding for evidence-based nursing practice in the UK. *Nursing Times Research*, 3, 2:100–7.

Dawson G, Lucocq B, Cottrell R and Lewison G (1998) *Mapping the Landscape: National Biomedical Research Outputs, 1988–1995* (London: The Wellcome Trust, London).

Department of Health (1992) *Research and Development Strategy* (London: Department of Health).

Department of Health (1999) *Making a Difference – Strengthening the Nursing, Midwifery and Health Visiting Contribution to Health and Healthcare* (London: Department of Health).

Department of Health (2000) *Towards a Strategy for Nursing Research and Development – Proposals for Action* (London: Department of Health).

Department of Health and Children (DoHC) (2003) *Research Strategy for Nursing and Midwifery in Ireland* (Dublin: Department of Health and Children).

Duffy K (2002) Choosing a research topic that has personal and professional significance. *Nursing Standard*, 17, 10:21.

Flaherty M J (1990) Nursing research: cornerstone of nursing practice in Canada. In: R Bergman (ed.) *Nursing Research for Nursing Practice – An International Perspective* (London: Chapman & Hall).

Hale C (2002) Nurses and doctorates. *Nursing Standard*, 16, 21:25.

Hannigan B (2001) A discussion of the strengths and weaknesses of 'reflection' in nursing practice and education. *Journal of Clinical Nursing*, **10**, 2:278–83.

Hayes L (2002) Research provides valuable skills that can be applied to everyday practice on the wards. *Nursing Standard*, **17**, 8:24.

Henderson V (1994) Quoted in G Lobiondo-Wood and J Haber, *Nursing Research: Methods, Critical Appraisal and Utilization*, 3rd edn (St Louis, MO: CV Mosby).

Higher Education Funding Council for England (HEFCE) (2001) *Research in Nursing and Allied Health Professions* (Bristol: HEFCE).

Jackson K (1994) So much for common sense. *British Journal of Midwifery*, **2**, 3:131–2.

Kenny C (1994) Nursing intuition: can it be researched? *British Journal of Nursing*, **3**, 22:1191–5.

Kirkham M J (1994) Using research skills in midwifery practice. *British Journal of Midwifery*, **2**, 8:390–2.

Laight S (2002) Research notes. Under the skin of any nurse researcher you will find a colleague quite like yourself. Nursing Standard, **16**, 33:20.

Laudan L (1996) *Beyond Positivism and Relativism: Theory, Method and Evidence* (Oxford: Westview Press).

Lee L Y K (2003) Evidence-based practice in Hong Kong: Issues and implications in its establishment. *Journal of Clinical Nursing*, **12**, 5:618–24.

Luker K A and Kenrick M (1992) An exploratory study of the sources of influence on the clinical decisions of community nurses. *Journal of Advanced Nursing*, **17**:457–66.

Mackintosh C (1998) Reflection: a flawed strategy for the nursing profession. *Nursing Education Today*, **18**:553–7.

Macleod-Clark J and Hockey L (1986) *Research for Nursing – Guide for the Enquiring Nurse* (Chichester: John Wiley & Sons).

Mancia J R and Gastaldo D (2004) Production and consumption of science in a global context. *Nursing Inquiry*, **11**, 2:65–6.

Mander R (1992) See how they learn: experience as a basis of practice. *Nurse Education Today*, **12**:11–18.

Mangay-Maglacas A (1992) Nursing research in developing countries: needs and prospects. *Journal of Advanced Nursing*, **17**:267–70.

McCutcheon H H I and Pincombe J (2001) Intuition: an important tool in the practice of nursing. *Journal of Advanced Nursing*, **35**, 5:342–8.

Moreno-Casba T and de Frutos-Sánchez D (2002) Developing a national strategy to promote and extend nursing research in Spain. *Nursing Times Research*, 7, 4:263–71.

National Institute of Nursing Research (NINR) http://ninr.nih.gov/ninr/research/diversity/mission.html; accessed 25 May 2004.

NHS Executive (1996) *Promoting Clinical Effectiveness: A Framework for Action in and through the NHS* (Leeds: NHS).

Nygren L and Blom B (2001) Analysis of short reflective narratives: a method for the study of knowledge in social workers' actions. *Qualitative Research*, **1**, 3:369–84.

O'Brien D and Davison M (1994) Blood pressure measurement: rational and ritual actions. *British Journal of Nursing*, **3**, 8:393–6.

Paget T (2001) Reflective practice and clinical outcomes: practitioners' views on how reflective practice has influenced their clinical practice. *Journal of Clinical Nursing*, **10**:204–14.

Polgar S and Thomas S A (1991) *Introduction to Research in the Health Sciences*, 2nd edn (Melbourne: Churchill Livingstone).

Rafferty A M, Bond S and Traynor M (2000) Does nursing, midwifery and health visiting needs a research council? *Nursing Times Research*, **5**, 5:325–35.

Rafferty A M, Traynor M, Thompson D R, Ilott I and White E (2003) Research in nursing, midwifery, and the allied health professions. *British Medical Journal*, **326**:833–4.

Richardson G and Maltby H (1995) Reflection on practice: enhancing student learning. *Journal of Advanced Nursing*, **22**:235–42.

Rolfe G (2001) *Knowledge and Practice* (London: Distance Learning Centre, South Bank University).

Romney M L and Gordon H (1981) Is your enema really necessary? *British Medical Journal*, **282**:1269–71.

Royal College of Nursing (1982) *Research-Mindedness and Nurse Education* (London: Royal College of Nursing).

Royal College of Nursing (1996) *Clinical Effectiveness. A Royal College of Nursing Guide* (London: Royal College of Nursing).

Royal College of Nursing (1998) *Guidance for Nurses on Clinical Governance* (London: Royal College of Nursing).

Royal College of Nursing (1999) *Doing the Right Thing: Clinical Effectiveness for Nurses* (London: Royal College of Nursing).

Royal College of Nursing (2003) *Promoting Excellence in Care through Research and Development: An RCN Position Statement* (London: Royal College of Nursing).

Sackley, C (1994) Developing a knowledge base: progress so far. *Physiotherapy*, 80(A), 24(a)–28(A).

Schon D A (1987) *Educating the Reflective Practitioner* (San Francisco: Jossey-Bass).

Stuart C C (1998) Concepts of reflection and reflective practice. *British Journal of Midwifery*, **6**, 10:640–7.

Thompson C, McCaughan D, Collum N, Sheldon T A, Mulhall A and Thompson D R (2001) The accessibility of research-based knowledge for nurses in United Kingdom acute care settings. *Journal of Advanced Nursing*, **36**, 1:11–22.

Tierney A J (1997) Organization report: the development of nursing research in Europe. *European Nurse*, **2**, 2:73–84.

Traynor M and Rafferty A M (2001) Need to know. *Nursing Standard*, **16**, 12:18–19.

Traynor M, Rafferty A M and Lewison G (2001) Endogenous and exogenous research? Findings from a bibliometric study of UK nursing research. *Journal of Advanced Nursing*, **34**, 2:212–22.

Tsai S (2000) Nurses' participation and utilization of research in the Republic of China. *International Journal of Nursing Studies*, **37**, 5:435–44.

Uys L (1998) Nursing research in a developing country: a different edge (Editorial). *Journal of Clinical Nursing*, 7:485–7.

Valizadeh L and Zamanzadeh V (2003) Research in brief. Research utilization and research attitudes among nurses working in teaching hospitals in Tabriz, Iran. *Journal of Clinical Nursing*, **12**, 6:928–30.

Walsh M and Ford P (1990) *Nursing Rituals, Research and Rational Action*s, 2nd edn (Oxford: Heinemann Nursing).

Waterworth D A (1995) Exploring the value of clinical nursing practice: the practitioner's perspective. *Journal of Advanced Nursing*, **22**:13–17.

Wood M J (2001) Canadian nursing research in the new millennium. *Clinical Nursing Research*, **10**, 3:227–32.

Wright C M, Davies C and Francis K (1995) The history of nursing research in Australia. *Reflections*, **21**, 1:17–18.

2 Knowledge, Science and Research

OPENING THOUGHT

We might have accumulated an immense amount of knowledge in what we regard as science but we have barely begun to understand what knowledge is.

M. DeMey

Introduction

Science has evolved as a dominant and legitimate mode of knowledge production in modern societies, and research plays an important part in the scientific enterprise. This chapter examines the relationships between knowledge, science and research. While there is agreement on the distinction between the supernatural, metaphysical and scientific belief systems, there is no consensus on a common definition of science. The traditional scientific method used in the natural sciences and alternative qualitative approaches are outlined and discussed in this chapter. It will be argued that they can both contribute to the understanding of social, health and nursing phenomena and that it is the research question which determines the design and method of the study.

The need for knowledge

Humans have always had a need for knowledge. Our prehistoric ancestors had to 'know' their environment in order to survive: to know what food to eat and where to get it. Knowledge brings with it a degree of power. Sometimes sheer force and numbers have not been enough to win battles; those with a superior knowledge of weapons and tactics often had the advantage. Authority and status are bestowed on people who possess knowledge. Those who appear on our television screens to display their knowledge on particular issues are referred to as 'experts'. Professionals are highly regarded because they possess a body of knowledge in their particular disciplines. Although some knowledge is sought for aesthetic reasons, most of us need to 'know' in order to make decisions in our daily lives.

We have come a long way since humans felt at the mercy of the environment. As Sigerist wrote in 1943 in his classic book, *Civilisation and Disease*:

We have created the means of lighting up the darkness and can heat our dwellings to the temperature of summer in the middle of winter. We have learned to produce food in the quantity and quality desired, sometimes even in complete disregard of the seasons.   (Sigerist, 1943)

Since then humans have invented the microchip and sent people to the moon. We seek knowledge to change not only our environment, but also ourselves. Behaviour therapy and genetic engineering are but some of the products of this quest for knowledge, which began with our ancestors' need to know how to adapt to their environment in order to survive. In 1927 Freud wrote that the 'principal task of civilisation, its actual raison d'être, is to defend us against nature'.

The knowledge we have acquired seems to have put nature at our mercy. Indeed, a mark of modern civilisation is how nature is protected by and from humans.

Belief systems

Knowing what happens only partly satisfies the thirst for knowledge; humans also need to know why things happen. For example, knowing how day follows night, that the tide comes in and goes out or that someone has abdominal pain is not enough. We need to know why these things happen. The first two phenomena can be explained by the movement of the planets, and the last could be food poisoning. However, the same phenomena would have been explained differently in the tenth century BC, in the Middle Ages or during the Renaissance. In the history of humans, different belief systems have provided the frameworks within which phenomena can be interpreted. These systems of belief have also provided rules governing what should or should not be questioned. Three belief systems that have been dominant in the West are the mythical or theological, the metaphysical and the scientific.

Mythical or theological beliefs

In primitive times, people predominantly believed that supernatural objects or beings had power over their lives. Thus gods, spirits, planets, mountains, rivers and trees were thought to possess magical powers, and everything that happened was determined by them. According to Sigerist (1943), 'primitive man found himself in a magical world, surrounded by a hostile nature whose every manifestation was invested with mysterious forces'.

Later, organised religions emerged and provided the framework for people to make sense of themselves and the world in which they lived. Judaism, Christianity and Islam seemed to have put some order into the mythical world by providing the notion of one supernatural being, God, instead of a number of gods or spirits, but they kept some of the elements of prereligious times (Sigerist, 1943).

Metaphysical beliefs

When people began to question and doubt the power of the supernatural and relied more on their own observation of the world around them, they began to put more faith in nature, which did not appear to be as threatening as they had previously thought. This was a time when armchair speculations were rife. Philosophers and others postulated theories to explain phenomena. One such theory, which illustrates the break from supernatural beliefs and the emphasis on the relationship between nature and human beings, is the theory of the four humours postulated by Hippocrates and later developed by Galen and the Arabs. As Sigerist (1943) explains:

> Each humor had elementary qualities. Thus blood was hot and moist like air; phlegm was cold and moist like water. Yellow bile was hot and dry like fire, and black bile was cold and dry like earth. Man was part of nature. Nature was constituted by the four elements, the human body by the four humors . . . When the humors were normal in quantity and quality . . . man was healthy . . . When, however, as a result of disturbances, one humor came to dominate in an abnormal way, the balance was upset . . . and the individual was sick.

Scientific beliefs

Metaphysical thoughts had elements of science and influenced earlier scientific theories, but they were limited because most of their explanations were based on speculation.

Polgar and Thomas (1991) place the origin of Western science in the metaphysical age:

> The beginnings of modern Western science are generally traced to the 16th century, a time in which Europe experienced profound social changes and a resurgence of great thinkers and philosophers. Gradually, scholars' interests shifted from theology and armchair speculation to systematically describing, explaining and attempting to control natural phenomena.

The next stage in the evolution of human thought was to put some of these theories to the test. We began to rely more on what we could observe in order to explain phenomena. However, casual observations were not enough: there was a need to observe systematically and rigorously so that the explanations offered could be verified by others. Experiments became the medium through which scientific knowledge was created, and this area of activity became known as research. The scientific age is characterised by the belief that nature can be controlled, that phenomena can be prevented and predicted. Epidemics were no longer thought to be a punishment for human transgressions of religious laws but were seen to be caused by the spread of infections. Therefore, by preventing the spread, the disease could be contained. In laboratory experiments, the infectious organisms could be identified, and the ways in which they were transmitted could be observed.

Belief systems and knowledge

The world is made up of more belief systems than can be described here. However, the three systems described above are believed to have dominated Western thought. Although they are presented here in chronological order, different belief systems have also coexisted throughout history. Scientists and philosophers worked and lived amidst primitive societies, and spiritual, religious and scientific beliefs coexist to this day. People are also eclectic in their beliefs. This means that they can borrow elements from different belief systems in order to make sense of their world. For example, some people who believe that AIDS is caused by a virus may believe at the same time that it is also a punishment for what they perceive as 'sin'.

By contrasting these three belief systems – the mythical, the metaphysical and the scientific – a number of issues can be raised. Firstly, each system seems to have evolved from the failure of the dominant system at the time to satisfy the curiosity of human beings, science being the latest attempt to explain natural phenomena. Secondly, they each have their own interpretation of the same phenomena. For example, in the mythical age, disease was explained by spirit possession or punishment from God or other supernatural beings. Metaphysical philosophers thought that the balance between the sick person and nature was disturbed, while science attempts to identify the causal agents using microscopes, X-rays and other scanning devices. Thirdly, their sources of knowledge differ. In the mythical or theological age, knowledge was thought to be acquired through divination, revelations or dreams. Knowledge was invested in witch-doctors, healers, prophets and religious leaders. Metaphysical knowledge was obtained through speculation, inspiration and no doubt as a result of some forms of limited observation. Scientific knowledge, on the other hand, is derived mainly from research. Finally, each of these systems has rules for what should or should not be questioned or studied. The knowledge of spiritual healers or religious leaders was not to be questioned. There was a mystique concerning where this knowledge came from and how it was passed down. By and large, religions were concerned with souls and forbade the study of the human body.

The metaphysical age, which can be thought of as a transition between the other two periods, opened the way for people to question everything. Philosophers speculated on the soul as well as the body. Science, on the other hand, dictates that only what can be observed can be studied: the body, not the soul, is now the central focus of study.

Referring to the interpretation of disease, Sigerist, in 1943, summed up for us the place of science in relation to other beliefs:

> The scientific interpretation of disease is still very young. We still have enormous gaps, and we know that the truth of today may appear as an error tomorrow. Yet we may face the future with confidence because we fill the gaps of our knowledge not with religious dreams or philosophical speculations but with scientific facts. And when we make use of working hypotheses, as we have to do all the time, we know that they are assumptions and we are ready to discard them whenever new facts warrant it.

Science and knowledge

The term 'science' is derived from the Latin word *scientia* meaning knowledge. However, it is difficult to find one definition of science that is acceptable to all. Dawkin's (1989) definition of science as 'a communal enterprise in which truths are established by appealing not to authority or private conviction but to public evidence and shared logic' would be acceptable to many people, but the notion of science as searching for universal laws to explain and predict human behaviour would be challenged by many who do not believe that the scientific methods used in the natural sciences can be applied to the study of man.

The aim of science is to produce a body of knowledge that can enhance our understanding of phenomena, and, where possible, to predict, prevent, maintain or change them. For example the theory of gravity was conceived or developed by Newton and built upon by other scientists. Through an understanding of such phenomena as gravity and speed it was possible, later on, to fly an aeroplane without it falling from the sky. Thus by understanding gravity it was possible to control it. The question is, can the methods used in the natural sciences produce the kind of theories or laws which can explain, predict and control human behaviour? This will be addressed further on in this chapter.

Science and research

Scientists construct knowledge through the process of induction and deduction. Induction means that after a large number of observations have been made, it is possible to draw conclusions or theorise about particular phenomena. A theory, simply defined, is an explanation of why certain phenomena happen (see Chapter 8). The inductive method consists of description, classification, correlation, causation and prediction. The scientific study of plants (botany), for example, initially necessitated a description of the different types of plant species. The next inevitable step was to classify these, according to whether they were trees, flowers or grass, or whether they were edible or poisonous, for example. Through observation, it was possible to discover that the same plants grew better in certain conditions. After a large number of observations, scientists were able to theorise that some plant species thrived better with adequate light and water, a suggestion that could then be tested in experiments. Scientists were able thereafter to predict the conditions under which plants would thrive or wither. According to Bronowski (1960), 'science puts order in our experience'. Without descriptions, classifications and theories, we would be exposed to a mass of information about plants which we would find difficult to make sense of. Wilson (1989) reminds us:

> in the natural sciences vast amounts of time and energy were – quite rightly – consumed in their early stages by way of simply observing and classifying and describing phenomena (think of zoology, for example): only much later, and with great difficulty, could scientists move toward anything like a theory.

Other scientists, however, formulate a theory or a hypothesis (a mini-theory) and then collect data in order to support or reject it. This approach to knowledge acquisition is called deduction. For example, if the proposed theory is that heat causes iron to expand, experiments will be carried out to put it to the test. This theory will be supported so long as no one shows, in one or more experiments, that heat does not cause iron to expand. If this happens, the theory is falsified, and a new theory may emerge. The testing process has been termed 'falsification' by Popper (1969). According to him, theories formulated by researchers must be 'put to the test' by the scientific community. As Chalmers (1980) explains:

> When an hypothesis that has successfully withstood a wide range of rigorous tests is eventually falsified, a new problem, hopefully far removed from the original solved problem, has emerged. This new problem calls for the invention of new hypotheses, followed by renewed criticism and testing. And so the process continues indefinitely. It can never be said of a theory that it is true, however well it has withstood rigorous tests, but it can hopefully be said that a current theory is superior to its predecessors in the sense that it is able to withstand tests that falsified those predecessors.

There is normally some form of generalisation from observations prior to the formulation of a theory. For example, casual observations made during the Napoleonic wars showed that injured servicemen left unattended for days were found to have higher survival rates if their wounds had been infested by maggots (*Sunday Times*, 1995). These observations, however unscientific, led to the hypothesis that maggots help wound healing. This could then be tested in laboratory-type experiments.

What is research?

In our daily lives, we use deductive and inductive approaches in gathering information, drawing conclusions, or having a 'hunch' about something, and we look for evidence to support our beliefs. For example, you may find that after taking a certain medication some patients always look drowsy. You may conclude (after finding that this has happened a number of times) that there is a connection between the drug and drowsiness. You have, therefore, used the inductive approach to collect this information. On the other hand, you may have a hypothesis or hunch that a particular form of treatment is ineffective. Subsequently, having found out that a number of patients who were given this treatment did not get better, you may conclude that your hypothesis is right. You have, therefore, used a deductive approach.

The 'scientific' research process consists mainly of formulating questions or hypotheses, collecting data using research methods such as observations, interviews or questionnaires, and analysing data. You may be right in thinking that this is what we do all the time. We always have questions to which we seek answers; we either observe or talk to others in order to gather our information and we process this information and come to some conclusions. There are, however, crucial differences between the way in which non-researchers and researchers find out about phenomena.

Researchers are rigorous and systematic in their approach. Suppose, for example, that a researcher is studying the 'effects of authoritarian management on the job satisfaction of nurses'. A literature review will be carried out to help her to arrive at definitions of 'authoritarian management' and 'job satisfaction' that are acceptable to others. It must be clear that what is being measured or observed is actually job satisfaction and not another concept. If, for example, the researcher observes nurses' interaction on the wards rather than asking them questions about their level of satisfaction, the data collected would not be valid because interactions in themselves do not tell us whether or not nurses are satisfied with their jobs. A method is valid when it measures what it sets out to measure.

The people from whom data are eventually collected must represent the population referred to in the research question. In the above example, the researcher is studying the job satisfaction of 'nurses'. Therefore she must draw a sample who will be representative of nurses, be objective in her choice and avoid selecting her friends or only those who volunteer to take part; she must be rigorous and systematic in her selection of respondents. If the sample is biased, the data will not be reliable because the answers may not reflect the views of those who did not have a chance to be selected. Similarly, if some nurses in the sample understand the questions differently from others, or have not all been asked the same questions, the answers may not be reliable. Reliability refers to the consistency of a particular method in measuring or observing the same phenomena.

Once the data are collected, the researcher will analyse them systematically. She cannot reject answers that do not reflect her views. Thus, the difference between lay people finding answers to questions in their daily lives and a researcher studying a particular phenomenon is that the latter is rigorous and systematic in her approach. She must not let her prejudice influence the decisions and actions she takes. She must describe in detail all the steps taken in order for others to follow what she has done and to verify her findings, if they so wish, by replicating the study. Replication refers to the process of repeating the same study in the same or similar settings using the same methods with the same or equivalent samples.

Research can be defined as the study of phenomena by the rigorous and systematic collection and analysis of data. Research is a private enterprise made public for the purpose of exposing it to the scrutiny of others, to allow for replication, verification or falsification. This is one definition of research which may not be acceptable to those who believe that, while it must be rigorously carried out, it does have to be systematic. Some researchers do not need to ask the same questions to all respondents, nor use large random samples, and do not subject their data to systematic statistical analysis. They use a flexible approach which they believe allows them to get closer to the truth or the essence of phenomena. One can still argue that they develop their own 'systems' of collecting and analysing data but that their systems are more flexible. The definition of research given above reflects the dominant approach in social and nursing research, although this is rapidly changing. This approach has been termed the 'scientific method'. But, as we shall see later on, other methods and approaches also claim to produce 'scientific' knowledge.

Science and non-science

So far we have distinguished science from other forms of beliefs such as the supernatural and the metaphysical. But where do other forms of knowledge production which do not use the traditional scientific method fit? According to Wolpert (1993), for a subject to qualify as science it needs at least to satisfy a number of criteria:

> the phenomena it deals with should be capable of confirmation by independent observers; its ideas should be self-consistent; the explanations it offers should be capable of being linked to other branches of science; a small number of laws or mechanisms should be able to explain a wide variety of apparently more complex phenomena; and ideally, it should be quantitative and its theories expressible by mathematics.

Wolpert (1993) goes on to question whether the social sciences can match the 'methods of the "hard" sciences – from physics to biology'. He concludes that because of the complexity of the subject matter in the social sciences, it is difficult to disentangle causal relationships.

Laudan (1996), on the other hand, quotes Aristotle, who stated that 'science is distinguished from opinion and superstition by the certainty of its principles'. One can ask if it is feasible and realistic to formulate laws and theories which can predict human behaviour and social phenomena with the same certainty that phenomena in the natural sciences can be described and predicted. Laudan believes that the 'quest for a specifically scientific form of knowledge, or for a demarcation criterion between science and non-science, has been an unqualified failure'. He adds:

> There is apparently no epistemic feature or set of such features which all and only the 'sciences' exhibit. Our aim should be, rather, to distinguish reliable and well tested claims to knowledge from bogus ones.

Laudan challenges 'traditional' scientists and social scientists to devise their own methods and criteria for testing their claims (knowledge). Whether one accepts (non-supernatural, non-metaphysical) knowledge as 'scientific' depends on the particular paradigms one believes in.

Paradigms

The term 'paradigm' was coined by Kuhn (1970). Paradigms can loosely be described as schools of thought, although it will be clear later that they are much more than that. Smith (1991) describes paradigms as:

> different scientific communities [who] share specific constellations of beliefs, values, and techniques for deciding which questions are interesting, how one should break down an interesting question into solvable parts, and how to interpret the relationships of those parts to the answers.

From this description, it seems that paradigms influence:

- the nature of phenomena (e.g., do they have an autonomous existence or do they depend on our interpretations?);

- the way they can be studied (e.g., should the researcher adopt a 'detached' stance or interact with participants?);

- the designs and methods which are the most appropriate to answer the research questions, taking the above into account.

In any era, one paradigm is likely to be dominant. When this paradigm, also called normal science, is no longer effective and influential in addressing topical research problems, a crisis occurs (Kuhn, 1970). According to Kuhn (1970), a 'scientific revolution' takes place in which the dominant paradigm is replaced by a new science, which in turn becomes normal and dominant until it is in turn challenged and replaced, and so the process continues. An analogy from the field of music will serve to illustrate the notion of paradigms.

Classical music was the dominant form in the West until replaced by jazz; this was then followed by rock and roll and pop music, which is itself challenged by newer forms of music. While different types of music coexist, there is always a dominant form that emerges as a response to the failure of the previous dominant type to reflect the views or musical taste of those who buy the records. The dominant form of music provides not only the current definition of what constitutes music, but also how it should be played.

Positivism

One paradigm that has influenced much research in the health and social sciences is positivism, a movement that evolved as a critique of the supernatural and metaphysical interpretations of phenomena. The name 'positivism' derives from the emphasis on the positive sciences – that is, on tested and systematised experience rather than on undisciplined speculation (Kaplan, 1968). Developments in the natural sciences, especially physics and chemistry, led early sociologists (in the mid-eighteenth century) to the belief that the methods of these sciences could be applied to the study of human behaviour. As Ayer (1969) explains:

> It was the belief of positivists [that] the empire of science was to be extended to every facet of man's nature; to the workings of men's minds as well as their bodies and to their social as well as their individual behaviour; law, custom, morality, religious faith and practice, political institutions, economic processes, language, art, indeed every form of human activity and mode of social organization were to be explained in scientific terms; and not only explained but transfigured.

Positivists believe in the unity of science. This means that the scientific method used in the natural sciences should equally be appropriate for the study of social phenomena (for example, why people commit suicide, life satisfaction or social solidarity). Equally they believe that it is possible to deduce universal laws to explain human and social phenomena in the same way as there are laws in physics, chemistry or biology. This is known as reductionism, which, in this case, means reducing complex phenomena (e.g. suicide) to simple laws. These laws predict with precision the probability of an event or phenomenon happening. The higher the degree of certainty, the more scientific the knowledge on which the prediction is based. Positivists believe that such laws can be uncovered for social phenomena as well.

Throughout history, mathematics was thought by philosophers to be the science potentially able to explain and predict human actions. Bertrand Russell

(1971) pointed out that positivists regarded mathematics as the pattern to which other knowledge ought to approximate, and thought that pure mathematics, or a not dissimilar type of reasoning, could give knowledge as to the actual world. Many phenomena or events in the physical world can be explained by mathematical formulae. Some physicists hope to discover a formula which explains how the world came into existence. Alchemists, the precursors of chemistry scientists, were preoccupied for centuries with finding a formula for mixing substances to produce gold or to develop a potion for eternal life. Taken to the extreme, positivists in the social sciences would aspire to develop mathematical formulae to explain human phenomena. For example, an editorial in the (British) *Daily Mail* newspaper (8 August 2003) made the following comments on the work of Professor James Murray of the University of Washington, who formulated equations to predict whether a couple will stick together or divorce.

> Wondering whether your financé is really the girl for you? Then wonder no longer. Simply sit her down, talk to her for 15 minutes about a subject on which you disagree, and then work out the following equation: $w(t + 1) = a + r1*w(t) + ihw[h(t)]$. If you are a woman, wondering whether the man you fancy is really Mr. Right, then you should adopt the same procedure, but apply a slightly different equation: $h(t + 1) = b + r2*h(t) + iwh[w(t)]$. The higher values you arrive at for $w(t + 1)$ and $h(t + 1)$ the better advised you will be to dump your intended and find someone else.

This formula claims it can predict with 94 per cent accuracy whether a couple will stick together or divorce. While this example may seem to portray an extreme form of the use of mathematics to understand human phenomena, Smith (1996) points out that from its very beginning, the Royal Statistical Society has sought to promote informed quantitative reasoning as 'the dominant modality in public debate, as well as in decision-making processes of government, business and individuals'.

Positivists take a 'realist' view of social phenomena. The world has an existence independent of our perception of it and there is an objective way of knowing what it is. They believe in the separation between researchers and their object of enquiry. If we take a social phenomenon such as the war in Vietnam; positivists believe that it actually happened whether we are conscious of it or not (independent of what we think). Only one true version of it exists and it is the task of historians to find this version. They can do so provided they take an 'objective' stance.

Another important characteristic of positivism is empiricism, according to which only what can be observed by the human senses can be called facts. Positivists also believe in the notion of cause and effect (determinism) and look for explanations in empirical data. They adopt the hypothetico-deductive approach of physics and chemistry. This means that hypotheses or theories are put to the test by the deductive process during the course of experiments.

Postpositivism

Positivist beliefs, in their original forms, lasted from the middle of the nineteenth century to the beginning of the twentieth century. The founding fathers – Auguste Comte and Herbert Spencer and their followers such as Emile Durkheim – through their fascination with the progress made in physics and chemistry, had what has been described as a 'naïve faith' in the ability and appropriateness of the scientific method to study social phenomena. This position came under criticism which led to a number of adjustments and revisions. There are different versions of these adaptations; however, the main beliefs described below represent what is called 'postpositivism'.

There was a realisation that the idea of 'reality' independent of the experience of people was thought to be 'naïve'. Using the above example of Vietnam, postpositivists might say that there are so many different ways to look at what happened that it is not possible to give one true account of it. Instead postpositivists believe that it is possible to get as close as possible to (an approximation of) the 'truth'. This position became known as 'critical realism'.

The positivist notion that social phenomena can be observed in a detached way was questioned. Observation is believed to be influenced by the researcher's frame of mind, and on social and cultural conditioning (Corbetta, 2003). According to postpositivists, these influences or biases can be avoided by devising strategies to make tools more objective.

Postpositivists seem to have abandoned the quest for universal laws to explain social phenomena. They realise that it is not possible to predict a social event with the same degree of certainty that natural scientists can with physical events. For example, if research shows that divorce affects the mental health of children involved, one cannot state with certainty that this will happen to every child whose parents go through a divorce. Postpositivists are more realistic and acknowledge the 'probable' nature of predictions in social science. The search for 'causes' and 'effects' in the study of human and social behaviour has, to a great extent, been replaced by efforts to establish 'correlations' (relationships) between variables. Postpositivist researchers still aim to produce generalisable findings but they are more cautious as to how this can be done. It must also be pointed out that the nature of all knowledge is probabilistic. Even though natural scientists can predict physical events, there is still a degree of uncertainty.

The positivist notion of empiricism whereby only what can be observed by the human senses (sight, hearing, touch, taste and smell) can be called social facts would exclude the study of such concepts as anxiety, well-being or life satisfaction. Postpositivists accept that these phenomena are not observable but can be studied by means of self-reports (provided tools to measure these concepts are valid and reliable).

Despite these adjustments, the legacy of positivism still persists. 'Naïve realism' has been replaced by 'critical realism', but the belief in the existence of 'one truth' is still there, although it is acknowledged that it cannot be accessed easily.

Corbetta (2003) explains that despite these changes, postpositivism has retained much of the original characteristics of positivism:

> The new positivism redefines the initial presuppositions and the objectives of social research; but the empirical approach, though much amended and reinterpreted, still utilizes the original observational language, which was founded on the cornerstone of operationalization, quantification and generalization . . . The operational procedures, the ways of collecting data, the measurement operations and the statistical analyses have not fundamentally changed. Conclusions are more cautious, but the (quantitative) techniques utilized in reaching them are still the same.

As can be seen from the above, postpositivistic research adopts the scientific process whereby research questions (or hypotheses) are formulated in advance, the key terms are operationalised (defined), the methods of data collection are selected prior to data collection and the analysis of data is mainly quantitative. Some qualitative methods can be included in the study and made to fit in this process. The designs of postpositivistic research are mainly surveys and experiments.

Interpretivism

Postpositivistic reaction to the limitations of positivism in its original form is to devise strategies to overcome them while keeping the positivistic principles. Interpretivists, on the other hand, reject these principles, as will be shown below.

Interpretivism has been put forward as an alternative to positivism. It 'is the belief that the social world is actively constructed by human beings' and that 'we are continuously involved in making sense of', or interpreting, our social environments (Milburn et al., 1995). They share the philosophical belief that human behaviour can only be understood when the context in which it takes place and the thinking processes that give rise to it are studied. These approaches also recognise that researchers have preconceptions that must either be 'bracketed' (i.e. prevented from influencing the research process) or discussed in relation to their implications for the data.

Interprevists focus on subjective experience, perception and language in order to understand intention and motivation which can explain behaviour. For example, when a man loses his job he may be depressed. It does not mean that he will be depressed each time he loses his job, nor can we say that everyone who loses their job becomes depressed. Therefore, not only does the same person not necessarily react the same way every time he is under the same pressure, but also different people may react differently when subjected to the same pressure. Apart from the loss of a job itself, there may be other factors, such as whether or not the man liked his job, that may precipitate or prevent the depression.

Humans can also be affected by the fact that they are being studied, and their actions cannot be understood without access to the thinking processes of the person. We do not always mean what we say nor do we always say what we mean, even when we are not lying or drunk. Sometimes we do not know if and why we behave the way we do. Therefore empirical observations only skim the surface of the behaviour being studied. The intentions and motivations of the person need to be examined if we are to make sense of a behaviour. Ayer (1969) pointedly asks:

> May it not be that there is something about the material on which these sciences have to work, something about the nature of men, which makes it impossible to generalize about them in any way comparable to that which has made the success of the natural sciences?

In order to study subjective perceptions and experiences, interpretivists know that they cannot behave as detached observers. Instead, through interactions, they can get insight into how and why people behave the way they do. Such interactions cannot be pre-planned and structured, as interactions between humans are not predictable in terms of process and outcome. Therefore the methods used by interprevists are interactive and flexible. The type of data collected are mainly in the forms of conversation and narratives. These are not normally analysed statistically. The findings have limited generalisation value and are not expected to lead to universal laws. This is because interpretivists believe that their findings are context-related.

It is possible for interpretivists to share the notion of 'critical realism' with postpositivists. This means that they see their (interprevist) methods and approaches as capable of producing findings which represent reality as closely as possible. However, not all interpretivists share these beliefs. Constructivists, for example, put forward the idea of 'multiple realities'. They do not believe that there is one reality but different perceptions of what the reality is. According to them, knowledge is constructed or co-created through interactions with others and with the environment. Such ideas sit uncomfortably with those who want to uncover the 'truth'. However, if we take the view that social phenomena and human behaviour are complex, dynamic, changeable, that participants and researchers bring their own prejudices to the research process and that the tools we use can reveal different aspects of the same phenomenon, then it is not diffi-cult to understand why research does not always provide unequivocal and uncontestable results.

Different perceptions of the same phenomenon are uncomfortable but can lead to reflection and negotiation. For example, if users and professionals view a particular service differently or different users have different perceptions of the same service, this could lead to discussions as to why this is so. In practice, it is likely that the perceptions which are given more credibility are the ones which the users of the findings find more acceptable and which serve the purpose for which the study was carried out. Different historian researchers would produce different accounts of the Vietnam war, and these accounts will be accepted or rejected according to how they match the perceptions of different groups in society. Multiple realities can also be heuristic (have a learning function) in that people would be made aware how others view the same phenomenon.

There are various strands of constructivism: social, physical and radical. For more understanding of constructivism see Wrigley (1995) and Colliver (2002).

Modernism and postmodernism

The beliefs about the nature of physical and social realities are not of relevance only to the fields of science and research. They reach and influence people's thoughts in different aspects of society including the arts, the humanities and politics. What is known as 'modernism' is a set of ideas that emerged during the enlightenment period (eighteenth century) as a reaction to earlier supernatural and metaphysical belief systems. Rational thinking began to take hold and people put faith in the ability of science to improve their lives. Knowledge based on science and rationality was seen as a liberating force. Scientific knowledge was supposed to increase as scientists built upon previous knowledge. The aim was to produce theories which could explain everything in the world.

By the end of the 1950s, intellectuals began to challenge some of these ideas for what they saw as the modernists' failure to improve the circumstances of people worldwide and the limitations of their scientific ideas and methods to produce meaningful findings. This new movement, called 'postmodernism' (which has a number of strands), rejected the notion of 'truth' or 'reality' as objective, and rationalism as the only way to think. They questioned how knowledge was created and for whose benefit.

Postmodernists support the notion that knowledge is socially constructed or co-created. Interpretation and meanings have a central place in knowledge production. According to Bouffard (2001) postmodernists 'repudiate' universal laws and they believe that the attempt to produce meta-narratives (grand theories) 'is misguided and should be replaced by smaller narratives that are local, contextual, and time-bound'.

There is by no means a consensus among proponents of the different strands as to what constitutes postmodernism. This brief outline hardly does justice to the ideas on which these two movements are based. For fuller discussions of modernism and postmodernism readers are directed to the works of Toulmin (1990), Lyotard (1992), Fox (1993), Cahoone (1996) and Rolfe (2001).

Qualitative research

Interpretivism and qualitative research are sometimes used interchangeably in the literature (Williams, 2000). Qualitative research is a broad umbrella covering a number of approaches which subscribe to the notion that phenomena can realistically be understood by studying the meaning that people give to them and the context in which they happen. It rejects the idea that researchers can remain detached (objective) and replaces it instead by interactive, flexible and inductive methods capable of gaining access to people's experiences and perceptions.

Beyond this, the different strands of qualitative research vary in many ways, including their focus, their process and the type of data which they produce. They draw upon different theories and conceptual frameworks from a wide range of disciplines including philosophy, sociology, anthropology, psychology and semiotics. Atkinson (1995) argues that there is too much diversity in the qualitative approach for it to constitute a paradigm. This will be further discussed in the chapter on qualitative research.

SUMMARY

Summary and conclusion

In this chapter, we have looked briefly at the need of humans for knowledge, and we have examined the relationship between knowledge, science and research. We have seen that each of the three main belief systems not only interprets phenomena differently, but also has its own ways of 'knowing'. Science is the latest attempt to produce and organise knowledge, and research plays an important part in generating and testing theories, which remain the ultimate goal of scientific endeavours.

There is, however, no consensus on what research is and how it should be carried out. The two main paradigms in social, health and nursing research (positivism and interpretivism) have their own assumptions of how phenomena should be studied and of what constitutes scientific knowledge.

The nature of science and knowledge is such that no one school of thought can have a monopoly on the definition and the production of knowledge, although the dominant or favoured paradigm tends to influence what is researched and how. Dzurec and Abraham (1993) sum up succinctly the relationship between knowledge and research:

All research is an effort to fulfill cognitive needs, to perceive, and to know. These needs emerge from curiosity about the world as expressed in a desire to understand it and from an incessant attempt to gain a sense of mastery over self and world. Consequently, if differences among researchers exist, it is not because they aspire to different ends, but because they have operationalized their methods for reaching those ends differently.

References

Atkinson P (1995) Some perils of paradigms. *Qualitative Health Research*, **5**, 1:117–24.

Ayer A J (1969) *Metaphysics and Common Sense*, 2nd edn (London: Macmillan).

Bouffard M (2001) The scientific method, modernism and postmodernism revisited: A reaction to Shephard (1999). *Adapted Physical Activity Quarterly*, **18**:221–4.

Bronowski J (1960) *The Commonsense of Science* (Harmondsworth: Pelican).

Cahoone L (ed.) (1996) *From Modernism to Postmodernism: An Anthology* (Malden, MA: Blackwell).

Chalmers A F (1980) *What Is This Thing Called Science?*, 2nd edn (Buckingham: Open University Press).

Colliver J A (2002) Constructivism: The view of knowledge that ended philosophy or a theory of learning and instruction? *Teaching and Learning in Medicine*, **14**, 1:49–51.

Corbetta P (2003) *Social Research: Theory, Methods and Techniques* (London: Sage).

Daily Mail (2003) The right formula. Editorial, 8 August 2003.

Dawkins R (1989) *The Selfish Gene* (London: Pelican).

DeMey M T (1982) Action and knowledge from a cognitive point of view. In D B P Kallen, H C Wagenaar, J J J Kloprogge and M Vorbeck (eds), *Social Science Research and Public Policy-Making: A Reappraisal* (Netherlands: NFER).

Dzurec L C and Abraham I L (1993) The nature of inquiry: linking quantitative and qualitative research. *Advances in Nursing Science*, **16**, 1:73–9.

Fox N J (1993) *Postmodernism, Sociology and Health* (Buckingham: Open University).

Freud S (1927) *The Future of an Illusion* (London: Hogarth Press).

Kaplan A (1968) Positivism. In D L Sills (ed.), *International Encyclopedia of the Social Sciences* (New York: Macmillan/Free Press).

Kuhn T (1970) *The Structure of Scientific Revolutions*, 2nd edn (Chicago, IL: University of Chicago Press).

Laudan K (1996) *Beyond Positivism and Relativism: Theory, Method and Evidence* (Oxford: Westview Press).

Lyotard J F (1992) *The Postmodern Explained to Children* (London: Turnaround).

Milburn K, Fraser E, Secker J and Pavis S (1995) Combining methods in health promotion research: some considerations about appropriate use. *Health Education Journal*, **54**:347–56.

Polgar S and Thomas S A (1991) *Introduction to Research in the Health Sciences*, 2nd edn (Melbourne: Churchill Livingstone).

Popper K R (1969) *Conjectures and Refutations* (London: Routledge & Kegan Paul).

Rolfe G (2001) Postmodernism for healthcare workers in 13 easy steps. *Nurse Education Today*, **21**:38–47.

Russell B (1971) *Logic and Knowledge: Essays 1901–1950*, 5th edn (London: George Allen and Unwin).

Sigerist H E (1943) *Civilisation and Disease* (Chicago, IL: University of Chicago Press).

Smith A F (1996) Mad cows and ecstasy: chance and choice in an evidence-based society. *Journal of the Royal Statistical Society*, **159**, 3:367–83.

Smith H W (1991) *Strategies of Social Research*, 3rd edn (St Louis, MO: Holt, Rinehart & Winston).

Sunday Times (1995) Hospitals use maggots to heal infected wounds. 21 January 1995, pp. 1, 20.

Toulmin S (1990) *Cosmopolis: The Hidden Agenda of Modernity* (Chicago, IL: University of Chicago Press).

Williams M (2000) Interpretivism and generalisations. *Sociology*, **34**, 2:209–24.

Wilson J (1989) Conceptual and empirical truth; some notes for researchers. *Educational Research*, **31**, 3:176–80.

Wolpert L (1993) *The Unnatural Nature of Science* (London: Faber & Faber).

Wrigley K M (1995) Constructed selves, constructed lives: a cultural constructivist perspective of mental health nursing. *Journal of Psychiatric and Mental Health Nursing*, **2**:97–103.

3 Quantitative Research

Aristotle maintained that women have fewer teeth than men; although he was twice married, it never occurred to him to verify this statement by examining his wives' mouths.

Bertrand Russell

Introduction

Quantitative research has a long tradition in nursing, dating back to the time of Florence Nightingale who collected statistical data to establish the causes of mortality during the Crimean War. For some, it produces 'hard', scientific knowledge, the highest form of evidence, vital for evidence-based practice. It is caricatured and vilified by others who reject it as a viable approach in nursing research. In this chapter the characteristics usually associated with quantitative research, its usefulness in advancing nursing knowledge, and the criticisms levelled at it, will be outlined and discussed.

What is quantitative research

It is important from the outset to differentiate between quantitative approach and quantitative methods. In this context the terms 'research', 'approach' and 'tradition' will be used interchangeably to designate a particular paradigm. An approach is the whole design, including the researcher's assumptions, the process of inquiry, the type of data collected and the meaning of the findings. The quantitative approach comes from a philosophical paradigm which views human phenomena as being amenable to objective study, in particular, to measurement. It has its roots in positivism, although most recent studies reflect a postpositivistic stance. According to Hammersley (1993), 'there are probably few social researchers today who would call themselves positivists, but the influence of positivism persists'.

The process of quantitative research mirrors that of the traditional scientific method used in the natural sciences. It consists of stating, in advance, the research questions or hypotheses, operationalising the concepts (see Chapter 9), and devising or selecting, in advance, the methods of data collection and analysis. Finally the findings are presented in numerical and/or statistical language.

The quantitative approach to research involves the use of data collection methods such as questionnaires, structured observations, structured interviews and a number of other measuring tools. On the other hand, in-depth interviews and unstructured observations are normally associated with qualitative research. Researchers have to choose methods which are appropriate for answering their research questions. Methods of data collection such as the questionnaire or the interview do not belong exclusively to particular paradigms; however, selecting them is not a neutral, value-free or haphazard exercise. Instead the choice reflects, consciously or unconsciously, the particular beliefs and values of the researcher in relation to the phenomenon she investigates. For example, an attitude scale is devised and used, based on the belief that attitudes can be measured. As Hughes (1980) claims:

> No technique or method of investigation . . . is self-validating: its effectiveness, its very status as a research instrument making the world tractable to investigation, is dependent, ultimately, on philosophical justification. Whether they may be treated as such or not, research methods cannot be divorced from theory; as research tools they operate only within a given set of assumptions about the nature of society, the nature of man, the relationship between the two and how they may be known.

Distinguishing between quantitative and qualitative research (whatever the merits of the exercise) is problematic. The popular notion that quantitative research deals with quantity and numbers and qualitative research deals with quality and description is too simplistic and unhelpful. According to Henwood and Pidgeon (1993):

> Part of this confusion comes from the narrow association of qualitative methodology either within particular modes of data gathering (typically interviews or fieldwork) or its non-numeric character (for example, verbal protocols, verbatim transcriptions of subjects' discourse . . .

Differentiating between these two approaches on the basis of data collection methods or sampling procedures alone can be misleading. The essential difference between quantitative and qualitative approaches lies in their philosophical assumptions which are inferred but not always stated. These assumptions in turn guide the data collection and analysis process. According to Blumer (1969), the kind of questions asked and the kind of problem posed determine the subsequent lines of enquiry and that 'the means used to get data depend on the nature of the data to be sought'.

The main purpose of quantitative research is to measure concepts or variables (e.g. attitudes) objectively and to examine, by numerical and statistical procedures, the relationship between them (e.g. attitudes and occupation). Blumer (1969) describes a quantitative researcher as 'someone who casts study in terms of quantifiable variables, who seeks to establish relations between such variables by use of sophisticated statistical and mathematical techniques, and who guides such study by elegant logical models conforming to special canons of the "research design"'.

It has been described as being reductionist, deterministic and deductive. Its findings are expected to be replicable and generalisable. Each of these characteristics is discussed below.

The role of measurement in quantitative research

Measurement has been defined as a systematic process which uses rules to assign numbers to persons, objects or events which represent the amount or kind of specific attribute (Strickland, 1998). Measurement occupies a central position in the traditional scientific method.

According to Strickland (1993), 'without accurate and precise measurements we cannot come to understand the nature of those things we want to study and ultimately control for the benefit of improving health care and society'. Bowker (1998) asks, 'How do we know that patients are getting better or worse without evidence?' According to him there must be some observable improvement or change which can be quantified. Bowker (1998) goes on to add that 'if outcome cannot be measured, it cannot be shown to have improved'. Quantitative researchers, therefore, try to achieve scientific status in their studies by aiming to measure the concepts and variables they deal with, as objectively and as accurately as possible. Objective knowledge, in the natural sciences, is the highest form of knowledge. For quantitative researchers, objective, valid and reliable measurements remain the goal although, in practice, this is not always possible.

It has been argued that qualitative researchers also use measurement in their studies. For example, such terms as 'most' or 'a few' (respondents) indicate 'quantity' although actual numbers are sometimes used. There is no reason, of course, why numbers cannot be used in qualitative research, as they are part and parcel of the language of communication and understanding. Sandelowski (2001) explains that while numbers generally have a less prominent place in qualitative research, they are, nevertheless, useful – for example in showing how samples are selected, in identifying patterns and themes and in generating hypotheses. Similarly 'words' are equally important to quantitative researchers. It is sometimes believed that the latter deal with numbers and do not understand that words can convey different meanings. The care and attention that is required in choosing the appropriate words and phrases for questionnaires and scales is evidence of the importance of words to quantitative researchers.

Numbers are used not only to describe the distribution of certain characteristics in a population but also to determine relationships between them. Most data in quantitative research are collected or converted in the form of numbers. These numerical data are analysed mathematically and/or statistically to produce answers to the researcher's questions. Although statistical findings can be interpreted in different ways, the figures tend to speak for themselves.

Objective and subjective measurements

Measurement in quantitative research can be objective or subjective, although in practice researchers may use a combination of both. Objective measurements are those which can be empirically observed, recorded and verified. Examples of objective measures include blood sugar levels, temperature readings or weight loss. The degree of error and bias in these measures is low (although instruments can be faulty and human errors can happen). Thus measuring the weight of person with a scale is high on objectivity because neither the researcher nor the person being measured can influence (alter) the outcome. This exercise can be repeated by the same or other researchers and the results should be the same. This type of measure is therefore verifiable and replicable.

Objectivity in the quantitative approach means that the researcher 'stands outside' the phenomena they study. The ways in which data are collected and analysed are expected to be free from bias on the part of the researcher and the participants in the study. The whole process of quantitative research should reflect objectivity. For example, in measuring the level of satisfaction with district nurses' services, the researcher hands out, or posts, questionnaires to the participants. The researcher will try to be as little involved with the participants as possible. In effect, it is the tool that does the measurement not the researcher (although later on we will discuss how the values and beliefs of researchers may influence the development of questionnaires or other measuring instruments). Objectivity is also shown by selecting samples through random techniques (see Chapter 12) and by analysing data using statistical tests which will show the same results no matter who performs them.

Quantitative researchers also engage in the study of human concepts which are often not amenable to objective measurement. For example, attitudes, pain, spirituality or fatigue are experiences or beliefs which can only be conveyed by the participants themselves. The task of quantitative researchers is to construct scales (or use existing ones) that can best capture these concepts. Typically researchers select and offer a number of responses (in the form of statements) which participants are asked to rate or indicate their agreement or disagreement with. An example of a subjective rating scale is the Rosenberg Self-esteem Scale (Rosenberg, 1965), consisting of ten statements (such as 'I feel I do not have much to be proud of' and 'I feel I have a number of good qualities'). Respondents are asked to indicate whether they 'agree', 'strongly agree', 'disagree' or 'strongly disagree' with these statements. Subjective measurements, therefore, are essentially responses by participants to structured questions or scales.

Subjective measures can be crude or rigorous. An example of a crude way to measure quality of life is by asking respondents to indicate if their self-esteem is either 'high', 'medium' or 'low'. On the other hand, researchers can go to great lengths to develop tools by carrying out interviews with people, reviewing the literature and consulting experts on the topic. These tools are then subjected to validity and reliability tests before they are used in projects. In time, other researchers will comment on the strengths and limitations of these instruments, thereby contributing further to their validity and reliability. Once developed, a tool represents the phenomenon it seeks to measure. For example, the self-esteem scale represents a definition of self-esteem. This is not to say that everyone agrees with this definition; those who will read and appraise the study have to decide whether they accept it or not.

Quantitative research is often described as being reductionist. To measure non-observable, subjective psychosocial concepts, researchers resort to measurement by proxy. For example, a complex concept such as self-esteem is reduced to ten statements. This reductionist approach is commonly used in measuring physical concepts such as density, gravity or speed. The latter, for example, is measured by the time it takes for an object to travel from A to B. Time itself is measured by the movements of the 'hands' on a clock. As explained in Chapter 2, reductionism also means reducing complex phenomena to universal laws.

Objective measures are considered to be more valid and reliable than subjective measures, as the latter depend on self-reports. McKnight and Cupples (1999), commenting on a study which used subjective measures for smoking abstention, concluded that 'self-reporting of quitting for 24 hours and smoking abstention for one month without biochemical validation are not reliable outcome measures and do not provide accurate evidence'. They suggested that urinary cotinine and breath carbon monoxide would have been effective measurements (McKnight and Cupples, 1999).

As pointed out earlier, some subjective measures are crude and others are robust, depending on how they are constructed and validated. Whether they are accepted as evidence or not depends on what else is available and how these are rated by the research community. In theory, valid, reliable, replicable and objective measures remain the ideal that quantitative researchers aim for. In practice this is not always possible. Therefore they use measures they believe are appropriate in the circumstances.

Types of quantitative data

Quantitative researchers collect a range of numerical data in their attempt to answer their research questions. Typically they use such terms as level, extent, frequency, number, amount, prevalence, incidence, trends, patterns and relationships. At its most basic, quantitative data are collected to classify, group and describe attributes and behaviour of populations, and activities within organisations. These attributes or variables can be classified as physical (e.g. height, weight, gender), physiological (e.g. blood sugar level, urinary pH, cortisol levels), psychological (e.g. anxiety, attitudes, dependency levels), social (occupation, education, social support) or behavioural (smoking status, self-care activities). Some of these attributes fall within more than one of these areas. For example, nutritional status is, at the very least, a physiological as well as a physical attribute. Data on activities, events, patterns or trends include, for example, hospital attendance rates, attrition rates, number of visits, and skill mix.

Studying relationships between concepts by the use of measurements and statistical tests is another characteristic of the quantitative approach. Researchers are interested in how variables or concepts are related. For example, a researcher may want to know if social support for carers is associated with their quality of life. Thus both 'social support' and 'quality of life' can be measured and their relationship can be tested statistically. For the findings of this study to have any influence on policy and practice, the researcher would have to show that these concepts (social support and quality of life) were adequately measured, that appropriate statistical tests were carried out and that the relationship between the two concepts was statistically significant (see Chapter 16).

Randomised controlled trials (see Chapter 11) rely on quantitative measures in order to determine whether interventions have the desired effects although qualitative methods can also be used to explore some issues related to the intervention or the outcomes. This type of approach is often termed 'deterministic' as it studies 'cause' and 'effect'. For example Dougherty et al. (2002) carried out a randomised controlled trial to evaluate the effectiveness of a behavioural management for continence programme (intervention) on the severity of urine loss (outcome). A number of tools were used to measure urine loss, micturation frequency, voiding interval and quality of life both at baseline and at 6-, 12-, 18- and 24-month follow-ups. Data analysis included a range of measures and statistical tests (Dougherty et al., 2002).

These examples show that quantitative research can provide data to describe the distribution of characteristics or attributes in populations, to measure variables and concepts, to explore correlations between them as well as to determine cause-and-effect relationships. Often the same study can collect data to perform all these functions, as in a study by Day et al. (2001) evaluating the effects of a teaching intervention on the practice of endotracheal suctioning in intensive care units (see Research Example 5).

An evaluation of a teaching intervention to improve the practice of endotracheal suctioning in intensive care units
Day et al. (2001)

This is an example of a study which measures concepts (knowledge and practice), relationships between them and tests the effectiveness of a 'research-based teaching intervention' on nurses' knowledge and practice of endotracheal suctioning in intensive care units.

The data collection tools used in this study were predetermined, structured and standardised. Knowledge was measured by a 'knowledge-based' questionnaire developed by the authors. Practice was observed using a 'structured observation schedule', which was 'developed from details included in the questionnaire, from published and unpublished instruments and from pilot work'.

Data were analysed by means of statistical tests. It was found that there were highly significant differences in knowledge scores between the control and the experiment groups four days after teaching ($p < 0.01$).

Quantitative approach as deductive

Quantitative research has also been described as 'deductive' – an approach which typically tests researchers' ideas or hypotheses. Quantitative studies which are correlational and deterministic can be described as using a deductive approach since researchers test whether variables are correlated or whether one variable causes change in another. For example, in a study on 'eating difficulties in stroke patients', the aim was to 'analyse the relationship between eating difficulties and nutritional status and subsequent pressure ulcer development' (Westergren et al., 2001). This type of research is deductive as it was the researchers who selected these variables (eating difficulties, nutritional status and pressure ulcer) and decided to find whether a relationship exists between them. Similarly when Oh and Seo (2003) carried out an experiment to test the effects of a sensory stimulation programme on the level of recovery in comatose patients, they were testing their idea that there may be a relationship between the programme and the recovery of patients.

Some quantitative studies can also be exploratory. Lewis et al. (2001) wanted to know which factors were related to tobacco use by adolescents. They included the following variables in their questionnaire: age, gender, ethnicity, self-esteem, physical activity, parental smoking and socioeconomic factors. An analysis of data may reveal relationships between those variables and smoking which the researchers did not anticipate. This may lead to the formulation of new questions for study. Therefore one can say that some quantitative studies can generate new hypotheses and can, in this sense, be described as inductive. However, the deductive approach seems to dominate in quantitative studies as it is the researchers who select, in advance, which variables they want to investigate.

Finally, quantitative research is described as producing findings which are generalisable to the setting where samples are drawn or to similar settings. The selection of representative samples by random and objective methods is expected to achieve this aim. In practice, it is not always possible to do so, so researchers also resort to non-random sample selection methods (see Chapter 12). However, a study is no less quantitative if a random, representative sample is not used.

Data collection and analysis

Questionnaires, observation schedules and other measuring tools – such as scales to measure knowledge, skills, competence – and instruments to measure physiological and biomedical indicators, comprise the main methods of data collection in quantitative research. What is common with these methods is that they are all *predetermined*, *structured* and *standardised*. A questionnaire is a predetermined tool (planned in advance) and constructed prior to the commencement of data collection. Ideally, it cannot be altered when data are collected, as it would mean that some participants may be asked different questions. In quantitative research, the selection or development of tools such as questionnaires is perhaps the most difficult task for researchers. An analogy to illustrate the importance of this aspect of quantitative research is the skill and precision involved in developing a scale to measure a person's weight. Constructing the scale involves testing and checking if indeed it can measure weight and if it can consistently do so. If the scale is well developed, valid and reliable, taking the measurements and analysing the findings are relatively simple tasks.

'Structure' in a questionnaire refers to the way the questions and answers are formulated so that respondents can 'tick' or 'circle' their preferred response. The more structured the questionnaire the less respondents have to write their answers in their own words. An example of a basic structure in a questionnaire is when respondents are asked their age. They may be offered the following responses:

under 18 ☐
18–25 ☐
26–45 ☐

Scales, such as those measuring attitudes, often offer respondents a choice between 'strongly agree', 'agree', 'neither agree nor disagree', 'disagree' and 'strongly disagree' to select in response to a number of items or statements. The purpose of structure, in quantitative research, is to contribute to the standardisation of responses, to facilitate the completion of questionnaires and data analysis. For example, the units (or aspects) of social support are specified in the form of a number of items. Respondents' task is to indicate on scale of 1 to 6, the degree with which they are satisfied or not with the items. All of them are given the same scale and the same instructions. Quantitative researchers collect data in the same way with all respondents in the study. Not only should questionnaires be the same but the circumstances in which they are administered should more or less be the same as well. For example, asking some patients to rate their satisfaction with nursing care while still in hospital and giving the same questionnaire to those who have been discharged home may give different results.

As explained earlier, values and numbers are central to the measurement of phenomena in quantitative research. The choice of techniques of data analysis goes hand in hand with the selection or development of data collection methods. Quantitative researchers carry out, wherever possible and appropriate, statistical tests to establish, among other things, the probability of certain phenomena occurring. For example, if the job satisfaction scores of male nurses are higher than those of female nurses, a statistical test may be performed to find out if these scores have been obtained by chance and, if so, what the chances of this happening are. Chapter 16 explains further the analysis of quantitative data.

The value of quantitative research to nursing

As we shall see in the next two chapters, quantitative research is not the only approach that can provide knowledge on which to base practice. Those who prefer, support, fund or do quantitative research believe that it provides hard and objective facts. However, there are those, like Schutz (1962), who maintain that:

> Strictly speaking, there are no such things as facts, pure and simple . . . They are, therefore, always interpreted facts . . . This does not mean that, in daily life or science, we are unable to grasp the reality of the world. It just means that we grasp merely certain aspects of it, namely those which are relevant to us for carrying on our business of living . . .

Therefore the type of data we collect depends on what we need to know. It is the 'business' of nurses to know whether their patients get better. There are a number of indicators such as symptom relief, self-report from patients or other signs to show whether they are satisfied or not with the care they receive. Quantitative researchers would say that with rigorously designed tools we should be able to 'grasp the reality' (in this case measure the indicators of symptom relief and/or other improvements in patients) that they are interested in.

Quantitative research is primarily concerned with measurement and, according to Strickland (1998), measurement is central to everything that nurses do.

The large number of tools that have been developed to measure physical, physiological, psychosocial and other concepts and phenomena of interest to nurses is a testimony to the value and importance of quantitative research to nursing. Many of these tools developed for research purposes are also used in clinical contexts to assess patients and to evaluate the care they receive.

Norbeck (1987) suggested that many of the questions nurses need to answer are consistent with the quantitative perspective. As she explains:

> When we plan for groups of patients, assess the acuity of a unit in the hospital, develop predictive models for at-risk groups or search for causal explanations, we rely on systematically gathered, objective data drawn from relatively large numbers of individuals.

Quantitative research provides data for many of the questions that arise out of nursing practice. It is useful in providing the means to measure single concepts or the relationships (correlations) between them. For example, quantitative research has provided tools to measure pressure sores (Dealey, 1999) and to examine the relationship between pressure sores and factors such as weight, mobility, activity, incontinence and nutritional status. This knowledge can help nurses to predict and prevent, to some extent, the occurrence of pressure sores.

Quantitative approaches have been used mainly in needs assessment, in measuring competence, knowledge, attitudes and beliefs, in the evaluation of interventions and in providing data on the organisation, delivery and use of services. Quantitative data are particularly useful in identifying trends and patterns, especially where large populations are involved, and for comparative purposes.

Needs assessment of patients and nurses is a preliminary but essential step in the delivery of care. An example of a quantitative study which focused on the needs of patients is that of Westergren et al. (2001), which measured the types and extent of eating difficulties, the need for assistance when eating, the nutritional status and pressure ulcers in patients admitted for stroke rehabilitation over a period of one year. There are a number of studies that have assessed the competence, knowledge, skills and attitudes of practitioners (Pelkonen and Kankkunen, 2001; Ahern and McDonald, 2002; Plant and Coombes, 2003). Other studies have explored, quantitatively, the roles and activities of nurses. For example, Blay et al. (2002) carried out a quantitative study into the workload and roles of oncology nurses within an outpatient oncology unit.

The evaluation of interventions has attracted increasing attention since the introduction of evidence-based practice policies, although nurses have always been concerned about the effects of their practice on patients. Studies on the evaluation of interventions have proliferated recently. An example of such a study is from Tsay et al. (2003), who evaluated the effectiveness of acupoints massage for patients with end-stage renal disease and experiencing sleep disturbances and diminished quality of life. Ideas for studies on intervention can come from nurses themselves, from research studies and from the literature. For example, McKinney and Melby (2002), after reviewing the literature on 'relocation stress in critical care', concluded that there is a need for 'more research on interventions that aim to reduce anxiety following transfer, such as structured teaching programmes and family conferences'.

Interventions designed to improve nurses' competence or skills have also been studied by means of quantitative research. Such data can be useful in informing the development of effective educational programmes. Adamsen et al. (2003) studied the effects of a one-year basic research methodology course on clinical nurses' own research activity and the commitment to research in general. There are numerous studies on the effects of courses, workshops and study days on nurses' knowledge, skills, attitudes, competence and other behaviour.

Quantitative data are useful to service purchasers and providers for informing policy decisions. This type of evidence can be used to justify expenditure or support claims for funding to support one service rather than another. Quantitative research can also provide a 'quick and ready' overview of the type and level of services provided. The survey method, with large samples, can provide valuable data within a short period of time, at relatively low costs. Surveys are also successful in 'feeling the pulse' of public opinion. They are not meant to study a phenomenon in any great depth. The *Oxford Dictionary* defines 'survey' as a 'general view, casting of eyes or mind over something'. Thus surveys provide a glimpse of, rather than a window into, human behaviour or practice. Sometimes this type of data is all that managers or policy makers need in order to find out what is happening. McDonnell et al. (2003) carried out a survey of all acute hospitals in England that performed adult in-patient surgery, 'in order to provide an accurate picture of the current level' of Acute Pain Teams' (APT) provision. They also explored associations between 'the presence of an APT and a number of organisational and clinical initiatives associated with clinical excellence in the management of postoperative pain' (McDonnell et al., 2003).

Quantitative research has a long tradition in nursing and the current emphasis on evidence-based practice has, to some extent, given it a new impetus.

Criticisms and limitations of the quantitative approach

Supporters of the quantitative approach have described it as the 'highest form of attaining knowledge that human beings have devised'; its critics 'have conceptualised it as ghost requiring exorcism from nursing'; as a barrier to nursing's 'scientific quest'; and 'as being non-congruent with nursing's philosophy' (Bargagliotti, 1983). Those who reject quantitative research point to the limitations of empirical observations in understanding human phenomena. For example, when concentrating on the manifestation of behaviour, it is possible only to study what is observable. Therefore only a partial glimpse of the phenomenon is revealed. By reducing complex phenomena such as stress, anxiety or hope to what can be observed, it is not possible to have a meaningful understanding of what it means to be stressed, anxious or hopeful. Even those defending empiricism admit to the differences between physical and human phenomena and the difficulties in measuring the latter, but they still believe that measurement is possible, as Norbeck's (1987) comments show:

> The inanimate objects in the physical world can be measured, melted down, fractioned and recomposed in predictable and repeatable ways. In contrast, human behaviour is difficult to measure, multideterminant and highly variable. But such difficulties do not necessarily imply that human behaviour defies objective observation.

What appears as objectivity does in fact reflect values and beliefs of researchers. Based on her own research experience, Burch (1999) wrote a paper in which she argued that 'standardised assessment instruments ignore the social dimensions of interviewing, decontextuative scores and contain implicitly individualistic biomedical ideology of health'. As she explains:

> It is naive to assume that people's 'real' response to a question can be prompted from them by detached interviewing. Many influences operate upon how one decides to answer a question. The 'choice' is not so much between true or false but between the varying aspects of experience and perception which commonly coexist.

Burch (1999) gave many examples of how items on standardised scales can be interpreted differently by participants than intended by those who developed them. She concluded that the structured interview (designed to obtain data objectively) 'cannot be assumed to be a neutral data-gathering exercise; scores are not generated in a context-free zone; implicit ideologies of what constitutes good and bad health mean that instruments may tell us more about what society requires of its members than whether interventions are effective for patients'. Similar views are expressed by Meredith and Wood (1996), who question 'whose agenda lies at the heart of the questionnaire survey: that of the patient or that of the researcher (or agency commissioning the research)?'

The view that if researchers do not measure they are not doing science has given rise to charges of 'scientism' against quantitative researchers. Scientism is the belief that only the scientific method can produce 'hard evidence' worthy to be called science and that other ways of producing knowledge are inferior. In evidence-based practice the highest status is given to objective, measurable outcomes. If quantitative data were taken for what they are instead of what they pretend to be, quantitative research would probably not have suffered the barrage of criticism which it has since the 1970s. Data in themselves are not pretentious; it is the claim that they provide 'hard evidence' which elevates the quantitative approach to a level far above others, a position highly contested by its critics.

SUMMARY

Summary and conclusion

In this chapter, the main characteristics of the quantitative approach were outlined and discussed. It was shown that its aim is to produce 'hard evidence' by means of objective and subjective measures. Concepts and variables are measured and, where relevant, the relationships between them are explored with the use of mathematics and statistics. Quantitative studies can be descriptive, correlational and deterministic; they adopt mainly a deductive approach to research. As far as possible, quantitative researchers aim to maintain objectivity throughout the whole process, which models itself on the traditional scientific method used in the natural sciences. It is acknowledged, however, that not all quantitative studies live up to this ideal type. In practice it is not always possible to measure objectively or to select random samples. However, if the aim is to measure, however crudely, and if the scientific method process is used, then these studies can claim to be quantitative.

Quantitative research has been instrumental in providing data for over half a century to inform nursing policy, practice and education. It remains a potent research approach to many of the problems, issues and concerns facing nurses and health professionals. It is still the favoured approach for those who provide funding for health research and it has been provided with a boost by the recent introduction of evidence-based practice. However, other approaches have, in the last two decades, stated their own claims to the production of knowledge for nursing and health practice.

References

Adamsen L, Larsen K, Bjerregaard L and Madsen J K (2003) Moving forward in a role as a researcher: the effect of a research method course on nurses' research activity. *Journal of Clinical Nursing*, 12, 3:442–50.

Ahern K and McDonald S (2002) The beliefs of nurses who were involved in a whistleblowing event. *Journal of Advanced Nursing*, 38, 3:303–9.

Bargagliotti L A (1983) Researchmanship: the scientific method and phenomenology: toward their peaceful coexistence in nursing. *Western Journal of Nursing Research*, 5, 4:409–11.

Blay N, Cairns J, Chisholm J and O'Baugh J (2002) Research into the workload and roles of oncology nurses within an outpatient oncology unit. *European Journal of Oncology Nursing*, 6, 1:6–12.

Blumer H (1969) *Symbolic Interactionism: Perspective and Method* (Englewood Cliffs, NJ: University of California Press).

Bowker P (1998) Instrumented measurement: its joys and sorrows. *Physiotherapy*, **84**, 4:187–9.

Burch S (1999) Evaluating health interventions for older people. *Health*, **3**, 2:151–66.

Day T, Wainwright S P and Wilson-Barnett J (2001) An evaluation of a teaching intervention to improve the practice of endotracheal suctioning in intensive care units. *Journal of Clinical Nursing*, **10**:682–96.

Dealey C (1999) Measuring the size of the leg ulcer problem in an acute trust. *British Journal of Nursing*, **8**, 13:850–6.

Dougherty M C, Dwyer J W, Pendergast J F, Boyington A R, Tomlinson B U, Coward R T, Duncan R P, Vogel B and Rooks L G (2002) A randomised trial of behavioural management for continence with older rural women. *Research in Nursing and Health*, **25**, 1:3–13.

Hammersley M (ed.) (1993) *Social Research: Philosophy, Politics and Practice* (London: Sage).

Henwood K L and Pidgeon N F (1993) Qualitative research and psychological theorising. In M Hammersley (ed.) *Social Research: Philosophy, Politics and Practice* (London: Sage).

Hughes J (1980) *The Philosophy of Social Research* (London: Longman).

Lewis P C, Harrell J S, Bradley C and Deng S (2001) Cigarette use in adolescents: the cardiovascular health in children and youth study. *Research in Nursing and Health*, **24**:27–37.

McDonnell A, Nicholl J and Read S M (2003) Acute pain teams in England: current provision and their role in postoperative pain management. *Journal of Clinical Nursing*, **12**, 3:387–93.

McKinney A A and Melby V (2002) Relocation stress in critical care: a review of the literature. *Journal of Clinical Nursing*, **11**, 2:149–57.

McKnight A and Cupples M (1999) Motivational consulting (letter). *British Journal of General Practice*, **49**, 447:837–8.

Meredith P and Wood C (1996) Aspects of patient satisfaction with communication in surgical care: confirming qualitative feedback through quantitative methods. *International Journal for Quality in Health Care*, **8**, 3:253–64

Norbeck J S (1987) In defence of empiricism. *Image: Journal of Nursing Scholarship*, **19**, 1:28–30.

Oh H and Seo W (2003) Sensory stimulation programme to improve recovery in comatose patients. *Journal of Clinical Nursing*, **12**, 3:394–404.

Pelkonen M and Kankkunen P (2001) Nurses' competence in advising and supporting clients to cease smoking: a survey among Finnish nurses. *Journal of Clinical Nursing*, **10**, 4:437–41.

Plant M and Coombes S (2003) Primary care nurses' attitude to sickness absence: a study. *British Journal of Community*, **8**, 9:421–7.

Rosenberg M (1965) *Society and the Adolescent Self Image* (Princeton, NJ: Princeton University Press).

Sandelowski M (2001) Real qualitative researchers do not count: the use of numbers in qualitative research. *Research in Nursing and Health*, **24**:230–40.

Schutz A (1962) *Collected Papers I: The Problem of Social Reality* (The Hague: Martinus Nijhoff).

Strickland O L (1993) (Editorial) Qualitative or quantitative: so what is your religion? *Journal of Nursing Measurement*, **1**, 2:103–5.

Strickland O L (1998) Practical measurement. *Journal of Nursing Measurement*, **6**, 2:107–9.

Tsay S, Rong J and Lin P (2003) Acupoints massage in improving the quality of sleep and quality of life in patients with end-stage renal disease. *Journal of Advanced Nursing*, **42**, 2:134–42.

Westergren A, Karlsson S, Andersson P, Ohlsson O and Hallberg I R (2001) Eating difficulties, need for assisted eating, nutritional status and pressure ulcers in patients admitted for stroke rehabilitation. *Journal of Clinical Nursing*, **10**, 2:257–67.

4 Qualitative Research

Not everything that can be counted counts, and not everything that counts can be counted.

Albert Einstein

Introduction

The traditional scientific method which relies heavily on measurement is one of a variety of approaches that can be used to answer research questions. In the 1970s nurse researchers began to realise that many of the core concepts and issues of direct relevance to practitioners and policy makers could not be adequately addressed by quantitative methods. This led to the adoption of approaches which could potentially provide in-depth understanding of people's thinking and behaviour. In this chapter we will examine the purpose of qualitative research, its main characteristics, and its potential contribution to nursing knowledge. Four main approaches (ethnography, phenomenology, discourse analysis and grounded theory) will be outlined. Finally, the limitations of qualitative research will be discussed.

What is qualitative research?

To care for people and to promote or change behaviour requires an in-depth understanding of concepts such as experience, belief, motivation and intention. Quantitative research with its adherence to the scientific method and its reliance on measurement only partially address these issues. The frustration with the failure of quantitative researchers to address adequately and meaningfully the core concepts and issues of relevance to those who need them most led to the adoption and development of new research approaches. Simply because some phenomena are not amenable to measurement does not mean that they cannot or should not be studied by other methods. Some researchers began to think that in order to understand people, one should listen to, and observe, them. Instead of sending out questionnaires, some thought they could learn more by interacting with those they wanted to study. More flexible strategies (than the ones used in quantitative research) to collect and analyse data were also thought to be necessary in order to 'get below the surface'.

What is qualitative research? It is an umbrella term for a number of diverse approaches which seek to understand, by means of exploration, human experience, perceptions, motivations, intentions and behaviour. They are based on the belief that interpretation is central to the exploration and understanding of social phenomena. They use interactive, inductive, flexible and reflexive methods of data collection and analysis in order to do so. Their findings are presented in a variety of formats including descriptions, themes, conceptual models or theories.

Main characteristics of qualitative research

What is often called qualitative research is in fact a collection of approaches which share some common characteristics although they have some distinct features as well. Hammersley (1993) explains that 'the time when qualitative research was an apparently unified movement ranged in opposition to quantitative research has largely gone' and that now they are 'free to disagree among themselves'. Some of the differences among qualitative approaches will become clear in the next section.

The essential distinguishing feature of qualitative approaches is exploration as a means to understand perceptions and actions of participants. It is not uncommon for quantitative researchers to claim that they also explore phenomena (by examining relationships between variables or the extent to which respondents possess some qualities). This type of exploration is quantitative in nature and is achieved by measuring the variables and by examining relationships through statistical tests. However, the main features of qualitative exploration are that it is inductive, interactive, holistic and it is mainly carried out by flexible and reflexive methods of data collection and analysis.

The term 'exploration' in qualitative research can best be understood using the analogy of an explorer in a strange land or in uncharted territory. The exploration is undertaken to 'discover' new lands, people or customs and to learn from them. The rationale for the use of exploration in this way is based on the assumptions that researchers can only understand perception and behaviour from participants' own perspectives, in their own words and in the context in which they live and work and that there can be different interpretations of the same phenomenon. Ultimately the purpose of exploration is to gain a better understanding of how people think and of their behaviour as individuals and as part of a group. For example, health professionals and patients may view the same situation, event or problem differently. This can affect the efficient use of services and expected outcomes. A qualitative study by Britten et al. (2000) uncovered 14 categories of misunderstandings between general practitioners and patients 'relating to patient information unknown to the doctor, doctor information unknown to the patient, conflicting information, disagreement about attribution effects, failure of communication about doctor's decision and relationship factors'.

Although to some people qualitative exploration can be perceived as conversation or observation without structure and purpose, in fact, if properly carried out, it is a difficult task requiring substantial training and experience. As Blumer (1969) explains:

> It is not a simple matter of just approaching a given area and looking at it. It is a tough job requiring a high order of careful and honest probing, creative yet disciplined imagination, resourcefulness and flexibility in study, pondering over what one is finding, and a constant readiness to test and recast one's views and images of the area.

Inductive approach

Inherent in the quantitative approach is the notion that the researcher knows in advance which variables to study and the answers to her questions. Typically a set of responses are offered from which participants are expected to choose those which best fit their views or situations. This deductive approach to research is used to test researchers' ideas or hypotheses. The purpose of qualitative exploration, on the other hand, is to develop concepts, conceptual frameworks and themes from observations, interviews and interpretation of discourses (diaries, letters, biographies, historical documents etc.). An inductive approach is used, in which the researcher is open to ideas which can emerge out of listening or observing people but also from examining and re-examining her own perspectives on the subject during and after data collection. Blumer (1969) explains that this type of approach is 'to move toward a clearer understanding of how one's problem is to be posed, to learn what are the appropriate data, to develop ideas of what are significant lines of relation, and to evolve one's conceptual tools in the light of what he is learning about the area of life'. So it is not just listening to people, but a constant reflection on, and analysis of, data from and between participants and of the researcher's preconceived ideas.

This inductive approach to research is particularly useful when little is known about the topics one wants to study or when existing conceptual definitions or theories are inadequate and do not reflect people's own experience.

Interactive and reflexive process

To avoid bias quantitative researchers try to study phenomena in a detached way. In qualitative studies, researchers use interaction between themselves and participants in order to get closer to the topic under study. The researcher becomes an instrument of data collection. This means that she has to think of questions during the interview or observation and of other strategies to get as close a view as possible of the perceptions, experiences and behaviour of participants. Using intuition she can decide when to continue probing, to stop or to steer the interview in other directions. The use of self to facilitate responses and to 'read' the situation is of vital importance.

The tone, hesitation, repetition in participants' responses and the presence of others are all relevant to the researcher who is trying to make sense of what is being said and the context in which it is said. Even silences have meanings (Mazzei, 2003). In order for participants to relate their experience, reveal their personal views or act in front of researchers the way they would normally, a degree of trust is required. Researchers have to use their contact with participants to build this trust and be accepted. A detached or disengaged stance is unlikely to achieve these results. This is succinctly described by Alderson (2001):

> Qualitative research involves being reflexive, which means examining not only what people say and do, but why they might be saying those words and how the interview setting, the questions and themes and the relationship between interviewer and the interviewee might influence how each person reacts, as together they construct and re-construct their conversation.

Holistic exploration

Although a number of variables can be studied in the same research project, quantitative researchers are constrained by the number of variables they can study at any one time. The variables selected for study also reflect what researchers believe are important to focus on. On the other hand, qualitative research allows participants to put their responses in context. For example, if a participant is asked how he is coping with back pain, he has the opportunity of explaining that there are times and circumstances when he can cope or not. This may reveal types, condition and extent of coping which the researcher may not have been aware of. The participant may also put his coping efforts in the context of his family or work. What is meant here by 'holistic' refers to participants' opportunity to talk about the totality of their experience of a particular phenomenon in their terms and not through the lens of researcher-generated variables.

Researchers also have the opportunity to put participants' responses in context. Participants' experiences can be historically, culturally and socially constructed.

Flexible methods

Qualitative research relies on methods that can allow researchers into the personal, intimate and private world of participants. Flexible, imaginative, creative and varied strategies are used to facilitate this process. These data collection methods include interviews, observations, group discussions, and the analysis of video recordings, letters, diaries and other documents.

In quantitative research the methods of data collection are selected or constructed in advance. Because they are structured, predetermined and standardised, researchers cannot change the structure or format of the questionnaires, scales or observation schedules. Instead the data are made to fit into these tools. For example, even if a respondent is not too sure whether he should choose to tick 'yes' or 'no', he has to provide an answer. In qualitative research, data collection methods can be bent and moulded in order to get close to people's perceptions and behaviour. In some ways, qualitative methods resemble everyday conversations and observations although researchers require considerable training or skills to use them effectively. Often researchers have to be creative and imaginative in order to achieve the understanding they look for. Oliver (1998) describes how, in her research on physical education in a school, she tried different ways to collect data:

> It was interesting to discover just how much I could learn about students and teachers by simply talking with them and listening. I tried all sorts of things with these students. I asked some students to write stories about why people their age like to exercise or what they liked about physical education. I asked others to draw pictures and describe what it looks like to be in shape or to be healthy. And I spent time talking with others in small groups. What I learned about the needs, interests, and concerns of students through their written, visual and oral stories was fascinating.

The flexible nature of qualitative exploration also applies to the size of samples and the sampling techniques. Because each interview or observation builds on previous ones, researchers can follow new 'leads' or check emerging ideas. They are not bound by a fixed sample size, decided prior to the study, as can sometimes be the case in quantitative research. Qualitative researchers can decide during the study to interview more participants, often 'hand picked' because of the particular experience or perspectives they bring to the topic being studied (see Chapter 12). On the other hand, a researcher can decide that no more interviews are necessary when she begins to experience the saturation of data (i.e. the same data are being repeated and nothing new is emerging).

The inductive, interactional and holistic goals of qualitative exploration are best achieved by flexible, creative and penetrative methods, as summarised in this extract from Alderson (2001):

> Qualitative interviews and observations can critically address long-held and possibly misleading assumptions: by asking open questions, rephrasing and dwelling on them, and approaching a topic from different angles; by encouraging extended replies during which people may arrive at new insights while they talk; by exploring examples through narrative during which people

voluntarily introduce rich examples and incidentally make passing comments that might not occur to them while quickly working through a questionnaire; by examining ambiguities and uncertainties, and reasons for holding stated beliefs; by exploring people's views and experiences through a range of research methods; and by understanding people's responses through the meanings invested in them by the context of their daily lives.

Common approaches in qualitative research

In this section we will briefly outline four common qualitative approaches in nursing research to illustrate their diversity of focus and process and the type of data they normally seek. These approaches are: ethnography, phenomenology, discourse analysis and grounded theory.

Ethnography

Ethnography is an approach relying on the collection of data in the natural environment. Ethnographers are interested in how the behaviour of individuals is influenced or mediated by the culture in which they live. According to ethnographers human behaviour can only be understood if studied in the setting in which it occurs. People can influence, and be influenced by, the groups they live in. They have shared meanings, perceptions, language, values and norms. By focusing on culture, the ethnographer gains a holistic understanding of their behaviour. It is not about individuals but how they interact in their groups. As Prus (1996) explains:

> ethnographers assume the task of achieving intersubjective understandings of the people participating in the settings under consideration. Ethnographic inquiry requires that researchers pursue and present the viewpoints of those with whom they have contact. Thus, ethnographers strive for intimate familiarity with the lived experiences of those they study and they attempt to convey as fully as possible the viewpoints and practices of these people to others.

Ethnography means a 'portrait of people'. It seeks to convey a cultural description of groups in society, and has its roots in cultural anthropology. It was adopted by early anthropologists such as Malinowski (1922) and Radcliffe-Brown (1964) who went to live in, and study, tribal communities. They immersed themselves in the culture and adopted the manners and habits of the people they studied, as well as taking part in their rituals and customs. Nowadays, ethnographic studies also take place nearer home: in hospitals, schools, prisons, clinics and nursing homes.

In its classical form, the researcher emerges herself in the culture of the group she wants to study, by living and/or working in their midst or spending significant time with them to begin to see the world from their (the participants') perspectives. The researcher is the main instrument of data collection and data are collected from as many sources as possible within ethical and legal boundaries. The main method is participant observation (see Chapter 15) where this is possible and feasible. Ethnography allows the researcher to study how and why people behave the way they do. Instead of just interviewing them, she can spend time to see for herself and try to put herself in their place. For example, in an Accident and Emergency (A&E) department, an ethnographer will experience the busy atmosphere, the noise, the smell, the 'heat', the frustration, the stress and the sense of achievement of the staff and everything as it normally happens. She can see the decisions and actions taken and is able to talk (when appropriate) with practitioners to explore their perspectives.

Thus ethnographers use inductive, flexible and interactive methods to understand the social realities of groups of people.

Phenomenology

Phenomenology as a research approach in the interpretivist tradition 'has its roots in philosophy' and was 'conceived by the German philosopher Husserl, at the beginning of the 20th century to investigate consciousness as experienced by the subject' (Baker et al.,1992). It focuses on individuals' interpretation of their experiences and the ways in which they express them. Unlike ethnography, which places particular emphasis on people's behaviour in relation to their cultural and social environments, phenomenology focuses on describing how the individual experiences phenomena.

Phenomenology as a philosophy stresses the notion that only those who experience phenomena are capable of communicating them to the outside world, and that the researcher's empirical observations are limited in understanding people's perceptions. It is concerned with the 'lived experience' of its respondents. As van Manen (1996) explains, phenomenology aims to explore the different ways in which people experience and understand their world and their relations with others and their environment.

The researcher's task is to describe phenomena as experienced and expressed. One of the main features of Husserlian phenomenology is the notion of 'bracketing'. Simply described, it means the 'suspension' of the researcher's preconceptions, prejudices and beliefs so that they do not interfere with or influence her description of the respondent's experience.

Phenomenology is also a method comprising a set of procedures and steps to guide the data collection and analysis processes (see Chapter 10).

A recent development in phenomenological research is the adoption of a Heideggerian hermeneutical approach to the study of nursing phenomena. Wilde (1992) describes hermeneutics as:

an ancient discipline, originally involving the interpretation of religious texts. It was initially a method for finding out the correct interpretation from several differing versions of the same text.

Heidegger, a student of Husserl, did not believe that getting to know and describing the experience of individuals was enough. Instead, he stressed the importance of knowing how respondents come to experience phenomena in the way they do. As Orne (1995) explains, 'meaning, in a hermeneutic sense, refers to how a socially and historically conditioned individual interprets his or her world within a given context'.

Heideggerian phenomenology seeks to find out how individuals' personal history, such as their education and social class, past events in their lives and their psychological make-up, influences the ways in which they experience phenomena. Its focus is not on social structures, as is the case in ethnography, but on the individual's background.

According to Koch (1995), Heidegger focuses on the experience of under-standing, while Husserl focuses on the 'experience' itself. An important difference between Heideggerian and Husserlian phenomenology is that the former rejects the notion of 'bracketing', because, as Koch (1995) puts it, 'one cannot separate description from one's own interpretation'. Both the researcher and the respondent have their own preconceptions and prejudices. Heideggerian phenomenology, far from rejecting or bracketing them, regards such preconceptions as essential to the understanding of how people experience phenomena differently. According to Gadamer (1990), who further developed the hermeneutical approach, a 'fusion of horizons' takes place as a result of the meetings of the preconceptions of the researcher and of the people she studies.

There are many different schools of phenomenology, mainly because they come from the work of many philosophers including Husserl (1970), Heidegger (1962), Gadamer (1990), Merleau-Ponty (1962) and Sartre (1993).

Discourse analysis

Compared to the other two approaches, discourse analysis is a relatively new method in nursing research. Like ethnography and phenomenology, it has a number of strands (and strands within strands). In essence it is the analysis of discourse. The latter is a term used to describe the systems we use in communicating with others. These include verbal (talk) and non-verbal (which accompany talk) and written materials. Discourse analysis approaches share the belief that language is not neutral in that it just conveys what we mean, but that it plays an active role in creating and changing our identities, social relations and our world (Phillips and Jorgensen, 2002). How we 'express' ourselves is not a neutral and passive medium. What we say, how we say it, our choice of words, tone and timing are full of values, meanings and intentions. The purpose of discourse analysis is to uncover them and thereby increase our understanding of human behaviour, in particular how, through language and interaction, we shape, and are shaped by, our world. In discourse analysis, what is spoken or written should also be analysed in its social, political and historical context.

The main sources of data are conversations (between participants) between participant and interviewer. Written materials in the form of policy documents, case notes, letters and educational programmes have also frequently been the object of discourse analysis (see e.g. Traynor, 1996; Spalding, 2000; Charles-Jones et al., 2003).

The various strands of discourse analysis draw from a range of philosophical and theoretical perspectives, which lead to particular aims, methods and focus (Phillips and Jorgensen, 2002). Discourse analysts have used frameworks based on the works of Garfinkel (1967), Cicourel (1964), Saussure (1960), Laclau and Mouffe (1985) and Foucault (1972) and others. One of the most common strands of discourse analysis is conversation analysis, which according to Corbetta (2003):

> starts from the premise that conversation is one of the most common forms of interaction between individuals, and that, like all forms of interaction, it does not take place haphazardly; rather, it follows a set of unspoken rules and standard patterns, of which the interlocutors themselves are unaware, and which are an integral part of the culture to which they belong.

The purpose of conversational analysis is 'to gain insight into questions about communication, social action and the construction of self; the Other and the world' (Phillips and Jorgensen, 2002). This type of analysis is illustrated in the work of Potter and Wetherell (1987). Conversational analysis uses social psychological concepts.

The work of Foucault (1972) has been very influential in the development and direction of discourse analysis. It is particularly used to provide critical frameworks for health and nursing research. According to Traynor (1996), 'Foucaultian analysis aims to unmask power for the use of those who suffer from it and is directed against those who seize power in their name'. This type of analysis has revealed how, through language, we acquire, exercise or lose power. Power relationships as exercised through language is the focus of the Foucaultian approach to discourse analysis in studies on consultation (between patients and professionals), negotiation (between health professions) and decision making.

There are similarities between discourse analysis and ethnomethodology (Garfinkel, 1967). In its original form, ethnomethodology is the study of social behaviour through interactions, in particular how language is used not only to convey but also to create meanings. The focus is on discourse and interactions which occur in natural settings (hence the use of the term 'ethno'). For a critical review of ethnomethodology see Atkinson (1988).

Discourse analysis is not just about power and dominance. It is also about how we convey and construct meanings in our daily lives through the content and structure of language and the context in which it is used.

Grounded theory

An alternative to the hypothetico-deductive approach of positivism was formulated by Glaser and Strauss (1967), who coined the term 'grounded theory' to mean an inductive approach to research whereby hypotheses and theories emerge out of, or are 'grounded' in, data. Grounded theory itself is not a theory but a description of theories developed in this way. Strauss and Corbin (1990) provide a clear answer to the question of 'what is grounded theory?':

> A grounded theory is one that is inductively derived from the study of the phenomenon it represents. That is, it is discovered, developed, and provisionally verified through systematic data collection and analysis of data pertaining to that phenomenon. Therefore, data collection, analysis, and theory stand in reciprocal relationship with each other. One does not begin with a theory, then prove it. Rather, one begins with an area of study and what is relevant to that area is allowed to emerge.

Grounded theory is based on the theory of 'systematic interactionism' (Blumer, 1969). This theory is useful in explaining social processes and has tremendous potential in increasing our understanding of human behaviour. Glaser and Strauss (1967) believed that existing theories were speculative and did not arise out of observations of behaviour.

The purpose of grounded theory is to generate hypotheses and theories, although, as Glaser and Strauss (1967) suggest, once hypotheses or theories have been formulated from observations, they can be tested deductively. Grounded theory, as a research approach, is particularly useful in nursing, an emerging science still seeking to clarify its concepts and to develop its own theories. In recent years there has been a split between Glaser and Strauss. Glaser (1992) believes that Strauss and Corbin's (1990) techniques and procedures 'force' concepts and theories, rather than allowing them to emerge. For a discussion of this split see Melia (1996) and Boychuk Duchscher and Morgan (2004). Other researchers, including Stern (1980) and Keady (1999), have modified and developed their own interpretation of grounded theory and its techniques. Grounded theory is further explained in Chapter 10.

Similarities and differences between approaches

What is common between the qualitative approaches discussed so far is that they are all interpretivist in the broad sense of the term, in that they place emphasis on interpretation (rather than on objective empirical observations).

They are interactive because researchers engage in conversations and with texts (for example in discourse analysis). These approaches collect data from the participants' perspectives and analyse data by taking into account their specific contexts.

These similarities can sometimes lead to 'method slurring' (Baker et al., 1992). Just because the views of individuals are sought does not mean that the study is phenomenological. In the same way, studying individuals in their own environment does not necessarily make it an ethnographic study. Since all four approaches seek to study individuals' experiences and perceptions in the context of their natural environment and at a particular point in time, it is difficult to differentiate between them. However, if one understands what the focus is for each of these approaches and their particular philosophical and theoretical premises, the differences between them may become clearer.

Ethnography focuses on culture, phenomenology on consciousness, discourse analysis on language, and grounded theory's aim is the development of theory through induction. However, the aim is the same: to understand the actions and reaction of individuals, groups and organisations. Each of these focal points (culture, consciousness and language) provides researchers access to the world of their participants.

These approaches have their own distinctive methods and procedures which researchers can use or adopt to collect and analyse data. These will be discussed further throughout the book and in particular in the chapter on Research Designs.

Finally, researchers also use two or more qualitative approaches in the same study. For example Maggs-Rapport (2000) combined ethnography and phenomenology in her study, while Swanson-Kauffman (1986) 'blended' phenomenological, grounded theory and ethnography in hers. Johnson et al. (2000) argues that this 'pluralistic' approach is 'not only sensible, it is increasingly inevitable', while Morse (1991) believes that such mixing 'violates the assumption of data collection techniques and methods of analysis of all the methods used'. Some of these approaches are difficult to understand singly, let alone to use combined in a study. To use more than one would require a good rationale and a thorough knowledge of their philosophical premises and their procedures and of the implications of mixing them.

Qualitative research and nursing

In the early years of the development of nursing research, quantitative approaches were dominant. In the 1970s researchers began to realise that many of the core concepts and issues of relevance to practitioners and policy makers could benefit from research approaches capable of providing in-depth understanding of nursing health phenomena.

With the emphasis, in recent years, on users' participation in decision making in their own care, the need to listen to them and understand their perspectives increased. While questionnaires and scales provide useful data to achieve this objective, qualitative methods are more appropriate for getting to know users' perspectives and experiences.

The increasing popularity of qualitative research in nursing in the last two decades has been noted by a number of authors. Morse et al. (1998) observed that qualitative research is proliferating and nursing and other health journals are increasingly publishing a higher proportion of qualitative research. Kirkevold (2000) believes that nursing has moved away from the traditional positivist research towards one which is 'based on human science assumptions'. The growing recognition of the value of qualitative research in addressing issues and problems of concern to practitioners is not confined to nursing. A crude search (using the term 'qualitative') of the *British Medical Journal* showed that from January 1994 to December 1999 (six years) there were 83 such items compared with 89 in just two years, from 2000 to 2002 (Parahoo, 2003).

Nursing's philosophy is perceived by some (Munhall, 1982; Kirkevold, 2000) as being congruent with qualitative approaches. Apart from being technical, nursing is also patient-centred, holistic and humanistic. Most qualitative approaches share some of these characteristics, which makes them suitable for the study of nursing phenomena. Qualitative research, with its focus on the experiences of people, stresses the uniqueness of individuals. In nursing, each patient is a unique individual for whom a specific care plan is developed.

Qualitative researchers collect data from respondents, often in their natural environments, taking into account how cultural, social and other factors influence their experiences and behaviour. Nursing care should ideally be holistic in that the patient and her illness are treated together, rather than the illness being treated separately. The environment in which the patient lives, her partner and her family, should all be taken into account in the planning and delivery of care. According to Holloway and Fulbrook (2001) qualitative research is now often favoured in nursing and midwifery because it emphasises a person-centred and holistic approach.

Qualitative approaches value respondents' views and seek to understand the world in which they live. Implicit in some approaches and explicit in others is the notion that respondents have experiences, wishes and rights that must be respected. Bailey (2001) explains that 'without knowledge of what illness and healthcare mean to people and of how lives are changed, we are left groping or insensitive about what it means to care for people'. As will be shown below, some researchers believe in the empowering potential of research for the participants. Nurses, too, are expected to adopt a humanistic approach to their work, which entails not letting their personal prejudices influence their professional judgement, and respecting and promoting their clients' rights.

Qualitative research is also perceived as contributing more towards ethical health care than quantitative research. Alderson (2001), referring to her work on ethical issues relating to the care and treatment of children, points out that 'each case is so individual that research about the elusive processes of children's competent decision making is understood more clearly through qualitative case studies rather than through standardised questionnaires'. However, it should be noted that quantitative methods also help to ensure that treatments are effective and do no harm, which is at the core of nursing philosophy itself.

The interactive process of qualitative approaches (more in some than in others) can also be perceived as being compatible with nursing's aims of achieving better care and creating more healthy conditions through patient participation. According to Cresswell (1994), researchers adopting a qualitative stance 'interact with those they study, whether this interaction assumes the form of living with or observing, informants over a long period of time or actual collaboration'. User participation in research studies 'is currently seen as an ethically appropriate way to proceed when researching disadvantaged groups and it is encouraged by funding agencies' (Parry et al., 2001).

Research produces knowledge and it has the potential to empower those who carry it out and those who fund it. Some sections of society benefit more than others. Some women in particular feel that research studies by men on women, considering topics chosen mainly by men, do not necessarily serve women's interests and in fact contribute to their domination. Thus feminist research emerged out of the failure of conventional research to address the issues of relevance and benefit to women. According to Seibold et al. (1994), 'feminist researchers share with critical theorists the need to make a difference through research; that is the desire to bring about social change of oppressive constraints through criticism and social action'. Seibold et al. (1994) cite Duffy's (1985) typical checklist of what characterises feminist research:

> the principal investigator is a women: the purpose is to study women and the focus of the research is women's experiences; the research must have the potential to help the subjects as well as the researcher; it is characterised by interaction between researcher and subject, non-hierarchical relations and expression of feelings and concern for values (one or all may be incorporated); the word feminist or feminism is used in the report; non-sexist language is used, and the bibliography includes feminist literature.

Although the qualitative approach, with its notion of interacting and collaborating with participants, is better suited to feminist research, there are those, like Oakley (1989), who believe that experimental research such as randomised controlled trials can be emancipatory in practice and can be of benefit to those involved in research and to women more generally. Jayaratne (1993) also advocates the use of quantitative methodology in feminist research. For an example of feminist research see Seibold (2000).

Finally, despite the popularity of qualitative research in nursing and in the professions allied to medicine, it still does not enjoy the same recognition from funders with their emphasis on interventions and outcomes research (Morse et al., 1998).

Qualitative studies in nursing and health research

In the previous chapter, ways in which quantitative research can enhance policy, practice and education in nursing and other health professions were highlighted. In this section we will look at examples of the types of problems or concerns of practitioners that can be addressed by qualitative approaches. For the sake of simplification these studies will be divided into those which:

- explore patients' experience and behaviour;
- explore the experience and behaviour of nurses and other health professionals;
- evaluate interventions and services;
- explore core concepts relevant to nursing and health.

Studies which explore patients' experience and behaviour

Nurses gain their understanding of their patients' experience mainly through direct care and from the literature. Qualitative studies can provide further insight into these experiences. For example Low et al. (2003) explored, through qualitative interviews, adolescents' experience of childbirth because very little was known about it. They found differences between women's interpretations of birth in the literature and 'the meanings assigned to childbirth experiences by the adolescents in this study'. They conclude that their results 'provide an entrée into understanding unique characteristics of giving birth as an adolescent and potential roles health care providers can play to provide a positive experience'.

To provide efficient, humane and ethical care nurses need to know why patients behave the way they do and about the personal and structural factors which influence the way they perceive health, illness and health services. One of the persistent problems in health care is the non-compliance of patients with prescribed treatment or advice of health professionals. Health professionals have their own beliefs and assumptions of why this happens. However, patients themselves have a lot to contribute towards an understanding of this problem. For example Tolmie et al. (2003) interviewed patients to find out why some patients, despite having established coronary heart disease and elevated cholesterol, do not comply with their prescribed statin regimen. They found that 'acceptance of and compliance with statin therapy appeared to be associated with the provision, interpretation and feedback of information during patient–practitioner consultation, and patients' beliefs about personal health status, cholesterol, and recommended cholesterol-lowering strategies'. These findings have implications for the assessment of patients prior to the initiation of therapy and at appropriate intervals thereafter (Tolmie et al., 2003).

Nurses need to know which factors facilitate or hinder their patients or clients to adopt healthy lifestyles or get better. Tod (2003) explored, by means of interviews, the barriers to pregnant women stopping smoking. The study uncovered a number of factors and barriers such as the role and meaning of smoking for women with a high caring burden and socioeconomic problems, the influence of family and friends, their perceptions of smoking risks and of the nature of smoking cessation service delivery (Tod, 2003). These findings have implications for those who provide such services. Another study investigated the barriers to good nutrient intakes during pregnancy (Begley, 2002). Researchers also want to know about the qualities of patients which contribute to positive outcomes. For example, King et al. (2003) examined the nature of resilience in people with chronic disabilities. They uncovered 'protective factors, processes, and ways in which people with disabilities draw sense and meaning in life' and concluded that these findings have important implications for service delivery.

Qualitative research has also been useful in exploring and assessing patients' knowledge of disease, illness, medication or health services. Steinberg et al. (2002) investigated the knowledge, attitudes and health care experiences of deaf women. Although the findings of such studies apply mostly to the population from which the samples are drawn, they can prompt those who read the report to reflect on their applicability to their own patients or clients.

Studies which explore the experience and behaviour of nurses and other health professionals

The experience, perceptions, knowledge, attitudes, beliefs and practice of nurses can also influence patients' outcomes. All these aspects have been studied with the use of qualitative research. Rubarth (2003) described the 'lived experience of nurses who care for newborns with sepsis'. They uncovered many different emotions, reactions and perceptions which they believe can assist nurses to have a better understanding of the role of the nurse and the emotional burden of working in the neonatal intensive care unit.

Nurses' perceptions of the concepts which they deal with on a daily basis have implications for their practice. Thunberg et al. (2001) carried out a grounded theory study of health care professionals' understanding of chronic pain. They found that while nurses talked about a biopsychosocial model of care of people with chronic pain, their practice reflected biomedical principles. Thus qualitative research, using the inductive process, can potentially reveal discrepancies between beliefs and practice.

Studies which evaluate interventions and services

Qualitative research has been used to compare the perceptions of the public with those of practitioners, as often there can be wide discrepancies between them. Examples of such studies include Gilmet and Burman's (2003) exploration of 'stroke perceptions of well lay persons and professional care givers' and

Britten et al.'s (2000) investigation of misunderstandings between patients and doctors associated with prescribing decisions in general practice.

Qualitative approaches can provide data on the effectiveness of tools and interventions which nurses and other health professionals use. For example, Cowley and Houston (2003) examined, by means of interviews and observations, the acceptability and effectiveness of a 'structured health needs assessment tool' from the perspective of health visitors. They found that the tool 'caused anxiety and distress to, particularly, the most vulnerable clients', the 'structured format of the tool appeared to encourage the health visitors to question instead of listen' and 'it did not help to identify all the needs and intruded into normal practice in an insensitive and unhelpful way' (Cowley and Houston, 2003). Jay (1996) reviewed the literature and found medical and nursing staff tend to respond to physiological needs without adequate consideration of psychological needs of seriously injured patients. However, her qualitative study showed that 'central to the delivery of emergency care is the individual's transitions from their normal independent existence through prehospital trauma and into the isolating experience of fear, dependence and the resuscitation room' (Jay, 1996). Other researchers have used qualitative research to explore nurses' knowledge of wound swabbing techniques on a plastic surgery unit (Starr and MacLeod, 2003) or to find out if 'touch is a valid therapeutic intervention' (Tune, 2001). Qualitative research can be useful to inform policy as well. For example, Parsons and Stonestreet (2003) identified through 'open-ended guided interviews' factors that contribute to nurse manager retention.

Studies which explore core concepts relevant to nursing and health

Many of the above examples are of studies which explored concerns of practitioners, and their findings are often of direct relevance to the population or setting where they have been carried out. However, qualitative research can also contribute to the development of concepts, conceptual frameworks and theories which can have wider applications. Glaus et al. (1996) explored the concept of fatigue/tiredness in cancer patients and in healthy individuals. They classified 'tiredness/fatigue into expressions of physical, affective and cognitive tiredness/fatigue' and offered, tentatively, 'a step-like theory, involving nociception, perception and expression of tiredness'. DeLaurentis Schultz (2000) studied the concept of 'dyspnea' in patients with chronic obstructive pulmonary disease. They produced a model which comprised three phases and three sub-types of the 'dyspneic' process and a set of preconditions and triggers that set the process in motion, as well as the consequences. According to DeLaurentis Schultz (2000), their study 'represents a first and necessary step towards concept refinement and theory development'. She explains that the notion of process in dyspnea 'represents a promising insight with potential nursing practice implications related to intervention' and that 'nurses can influence patient thinking, their responses and ultimately patient outcomes'.

Often, as acknowledged by the researchers themselves, one study can only tentatively develop a conceptual framework or theory. Further research is recommended to build upon these preliminary findings. Combining results of a number of studies can also contribute towards the development of theories. Kearney (2001) systematically analysed and combined the findings of 13 studies in order to develop a theory of women's experience in violent relationships.

While theories can broaden practitioners' thinking, they can enhance practice directly or indirectly. Morse et al. (1998) describe in detail how theories derived from qualitative research were used to develop the Hope Assessment Guide (Penrod and Morse, 1997) and the Assessment Guide for Bi-polar Disorders (Hutchinson, 1993, 1998). Both guides were implemented and evaluated using qualitative methods in order to modify and strengthen them. The direct application of findings from qualitative research is not evident enough in the literature. Morse et al. (1998) suggest that 'it is time for qualitative researchers to consider how their research can be used directly to guide clinical practice'.

The examples in this section show the relevance and potential contribution of qualitative research to practice, policy, education and theory development. It should, however, be obvious by now that both quantitative and qualitative research can be used to study the same phenomena: views of patients and nurses, barriers to positive health, knowledge, attitudes, effectiveness of intervention and similar issues. The difference, however, is *how* they study these phenomena. For example, a quantitative researcher may give respondents a list of barriers to a healthy diet and ask them to tick those which apply to them, while a qualitative researcher will explore with them what they think the barriers are without imposing their own views on them. Quantitative researchers study these problems using questionnaires and scales with the purpose of measuring them. Qualitative researchers, on the other hand, explore phenomena by using inductive, flexible and interactive processes. For an example of a qualitative study see Research Example 6.

Criticisms and limitations of qualitative research

The main criticisms of qualitative research are that it is anecdotal, unscientific and produces findings that are not generalisable. Qualitative research has been described as anecdotal, journalistic, impressionistic and subjective. Green and Britten (1998) point out that there are important differences

> between anecdotes (stories told for their dramatic or other qualities, without analysis or critical evaluation) and qualitative research. Rigorously conducted qualitative research is based on explicit sampling strategies, systematic analysis of data, and a commitment to examining counter explanations.

Nurse–patient relationships in palliative care

Mok and Chui (2004)

A qualitative study.

Mok and Chui carried out a qualitative study to explore aspects of nurse–patient relationships in the context of palliative care.

Comments:

1   They wanted to focus on 'several dimensions of this relationship, including its context, relational qualities and patients' and nurses' interpretations and meanings of the relationship'. The rationale for doing so was based on the lack of research that focused on nurse–patient relationships in the context of palliative care, in particular in the Chinese context.

2   Data were collected by means of open-ended, unstructured interviews. The emphasis was on obtaining participants' views rather than testing the researchers' ideas. Mok and Chui (2004) explain that they tried 'to strike a balance between allowing the story to emerge and directing the interview'.

3   The purpose of qualitative studies is to gain an insight into phenomena. In this study the data revealed four major categories: 'forming a relationship of trust', 'being part of the family', 'refilling the fuel among the journey of living and dying', and 'enriched experience'. These categories were then used to develop a nurse–patient relationship within a palliative care context.

All research involves the systematic and rigorous collection and analysis of data, and qualitative research is no exception. All researchers, including qualitative ones, have to demonstrate how they collect and analyse data, justify their decisions and be aware of the strengths, limitations and implications of their selected approach for studying a particular topic or phenomenon.

Qualitative research has been charged with being unscientific in that it does not use methods which have been shown to be valid or reliable (two concepts which are at the heart of quantitative approaches). In particular it is suggested that researchers get so involved that they cannot be objective. Reliability in quantitative terms is the consistency with which a tool measures what it is supposed to measure. This interpretation of reliability is rejected in qualitative research since it is believed that an interaction between a researcher and a participant (such as in an interview situation) is a unique encounter which happens at a specific point in time and space. Neither the same researcher nor others can reproduce this interaction and the data collected from it. Far from seeing this as a weakness, qualitative researchers point out that it is necessary not to remain detached, otherwise it is not possible to obtain an in-depth understanding of whatever is being studied.

The problem of knowing whether participants tell us what they really think and believe applies to both quantitative and qualitative approaches. The latter involves social interactions of a kind that are conducive to disclosure, in particular if there is a degree of 'cosiness', trust and intimacy. On the other hand, one can argue that intimate, embarrassing and personal details can best be collected by means of questionnaires which can guarantee anonymity.

Qualitative research also allows for questioning, probing and for clarification of contradictions and inconsistencies in responses, in particular when there is more than one contact with the same participants and if data are collected from a number of sources (as happens in grounded theory and ethnographic research).

In quantitative research the focus is on producing reliable and valid tools. If a tool is reliable it is assumed that it will produce reliable findings. While this is usually true of tools measuring physical concepts such as temperature or weight, it is not necessarily so with the measurement of attitudinal or behavioural concepts, since humans can react to tools the way that temperature cannot do to a thermometer. For example even if a reliable and valid scale is used to measure research utilisation in clinical practice, one cannot be certain that respondents are giving an accurate account of their practice. It is possible that they consistently give socially desirable answers. One can conclude that no method or approach has a monopoly on collecting reliable data. It is not a question of whether qualitative or quantitative methods are reliable or not, but rather the degree to which one can assume that they are reliable. This depends on the type of data, the context in which, and the people from whom, data are collected. Both approaches have devised appropriate and relevant strategies to try and ensure that their findings are reliable.

The concept of validity reflects the accuracy with which the findings reflect the phenomenon being studied. In the final analysis, the findings must be credible to be of any value. Data collection in qualitative research carries with it an in-built process whereby as the first tentative findings emerge, they are rigorously examined, compared with other participants' responses, viewed within the context of existing knowledge, confirmed, modified or rejected in further interviews or observations until the researcher is confident that the final findings represent the phenomenon as accurately as possible. As Morse (1999) reminds us, 'the most significant feature of all qualitative methods (except the semi-structured interview) is the pattern of data collection – analysis – collection – analysis, ad infinitum'.

Perhaps the most frequent criticism of qualitative studies is that their findings are not generalisable because small, 'hand-picked', localised, unrepresentative samples are used. Most studies that are carried out well can be of value beyond the sample studied. For example, Britten et al. (2000) conducted an exploration of patients' expectations before consulting a general practitioner and related these expectations to the behaviour of both patients and doctors in the consultation and to subsequent use of medicine. They identified 14 categories of 'misunderstandings'. Doctors reading the paper will be able to compare these findings with their own experience and identify which, if any, of those 'misunderstandings' apply to their own practice. Many qualitative studies are in the form of case studies, the findings from which are often criticised as only applicable to the case or group being studied. Sandelowski (1997), on the other hand, points out that generalisations can be drawn from and about cases and that 'entire fields of knowledge, such as ethics, law, and several domains in psychology, have been constructed from case generalizations'.

In quantitative research the findings from large, random, representative samples, are expected to be generalisable to the population from which the samples are drawn. This is appropriate for studies, for example, which seek to know how many people are satisfied with the care they receive or how they score on a 'quality of life' scale. In qualitative research the aim would be to explore what the concept 'quality of life' means to the participants. For this task the number of participants is of little relevance. The aim is to find out who can help the researcher to gather as many different perspectives as possible. She has to rely on her knowledge of participants and on the advice of health professionals to explore this concept. A random, representative sample would most likely reveal more of the same. The focus, therefore, is not on generalising to the sample but on developing a concept or theory that represents the phenomenon. As Green and Britten (1998) put it, 'the generalisability of qualitative research is likely to be conceptual rather than numerical'.

Qualitative research, like other approaches, has its limitations as well. Since it is believed that one interpretation is as valid as any other, the problem of choosing between them when presented with conflicting ones remains a challenge. Researchers have devised ways such as asking participants if they recognise the researcher's interpretation of what they said, or finding out if other researchers would interpret the data in the same way as the researcher. These strategies are not without challenges and problems.

These and other criticisms have been addressed in detail as far back as a quarter of a century ago by Halfpenny (1979) and more recently by Sandelowski (1997). It is important to note that research paradigms have different philosophical assumptions, rules and norms which researchers follow in order to produce scientific knowledge. It is not helpful to use the rules and criteria of one paradigm to evaluate the process and outcomes of other paradigms. To use an analogy, one cannot use the beliefs of one religion to judge another. Each has its own criteria and rules of what is 'good' or 'bad' and how people should live their lives.

Although the term 'scientific method' is usually associated with quantitative research, other approaches are not less scientific since they do not explain phenomena in supernatural or metaphysical terms. Alternative approaches to quantitative research recognise that human beings think and act rationally but that they do not do so all of the time and in all circumstances, and in a mechanical way. They have feelings, emotions, motivations, beliefs, customs, environmental constraints which are difficult for quantitative approaches, with their emphasis on objectivity and measurement, to access in a meaningful way.

SUMMARY

Summary and conclusion

In this chapter we have discussed the meaning, characteristics and purpose of qualitative research. It is a broad term comprising a number of diverse approaches which share the belief that subjective interpretation is central to the exploration of human and social phenomena. Qualitative researchers use interactive, inductive, flexible and reflexive methods in their studies. Beyond this some of the main qualitative approaches, such as ethnography, phenomenology, discourse analysis and grounded theory, have their own procedures to collect, analyse, interpret and present data. They are based on theories from diverse disciplines such as philosophy, sociology, psychology, semiotics or a combination of these.

Qualitative research is particularly useful in exploring users' and professionals' experience, behaviour and practice, and for contributing to the definition of core nursing and health concepts.

Both qualitative and quantitative research have their strengths and limitations. In the next chapter we will explore how these two approaches and methods can be combined in the same study.

References

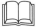

Alderson P (2001) *On Doing Qualitative Research Linked to Ethical Healthcare*. Vol. 1 (London: The Wellcome Trust).

Atkinson P A (1988) Ethnomethodology: A critical review. *Annual Review of Sociology*, 14:441–65.

Bailey C (2001) Revisiting qualitative inquiry: Interviewing in nursing and midwifery research. *Nursing Times Research*, 6, 1:551.

Baker C, Wuest J and Stern P N (1992) Method slurring: the grounded theory/phenomenology example. *Journal of Advanced Nursing*, 17:1355–60.

Begley A (2002) Barriers to good nutrient intakes during pregnancy: a qualitative analysis. *Nutrition and Dietetics*, 59, 3:175–80.

Blumer H (1969) *Symbolic Interactionism: Perspective and Method* (Englewood Cliffs, NJ: University of California Press).

Boychuk Duchscher J E and Morgan D (2004) Grounded theory: reflections on the emergence vs. forcing debate. *Journal of Advanced Nursing*, 48, 6:605–12.

Britten N, Stevenson F A, Barry C A, Barber N and Bradley C P (2000) Misunderstandings in prescribing decisions in general practice: qualitative study. *British Medical Journal*, **20**:481–4.

Charles-Jones H, Latimer J and May C (2003) Transforming general practice: the redistribution of medical work in primary care. *Sociology of Health and Illness*, **25**, 1:71–92.

Cicourel A V (1964) *Method and Measurement in Sociology* (New York: Free Press).

Corbetta P (2003) *Social Research: Theory, Methods and Techniques* (London. Sage).

Cowley S and Houston A M (2003) A structured health needs assessment: acceptability and effectiveness for health visiting. *Journal of Advanced Nursing*, **43**, 1:82–92.

Creswell J W (1994) *Research Design* (Newbury Park, CA: Sage).

DeLaurentis Schultz D M (2000) Dyspnea as a perceptual-interpretive response process: a qualitative inductive study of the concept in patients with chronic obstructive pulmonary disease. University of Rhode Island Ph.D. (258 pp.).

Duffy M (1985) A critique of research: a feminist perspective. *Health Care for Women International*, **6**:341–52.

Foucault M (1972) *The Archaeology of Knowledge* (London: Routledge).

Gadamer H G (1990) *Truth and Method*, 2nd rev. edn (New York: Crossroad).

Garfinkel H (1967) *Studies in Ethnomethodology* (Englewood Cliffs, NJ: Prentice Hall).

Gilmet K and Burman M E (2003) Stroke perceptions of well laypersons and professional caregivers. *Rehabilitation Nursing*, **28**, 2:52–6.

Glaser B (1992) *Basics of Grounded Theory Analysis: Emergence versus Forcing* (Mill Valley, CA: Sociology Press).

Glaser B and Strauss A (1967) *The Discovery of Grounded Theory* (Chicago, IL: Aldine).

Glaus A, Crow R and Hammond S (1996) A qualitative study to explore the concept of fatigue/tiredness in cancer patients and in healthy individuals. *European Journal of Cancer Care*, 5 (Suppl 2):8–23.

Green J and Britten N (1998) Qualitative research and evidence based medicine. *British Medical Journal*, **316**:1230–32.

Halfpenny P (1979) The analysis of qualitative data. *Sociological Review*, **27**, 4:799–825.

Hammersley M (ed.) (1993) *Social Research: Philosophy, Politics and Practice* (London: Sage).

Heidegger M (1962) *Being and Time*, trans. J Macquarrie and E Robinson (New York: Harper and Row.

Holloway I and Fulbrook P (2001) Revisiting qualitative inquiry: Interviewing in nursing and midwifery research. *NT Research*, **6**, 1:539–51.

Husserl E (1970) *Logical Investigations*, Vol. 2, trans. J N Findlay (London: Routledge and Kegan Paul).

Hutchinson S A (1993) People with bi-polar disorders quest for equanimity: Doing grounded theory. In: P L Munhall and C Oiler Boyd (eds), *Nursing Research: A Qualitative Perspective* (pp. 213–36). (New York: National League for Nursing).

Hutchinson S A (1998) An assessment guide for bi-polar disorders (unpublished). Cited in Morse et al., From theory to practice: the development of assessment guides from quality derived theory. *Qualitative Health Research*, **8**, 3:329–40.

Jay R (1996) Reassuring and reducing anxiety in seriously injured patients: a study of accident and emergency interventions. *Accident and Emergency Nursing*, **4**, 3:125–31.

Jayaratne T E (1993) The value of quantitative methodology for feminist research. In M Hammersley (ed.), *Social Research: Philosophy, Politics and Practice* (London: Sage).

Johnson M, Long T and White A (2000) Arguments for 'British Pluralism' in qualitative health research. *Journal of Advanced Nursing*, **33**, 2:243–9.

Keady J S (1999) The dynamics of dementia: a modified grounded theory. Bangor University of Wales, unpublished thesis.

Kearney M H (2001) Enduring love: a grounded formal theory of women's experience of domestic violence. *Research in Nursing & Health*, **24**, 4:270–82.

King G, Cathers T, Brown E, Specht J A, Willoughby C, Polgar J M, MacKinnon E, Smith L K and Havens L (2003) Turning points and protective processes in the lives of people with chronic disabilities. *Qualitative Health Research*, **13**, 2:184–206.

Kirkevold M (2000) Qualitative methods in the caring sciences: time for critical reflection and dialogue. *Scandinavian Journal of Caring Services*, **14**, 1:1–2.

Koch T (1995) Interpretive approaches in nursing research: the influence of Husserl and Heidegger. *Journal of Advanced Nursing*, **21**:827–36.

Laclau E and Mouffe C (1985) *Hegemony and Socialist Strategy: Towards a Radical Democratic Politics* (London: Verso).

Low L K, Martin K, Sampselle C, Guthrie B and Oakley D (2003) Adolescents' experiences of childbirth: contrasts with adults. *Journal of Midwifery & Women's Health*, **48**, 3:192–8.

Maggs-Rapport F (2000) Combining methodological approaches in research: ethnography and interpretive phenomenology. *Journal of Advanced Nursing*, **31**, 1:219–25.

Malinowski B (1922) *Argonauts of the Western Pacific* (London: Routledge and Kegan Paul).

van Manen M (1996) Phenomenological pedagogy and the question of meaning. In: Donald Vandenberg (ed.), *Phenomenology and Educational Discourse* (Durban: Heinemann).

Mazzei L A (2003) Inhabited silences: In pursuit of a muffled subtext. *Qualitative Inquiry*, **9**:355–68.

Melia K M (1996) Rediscovering Glaser. *Qualitative Health Research*, **6**, 3:368–78.

Merleau-Ponty M (1962) *Phenomenology of Perception*, trans. Colin Smith (London: Routledge and Kegan Paul).

Mok E and Chui P C (2004) Nurse–patient relationship in palliative care. *Journal of Advanced Nursing*, **48**, 5:475–83.

Morse J M (1991) Qualitative nursing research: a free for all? In: J M Morse (ed.), *Qualitative Nursing Research: A Contemporary Dialogue* (Newbury Park, CA: Sage).

Morse J M (1999) Editorial: Myth 1: Qualitative inquiry is not systematic. *Qualitative Health Research*, **9**, 5:573–4.

Morse J M, Hutchinson S A and Penrod J (1998) From theory to practice: The development of assessment guides from quality derived theory. *Qualitative Health Research*, **8**, 3:329–40.

Munhall P L (1982) Nursing philosophy and nursing research: in apposition or opposition. *Nursing Research*, **31**, 3:176–7.

Oakley A (1989) Who's afraid of the randomised controlled trial? Some dilemmas of the scientific method and 'good' research. *Women Health*, **15**:25.

Oliver K L (1998) A journey into narrative analysis: a methodology for discovering meanings. *Journal of Teaching in Physical Education*, **17**:224–59.

Orne R M (1995) The meaning of survival: the early aftermath of a near-death experience. *Research in Nursing and Health*, **18**:239–47.

Parahoo A K (2003) Guest editorial: Square pegs in round holes: reviewing qualitative research proposals. *Journal of Clinical Nursing*, **12**, 2:155–7.

Parry O, Gnich W and Platt S (2001) Principles in practice: reflections on a 'postpositivist' approach to evaluation research. *Health Education Research*, **16**, 2:215–26.

Parsons M L and Stonestreet J (2003) Factors that contribute to nurse manager retention. *Nursing Economics*, **21**, 3:120–6.

Penrod J and Morse J M (1997) Strategies for assessing and fostering hope: the hope assessment guide. *Oncology Nursing Forum*, **24**, 6:1055–63.

Phillips L and Jorgensen M W (2002) *Discourse Analysis as Theory and Method* (London: Sage).

Potter J and Wetherell M (1987) *Discourse and Social Psychology* (London: Sage).

Prus R C (1996) *Symbolic Interaction and Ethnographic Research* (Albany: State University of New York Press).

Radcliffe-Brown A R (1964) *The Andaman Islanders* (New York: Free Press).

Rubarth L B (2003) The lived experience of nurses caring for newborns with sepsis. *Journal of Obstetric, Gynaecologic & Neonatal Nursing*, 32, 3:348–56.

Sandelowski M (1997) To be of use: Enhancing the utility of qualitative research. *Nursing Outlook*, 45:125–32.

Sartre J P (1993) Freedom and responsibility. In: W Baskin (ed.), *Essays in Existentialism* (pp. 63–8) (New York: Kensington).

Saussure F de (1960) *Course in General Linguistics* (London: Fontana).

Seibold C (2000) Qualitative research from a feminist perspective in the postmodern era: methodological, ethical and reflexive concerns. *Nursing Inquiry*, 7:147–55.

Seibold C, Richards L and Simon D (1994) Feminist method and qualitative research about midlife. *Journal of Advanced Nursing*, 19:394–402.

Spalding N (2000) The empowerment of clients through preoperative education. *British Journal of Occupational Therapy*, 63, 4:148–54.

Starr S and MacLeod T (2003) Wound care: Wound swabbing technique. *Nursing Times*, 99, 5:57–9.

Steinberg A G, Wiggins E A, Barmada C H and Sullivan V J (2002) Deaf women: experiences and perceptions of health care system access. *Journal of Women's Health*, 11, 8:729–41.

Stern P N (1980) Grounded theory methodology: Its uses and processes. *Image*, 12, 1:20–3.

Strauss A and Corbin J (1990) *Basics of Qualitative Research: Grounded Theory, Procedures and Techniques* (Thousand Oaks, CA: Sage).

Swanson-Kauffman K M (1986) A combined qualitative methodology for nursing research . . . the human experience of miscarriage. *Advanced in Nursing Science*, 8, 3:58–69.

Thunberg K A, Carlsson S G and Hallberg L R (2001) Health care professionals' understanding of chronic pain: a grounded theory study. *Scandinavian Journal of Caring Sciences*, 15, 1:99–105.

Tod A M (2003) Barriers to smoking cessation in pregnancy: a qualitative study. *British Journal of Community Nursing*, 8, 2:56–60, 62–4.

Tolmie E P, Lindsay G M, Kerr S M, Brown M R, Ford I and Gaw A (2003) Patients' perspectives on statin therapy for treatment of hypercholesterolaemia: a qualitative study. *European Journal of Cardiovascular Nursing*, 2, 2:141–9.

Traynor M (1996) Nursing documentation and nursing practice: a discourse analysis. *Journal of Advanced Nursing*, 24:98–103.

Tune D (2001) Is touch a valid therapeutic intervention? Early returns from a qualitative study of therapists' views. *Counselling and Psychotherapy Research*, 1, 3:167–71.

Wilde V (1992) Controversial hypotheses on the relationship between researcher and informant in qualitative research. *Journal of Advanced Nursing*, 17:234–42.

5

Combining Quantitative and Qualitative Methods

OPENING THOUGHT ▶ Humans are both rational calculating beings . . . and they also operate on a deeper level of feelings, drivers and irrationality.

H. Mariampolski

Introduction

In the last two chapters, quantitative and qualitative research have been presented as having different characteristics and purposes although they also share some similarities. The debate about how different or similar they are and which one best serves the discipline of nursing has been going on for decades. More recently the focus has shifted to the combination of quantitative and qualitative methods in the same study. In this chapter we will explore the rationale for mixing methods and identify ways in which methods can be combined and the purposes for which this is done. We will also discuss the meaning of triangulation and the arguments for and against the mixing of methods from the two paradigms.

The quantitative–qualitative debate

For more than three decades nursing has been discussing which of these two approaches has a more useful contribution to make towards developing and increasing its body of knowledge. The quantitative–qualitative debate is not confined to nursing and it can be traced back to the two 'opposed Greek philosophical visions of human science that emphasise number (Pythagoras) and meaning (Socrates) as the essence of mind' (Wakefield, 1995). A revival of the debate about quantitative and qualitative research took place in the mid-nineteenth century when there was much argument about the scientific status of history and the social science (Hammersley, 1992).

Other professions and disciplines such as occupational therapy (Creek, 1997), social work (Wakefield, 1995), sociology (Halfpenny, 1979) and education (Smith and Heshusius, 1986) have also been wrestling with this issue for a number of years. The discussions have sometimes been at a lower level than one expects of intellectuals. Barber (1996) points out that qualitative research has been portrayed as 'noble, good and empowering', and quantitative methods as 'evil and oppressive'. On the other hand, qualitative research is often described as 'touchy-feely', story telling and anecdotal. Referring to the field of education, Smith and Heshusius (1986) point out that until the mid-1980s, the relationship between qualitative and quantitative researchers was one approaching 'mutual disdain'. Proponents of the two approaches have also been described 'as religious zealots who cannot perceive but one way to get to heaven' (Strickland, 1993).

The main (serious) arguments put forward for rejecting quantitative research are that it is limited in researching 'meaning', 'experience' and 'behaviour' (key concepts in understanding patients) and that it 'strips' data of their context. Qualitative research is criticised for being biased, subjective and lacking in reliability, validity and generalisability. In fact, each approach uses its own criteria to criticise the other. While there are some researchers who would totally reject one or the other approach, there are many who would acknowledge that each approach has a contribution to make to nursing knowledge. The following examples show how different questions can be addressed by different methods. Example A is about a study on social support for, and coping among, people diagnosed with heart disease. The researcher may want to use quantitative methods to measure the presence and level of social support, the degree of coping and the relationship between these two variables. In example B, a researcher may want to study, by means of in-depth interviews, the meaning of social support, how it operates in practice and how it helps people cope. The choice of approach (qualitative or quantitative) depends on the type of data which the researcher requires in order to answer the research questions. Although qualitative research can still be used to answer the questions in example A, it is unlikely to satisfy those who require a degree of precision expressed in numerical and statistical terms. Similarly the questions in example B, if studied by quantitative methods, would not satisfy those who want to understand what social support and coping means for those people with heart disease. Therefore it is the type of data the researcher seeks which determines the choice of methods.

More recently a new perspective has been added to the quantitative–qualitative debate. Instead of discussing which approach is best and pointing out the differences, it argues that the two approaches should not be seen as dichotomous (divided into two opposing camps) but rather as sharing many similar characteristics (Hammersley, 1992). Those who argue for this position point out that both quantitative and qualitative researchers use numbers, that both approaches can be inductive and that some researchers on both sides even share the same vision of reality. Paley (2000) argues that the terms 'qualitative' and 'quantitative' refer 'not to different types of research, but to various tools . . . and nothing more'. (For a response to this position, see Sandelowski,

2000a.) Clark (1998) also points out that postpositivist research takes into account many of qualitative researchers' concerns. In sum, some people argue that the differences between qualitative and quantitative approaches have been oversimplified (Hammersley, 1992); that there is a great deal of overlap between the two (Greenhalgh and Taylor, 1997); that the boundaries are fuzzy (Risjord et al., 2001); and that they should be seen as 'on a continuum with each approach at the opposite ends of the same pole' (Strickland, 1993).

There have been many calls to end the quantitative–qualitative debate and to concentrate efforts on combining both approaches (see e.g. Morgan, 1998; Barbour, 1999). Others believe that it is unfortunate that the debate is being closed down because this will prevent discussions of issues which are at the core of the researcher enterprise (Sale et al., 2002). There is little sign, however, that this is happening just yet, judging by the publication of new articles on this topic (see e.g. Watson, 2003; Payne et al., 2003; Draper and Draper, 2003).

The antagonism between the two approaches is, however, about more than methodology; it has implications in terms of funding and status. It is a battle for the 'soul' of nursing research and about which one produces legitimate knowledge for nursing practice. This is one of the issues at the heart of evidence-based practice, which in its traditional form puts randomised controlled trials and measurable outcomes on a pedestal far above qualitative research.

To some extent this debate has been overtaken by a new development: the combination of quantitative and qualitative methods in nursing, health and social studies. This gave rise to a different but related debate, in particular on the reasons why they should or should not be mixed and the implications of mixing. We now turn to the main arguments for this new approach.

Rationale for combining quantitative and qualitative methods

Combining evidence from different sources and by different methods to make decisions is nothing new. In such fields as archaeology, navigation or forensic medicine a number of methods and sources of data are used to answer single questions. For example, in archaeology when a skeleton is found, different data are collected in order to find out the time when the person died. Bones are examined (by visual and laboratory tests), samples of the soil are analysed and clothing and other artefacts found near the body are examined to provide clues to construct a profile (with the help of experts from different disciplines) of the person to which this skeleton belongs. Roberts (2003), a palaeopathologist, explains that in order to interpret abnormalities in skeletons a number of approaches including visual observation, radiography, histology and molecular methods of analysis are used. In the legal field, evidence from a number of sources such as witnesses' accounts, forensic tests and other circumstantial factors are considered in court. Together they help the jury or the judge to decide if the accused is guilty or not. Doctors and nurses, too, rely on information from a number of sources such as signs and symptoms, self-reports, X-ray and laboratory results when making a diagnosis or assessment.

Different methods bring different perspectives to what one studies. A single method is often incapable, on its own, of unravelling complex phenomena. According to Barbour (1999) the health field is often faced with problems that are multi-dimensional and multi-disciplinary which can best be studied with the use of a range of methods available to researchers. Nursing, in particular, is viewed as multi-layered and multi-faceted (Maggs-Rapport, 2000) and nursing research uses approaches from the natural as well as the social sciences.

Combining quantitative and qualitative methods in the same study can be perceived as an attractive and acceptable strategy to practitioners who aspire to valid, reliable and generalisable knowledge, with the added bonus of data reflecting patients' and clients' views. Government policies promoting users' participation in research and decision-making relating to their own care seem to be congruent with approaches which are more suitable for accessing patients' and carers' views while providing data from which one can also generalise.

Every method has its weaknesses. For example, interviewing people about what they eat does not necessarily describe what they actually eat. Observing them may be more accurate, but one observer (or even two) may miss important data. Observation, itself, may make people behave differently from usual. These two methods, together, can provide more accurate information than if only one method is used. In theory the limitations and biases of a single method can be overcome by the use of multiple methods (Brewer and Hunter, 1989). This supports Morgan's (1998) claim that such a strategy uses the strength of one method to enhance the performance of the other method. The combination of methods is expected to strengthen confidence in the validity of the findings. While this may be the goal in some studies, problems arise when the findings of different methods are either inconsistent or contradictory. This will be discussed later in this chapter.

Types and purpose of combining methods

Researchers have combined methods in a number of ways in order to achieve one or more of these objectives:

1. To develop and enhance the validity of scales, questionnaires and other instruments.

2. To develop, implement and evaluate interventions.

3. To further explore or test the findings of one method.

4. To study different aspects of the same topic.

5. To explore complex phenomena from different perspectives.

6. To confirm or cross-validate data.

Researchers can, of course, combine methods to achieve more than one of these purposes in the same study. For a fuller discussion on why and how researchers combine qualitative and quantitative sampling, data collection and analysis techniques, see Sandelowski (2000b).

1 Developing and enhancing the validity of scales and questionnaires

Qualitative methods, in particular semi-structured and in-depth interviews and focus groups, are frequently used to develop and enhance the validity and reliability of quantitative scales and other measuring tools. Scales and questionnaires are often criticised for being 'researcher-oriented'. They tend to reflect researchers' values, concerns and even their wordings. Qualitative methods are therefore ideal for generating items for these tools. For example, Stokes and Gordon (1988) developed an 'instrument to measure stress in the older adult' by first identifying stressors from a literature review and then conducting qualitative interviews with a sample of older people, before finally submitting the resulting list to two 'experts in gerontologic nursing'. Wilde et al. (1994) developed a patient-centred questionnaire based on a grounded theory model. They carried out in-depth interviews with patients and followed the grounded theory method to code the data. Their questionnaire benefited from the fact that it was based on the patients' perspectives and, because 'the wordings were inspired by the patients' interview responses', most patients found the questions easy to comprehend (Wilde et al., 1994).

Qualitative methods can be useful at every stage of scale development, validation and evaluation. Mahoney et al. (1995) proposed a model for scale development integrating qualitative and quantitative methods. They showed that qualitative methods can be used not only to develop items and statements but also to pre-test the draft scale. After data are collected the validity of the scale can be further enhanced through the use of focus groups. Finally qualitative interviews can help to interpret the quantitative findings from the scale. Feedback from this qualitative phase may 'stimulate revision' of the scale (Mahoney et al., 1995).

There are numerous examples of the use of qualitative methods in scale and questionnaire construction, validation, implementation and evaluation in the nursing literature. This is an area where the integration of qualitative and quantitative methods seems to work well. Research Example 7 shows how a qualitative approach was used to develop a scale.

2 Developing, implementing and evaluating interventions

Quantitative methods within a randomised controlled trial design have traditionally been the premier method to evaluate the effectiveness of interventions. Practitioners and policy makers put greater emphasis on measurable outcomes

Development of an instrument to measure the responses and management of Chinese primary caregivers in caring for children with minor upper respiratory disorders   *Tse and Fok (2003)*

An example of a study using a qualitative method to develop a quantitative instrument.

In this study, Tse and Fok (2003) carried out 32 semi-structured interviews 'to explore the phenomenon of primary caregivers caring for children with minor upper respiratory disorders' and to identify the items in the survey instrument. Five categories and 29 sub-categories were generated. The results of the interviews were used to develop the instrument.

The main reason given by the authors for using a qualitative method is that there is 'a paucity of information mentioned in the literature on this phenomenon, including in the local context'. Also, qualitative methods 'can effectively generate more culturally relevant instrument items directly from primary caregivers' (Tse and Fok, 2003).

on which to base their practice and develop policies. However, the need to develop outcomes which are patient-centred and the emphasis on involving patients in their own care have led to increasing recognition of the value of qualitative research in intervention studies.

Quantitative methods, on their own, cannot answer questions such as why an intervention works for some people and not for others and what types of interventions work best (from patients' perspectives). The Medical Research Council (MRC) (2000), in *A Framework for Development and Evaluation of RCTs for Complex Interventions to Improve Health* acknowledges the contribution that qualitative methods such as focus groups, individual in-depth interviews and observations can make towards addressing some of these questions. In particular qualitative research is suggested as potentially useful for developing and defining interventions which are patient-centred and for testing the underlying assumptions relating to an intervention. Ways in which interventions can be modified to suit different groups or types of people can also be studied by qualitative methods (Medical Research Council, 2000).

Sandelowski (1996) has provided a detailed discussion of the variety of uses of qualitative research in intervention studies. Some of her suggestions include the use of qualitative methods to interpret statistical findings, to 'detect subtleties in the intervention process that may better account for research findings and help researchers specify the circumstances in which their findings may be generalisable to other patients and care giving situations' (Sandelowski, 1996).

Crawford et al. (2002) also recognise the value and potential uses of qualitative research in 'exploring and describing the process and outcomes of psychological and other complex interventions used to treat mental disorders'. They suggest ways in which qualitative research can be of benefit in the pre-trial, during a trial and post-trial stages in the evaluation of complex interventions. They pointed out, however, that issues concerning the synthesis and interpretation of data are yet to be considered, in particular when one set of data (qualitative) challenges another (quantitative) or vice versa.

For an example of the development, implementation and evaluation of an intervention by combining a number of research methods, see Research Example 8.

RESEARCH EXAMPLE 8

Research methodology for developing efficient handwashing options: an example from Bangladesh

Hoque et al. (1995)

A study using multiple methods to develop, implement and evaluate an intervention.

Effective handwashing after defecation is vital in reducing bacterial concentration and transmission. Hoque et al.'s (1995) aim was to understand the factors related to handwashing behaviour and, thereafter, develop and test the effectiveness of an intervention designed to reduce bacterial concentration. As they explain:

> The components of handwashing practices after defecation of 90 rural women were studied (phase 1). During phase 1 an in-depth interview was used to design the observational and questionnaire surveys. Behaviour was observed using a semi-structured record form and the effectiveness of the acts was measured by means of bacteriological tests. A questionnaire survey was undertaken on socio-economic and water sanitation-related variables since they influence behaviour. Then, to develop efficient handwashing options, an experimental phase (phase 2) tested the bacteriological efficacy of the components found appropriate in phase 1.

The authors conclude that:

> The use of multi-method techniques in the study helped to understand and develop efficient handwashing options.

3   Exploring further the findings of one method by means of another

Qualitative methods can further explore quantitative findings to put them in context or to provide more in-depth understanding. This is because in researching large samples with structured methods such as questionnaires, it is not always possible to capture the particular contexts in which the responses are made. For example, in a survey on HIV, one of the items asked respondents if their relationship with their relatives had changed since being diagnosed with the disease. Most indicated that it had not. However, qualitative interviews revealed later that relationships did not change because they did not tell their relatives that they had HIV (Melby, 2004, personal communication).

Burch (1999) gives an example of the 'decontextualization' of responses which may distort the score on a scale:

> Instruments in general use commonly asked questions about activities of daily living on the assumption that any limitation will be imposed by the physical inability to carry out the task in question. Thus whether one gets in or out of a car, an item in the Nottingham Extended Activities of Daily Living Scale, is assumed to be due to one's mobility. In reality, it may also be due to the fact that an older person or their carers cannot afford a car, cannot drive a car or that they are so isolated – by choice or compulsion – that they never have the opportunity to carry out this manoeuvre.

Individual interviews or focus groups with a smaller sample of respondents can help to clarify results collected in the quantitative phase of a study. On the other hand, qualitative methods can reveal patterns, trends and relationships which can lead to the formulation of hypotheses. These can then be tested further by quantitative methods. For example, if qualitative interviews in phase one of a study identify gender differences in ways of coping among people with depression, this can be tested with a larger population by means of a survey. Meredith and Wood (1996) explain that in patient satisfaction research it is necessary to interview patients to identify issues of concern to them, in particular, their perceptions and interpretation of services. Once this is done, it is necessary to discover 'how pervasive these attitudes are, and how their incidence might differ according to, for example, the socio-demographic characteristics of representative population of patients' (Meredith and Wood, 1996). Research Example 9 shows how quantitative findings were further explored by means of qualitative methods.

4   Studying different aspects of the same topic

Different aspects of the same topic can be explored by different methods in the same study. For example, in studying 'non-compliance with professional advice',

The distress experienced by people with type 2 diabetes   *West and McDowell (2002)*

A study using qualitative methods to further explore quantitative findings.

West and McDowell (2003) explain:

> This study aimed to investigate the distress associated with type 2 diabetes, whether gender differences existed in the impact of type 2 diabetes and how men and women viewed dietary management. A multi-method, two-stage research approach was taken. Quantitative data were obtained using the Problem Areas in Diabetes (PAID) questionnaire, and no statistically significant gender difference was identified. Worrying about the future, the possibility of complications and feelings of guilt or anxiety when 'off-track' with diabetes management were sources of significant distress. Treatment mode, length of time diagnosed with diabetes and age were significant factors which impacted on the emotional distress experienced by the individual. A subsample of respondents took part in gender-specific focus group interviews which explored issues identified in the survey. Behavioural impact, emotional impact and fear of complications were major themes identified in the interviews. Views of the dietary management of diabetes were also explored within the focus groups and three broad categories identified: dietary restrictions, value judgments and the influence of others.

the survey method can provide data from a large number of clients to explore links between non-compliance and such variables as gender, occupation, education or age, and trends such as how often, when and in what circumstances people do not comply. At the same time it is possible to use a qualitative method such as an in-depth interview to explore the meaning and experience of non-compliance of some of the respondents in order to gain an understanding of their way of thinking, their priorities, their motivations and their beliefs. In this way a broader picture of non-compliance can emerge. It is not, and cannot ever be, the complete picture since there is more to compliance than these aspects described above. However, the findings will provide practitioners with valuable data to understand both the 'thinking' and 'experience' of participants and the broader demographic profile of those who comply and those who do not.

With this type of combination of methods, it could appear that these are in fact two studies, each looking at different aspects of the same phenomenon (non-compliance). Researchers undertaking this type of study will have to explain why these two aspects were selected for study and how the two methods were integrated.

The use of different methods to study different aspects of the same phenomenon is illustrated in Research Example 10.

RESEARCH EXAMPLE 10

The food consumption patterns and perceptions of dietary advice of older people *McKie et al. (2000)*

A study using different methods to study different (but related) aspects of the same phenomenon.

In this study semi-structured interviews were carried out with 152 people aged over 75 in order to explore dietary beliefs and perceptions of advice. The same sample was also administered a 24-hour food recall questionnaire.

Together these methods allowed for a better understanding of the relationships between beliefs and actual behaviour than would have been possible by using a single method. As McKie et al. (2000) explain:

> This study has demonstrated a more complicated, fragmented picture of the diet of people aged 75 years and older. Interview material indicates the historical basis to beliefs and, when combined with a consideration of the food recall data, demonstrates how practices and beliefs may be compromised by local and personal circumstances, as well as structured factors such as physical access to food, the cost, quantity and quality of food. These findings reinforce the need for a diet action plan to work across all sectors of the food, retail and health services.

5   Exploring complex phenomena from different perspectives

To understand the complexity of concepts such as caring or the roles of health professionals requires data from a number of sources. To study the effects of care and services is equally daunting and often not possible by the use of a single research method. In a study of the views of patients and carers on one palliative care service, Ingleton (1999) explains:

> Palliative care is not a discrete activity but a complex nexus of interventions which may be implemented over time, in a wide array of settings and by a wide range of people. Any attempt to measure or assess the quality of a palliative care service is conceptually and methodologically fraught with difficulties.

She responded to the challenge by employing a variety of methods such as non-participant observation, a questionnaire survey and interviews using 'a variant of the Critical Incident Technique'. Ingleton (1999) pointed out that while the survey 'concentrated on professionally determined behavioural components of care', the critical incident interview facilitated 'access to client-generated and less tangible aspects of care'.

This type of approach is commonly used in evaluation studies. In order to carry out a 'holistic' evaluation researchers seek data from the main groups involved in the service – patients, carers and health professionals – and by means of a variety of methods. There is no attempt to construct a consistent picture of patients', carers' and professionals' views. In fact it is likely that each of these groups may perceive the service differently. See Research Example 11 for an example of a study combining multiple methods to study a complex phenomenon.

RESEARCH EXAMPLE 11

An overview of sperm cryopreservation services for adolescent cancer patients in the United Kingdom
Wilford and Hunt (2003)

A study combining multiple methods to study a complex phenomenon.

Describing or evaluating any service requires data from a number of sources by means of multiple methods. In this study, Wilford and Hunt (2003) set out to provide an overview of sperm cryopreservation services for adolescent cancer patients in the UK with the use of three methods in three discrete stages. These included:

- A self-completion questionnaire to explore, among other things, availability of sperm cryopreservation services, the number of patients at each centre for whom such services could potentially be provided, the availability of patient/parent information literature and funding sources.

- Documentary analysis to identify the availability and nature of information given to patients. This phase included an analysis to determine the quality and readability of the information.

- Focused telephone interviews with nurses to examine the degree to which such services and information were standardised. As the authors explain, these interviews complemented and built upon data collected during the previous two stages of the research.

6   Confirming or cross-validating findings

Two or more methods can be used simultaneously in order to answer the same question. It is thought that if the answers are similar, confidence in the validity of the findings is increased. These methods can all be quantitative, qualitative or a combination of both. For example, to find out what student nurses eat at lunch-times, they can be asked to complete a questionnaire and they can be observed during lunch. If both methods reveal similar findings, the researcher will have greater confidence in their validity than if only one method was used. In a study of patient satisfaction with communication in surgical care, Meredith and Wood (1996) used a number of methods including qualitative interviews and observations, and a questionnaire. Their aim was to confirm qualitiative findings through the quantitative method. Some of their findings were similar and some were different. For example, 'evidence that a long wait at the outpatient clinic led patients to take this dissatisfaction with them into the meeting was not forthcoming from the questionnaire survey' (Meredith and Wood, 1996).

To cross-validate findings, self-reports are often compared with biochemical measurements (e.g. in studies on smoking) and instruments' scores are compared with data from semi-structured interviews (e.g. in studies on quality of life). For an example of a study using qualitative and quantitative methods to answer the same question see Research Example 12.

In summary, researchers combine methods to achieve one of the following:

- complementarity
- completeness
- confirmation.

Complementarity is achieved when a different method from the one used in the main study is used to help in the construction and validation of tools, to develop, implement and evaluate interventions, and to put findings in context. Usually the methods in these types of studies are fully integrated and each one plays an important part in assisting the other methods by making their tools more valid or their findings more understandable. There is a division of labour and each method has clear roles to perform. In this case paradigms are not mixed, only methods.

Completeness (Knafl and Breitmayer, 1991) is expected to be achieved when different methods are employed to look at different aspects of the same phenomenon. It is similar to the construction of a whole picture by putting 'jigsaw pieces' together. It is believed that some research methods are more appropriate for the study of some aspects of phenomena than others, and that together they can provide a broader, more meaningful picture, than one single method can. For example, a researcher aiming to offer a broad understanding of

RESEARCH EXAMPLE 12

Methodological triangulation in researching families: making sense of dissonant data   *Perlesz and Lindsay (2003)*

A study cross-validating data.

In this paper Perlesz and Lindsay (2003) argue that triangulation enables analysis which is both more complex and more meaningful. They gave two examples (from their own research) where dissonant findings (from quantitative and qualitative methods) contributed to a better understanding of the issues which they studied. One of the examples is described below.

Lindsay's (1996) research 'was a predominantly qualitative study of 15 heterosexual, unmarried childless couples who had been living together for less than four years'. The participants were also administered a scale to measure 'egalitarianism' among the partners. As they explain:

> The qualitative and quantitative data on gender equality were strongly dissonant. On the one hand, the qualitative data (both from conjoint and individual interviews) showed the couples avoiding an assessment of how equal their relationships were; equality was rarely mentioned. On the other hand, the quantitative data showed an extremely strong commitment to equality: the cohabiters' scores on the egalitarianism scale were very high.

Perlesz and Lindsay (2003) found that the general statements in the egalitarianism scale elicited a particular type of data by inviting them to take a position on abstract principles about general equity and to give general views on how society should operate. In the qualitative interviews notions of equality were largely absent in the domestic context.

By examining the context of data gathering (in particular the relationship between the researcher and the researched) and having an awareness of family context such as sociocultural beliefs and intrafamiliar loyalties, they were able to make use of both sets of data.

The researchers were able to differentiate between 'public and domestic discourses on gender relations and equality'. As they conclude:

> The dissonant data opened up new theoretical insights and provided a richer understanding than would have been possible without triangulation.

the problem of incontinence may carry out a survey on the incidence of incontinence, the types of pressure sores and the demographic variables associated with it. She may also carry out in-depth interviews to explore patients' experience of incontinence. Each method provides understanding and insight into different aspects of the same phenomenon. These methods can be used side by side in the same study. Alternatively they could have been carried out as two separate studies. There is little danger of mixing paradigms.

Finally, researchers use different methods to answer the same question or study the same aspect of a phenomenon. If the findings are similar, confirmability is achieved (Knafl and Breitmayer, 1991) and researchers may assume that their findings are valid. It is this type of combination of methods which is often described as triangulation.

Triangulation

A number of terms are used interchangeably in the literature to describe the combination of methods in the same study. Some of the common ones are: mixed methods, multiple methods, multi-method, methodological pluralism and triangulation. The latter is often an abused term to describe any study which uses more than one method or a study which combines qualitative and quantitative methods. From the examples given above, one can see that two or more methods can be used in the same study to do different, but related tasks. Therefore triangulation is one form of combining more than one method in the same study.

Triangulation has different meanings depending on the perspectives one adopts. In quantitative research, its purpose is to cross-validate findings. Webb et al. (1966), representing this view, refer to triangulation as 'a series of complementary methods' to test a hypothesis. If the hypothesis is confirmed or rejected then, according to Webb et al. (1966), it contains a degree of validity unattainable by one tested by a single method. This type of triangulation can involve methods within the same approach (quantitative) or from different approaches (quantitative and qualitative).

The view that triangulation is carried out for cross-validation or confirmation purposes is not universally shared (see e.g. Denzin, 1989; Sale et al., 2002). From a qualitative perspective, a variety of methods can be used in the same study, not to seek validity, but to gain in-depth understanding as each yields a different picture and slice of reality (Denzin, 1989).

In qualitative studies, researchers actively seek diversity and 'negative' cases in order to present phenomena in all their different facets and from different perspectives. Richness of data comes from diversity. When data from one method are different from those of another, it raises more questions, which can be further explored due to the flexible nature of qualitative enquiry.

Denzin (1989) defines triangulation as the combination of two or more theories, data sources, methods or investigators in the study of a single phenomenon. Kimchi et al. (1991), drawing on Denzin's work, list six types of triangulation:

- *theory* – an assessment of the utility and power of competing theories or hypotheses;

- *data* – the use of multiple data sources with similar foci to obtain diverse views about a topic for the purpose of validation;

- *investigator* – the use of two or more 'research-trained' investigators with divergent backgrounds to explore the same phenomenon;

- *analysis* – the use of two or more approaches to the analysis of the same set of data;

- *methods* – the use of two or more research methods in one study;

- *multiple* – the use of more than one type of triangulation to analyse same event.

Although methods triangulation is by far the most common, there are studies using other types of triangulation (see e.g. Maggs-Rapport, 2000).

Implications of triangulation

Methods usually associated with different paradigms are increasingly being used in the same study. In the 1980s, Myers and Haase (1989) emphasised the importance of different data sources by pointing out how, in studies of bonding between mother and infant, 'the subjective descriptions of mothers' progressive ability to anticipate their infants' need' can be contrasted with objective observations of the mother–infant interaction. Not everyone agrees, however, that methods from different paradigms can be mixed in the same study. Cresswell (1994) identified three schools of thought on the subject: 'purists' are described as those who are against the mixing of paradigms; 'situationalists' believe in certain methods being appropriate for specific conditions; and 'pragmatists' are actively involved in using methods from different paradigms.

Triangulation for cross-validation purposes can raise more questions than it can solve. Three outcomes are possible: the findings can be similar, inconsistent or divergent. What to do with findings which are inconsistent (some are similar, some are not) or divergent (not at all similar) is a serious problem. This is an issue which has received little attention in the research literature (Perlesz and Lindsay, 2003). As Maggs-Rapport (2000) explains, if multiple findings are produced by multiple methods, 'it may be impossible to make a case for the validity of one set of findings over another'.

Assessing the validity or worth of research findings in mixed-methods studies depends on whether one uses quantitative or qualitative criteria (see Chapter 17). Those who believe that validity and reliability are achieved by being 'objective' and 'detached' will, by definition, believe that qualitative interviews are subjective and, thus, biased. It is not possible for the same researcher to subscribe to quantitative and qualitative notions of what constitute rigorous, unbiased and valid research. In practice, deciding which of the divergent findings are acceptable could depend on whether the researcher or the team are more quantitative- or qualitative-minded. It is likely that within a postpositivist framework, the quantitative approach is the anchor or in a more dominant position than the qualitative one. Wakefield (1995) contends that, in such a scenario, quantitative findings would be preferred because they are considered to be superior for establishing validity and generalisability. On the other hand, qualitative-minded researchers can adopt the opposite view. Rose and Webb (1997), reflecting on their study of informal carers of terminally ill cancer patients, explain how they reacted when mixing paradigms became problematic.

> Logically, although it is possible to use tools from both paradigms, there can be only one underlying philosophical approach. In my study, the conflict in paradigms was apparent, but because I was certain that the study was essentially hermeneutically based, I always allowed the qualitative, hermeneutic research paradigm to prevail.

In practice, it is probably rare that researchers reject the findings of one approach without seriously considering why findings are divergent. It is possible that such differences can be explained by the characteristics of researchers, the process of data collection, including the methods, and the context in which data are collected and analysed. Such critical reflection is likely to raise further questions.

Researchers combining methods and approaches need to appreciate the context, nature and implications of data obtained from different methods and not take them at face value. For example, data obtained in focus groups should be interpreted within the context of the group dynamics, the type of discussions which took place, the role of the researcher and how the participants perceived the whole exercise. This is different from that of 'one-to-one' interviews where privacy and intimacy provide the context in which the exchange takes place. The completion of self-administered questionnaires takes place in yet another context.

Combining methods and approaches should be a well thought-out process backed by a strong rationale discussing the purpose and benefits of such decisions and the choice of methods. Sale et al. (2002) believe that 'mixed-methods research is now being adopted uncritically by a new generation of researchers who have overlooked the underlying assumptions behind the qualitative–quantitative debate'. Barbour (1999) points to 'the need to ensure that our combining of methods is driven by the research question rather than the perceived preference of funders of multi-method approaches or the diverse backgrounds of those who are collaborating'.

SUMMARY

Summary and conclusions

The quantitative–qualitative debate has been, to some extent, overtaken by discussions about the feasibility, benefits, limitations and implications of combining more than one method in the same study. The complex and multi-dimensional nature of nursing and health phenomena has led an increasing number of researchers to use a variety of methods and approaches, sometimes singly and sometimes in combination. This chapter has outlined the different types and purposes of combining methods to achieve complementarity, completeness and confirmation.

While some researchers find the combination of qualitative and quantitative approaches useful for complementary purposes, they reject the notion that these approaches can be used in the same study for validation or confirmatory purposes. In practice, when findings from qualitative and quantitative research are divergent, the methodological orientation of researchers often determines which sets of findings they can trust more.

Mixed-methods studies are on the increase and are well accepted in nursing, health and social research. It is important that researchers are fully aware of why and how they combine methods and address issues raised when the different methods do not produce similar findings. As Mechanic (1989) explains:

> In our efforts to understand our world around us we recognise many technical barriers, but we use the best methods we can . . . but it does us well to re-examine our assumptions periodically and to inquire more deeply about the meaning of the information which serves as a source of our interpretations of reality. By inquiring more carefully about what the data mean, we can also bridge gaps between the research culture of those committed to varying types of methods.

References

Barber J G (1996) Science and social work: Are they compatible? *Research on Social Work*, **6**, 3:379–88.

Barbour R S (1999) The case for combining qualitative and quantitative approaches in health services research. *Journal of Health Services Research and Policy*, **4**, 1:39–43.

Brewer J and Hunter, A (1989) *Multimethod Research – A Synthesis of Styles* (Newbury Park, CA: Sage Publications).

Burch S (1999) Evaluating health interventions for older people. *Health*, **3**, 2:151–66.

Clark A M (1998) The qualitative–quantitative debate: moving from positivism and confrontation to post-positivism and reconciliation. *Journal of Advanced Nursing*, 27:1242–9.

Crawford M J, Weaver T, Rutter D, Sensky T and Tyner P (2002) Evaluating new treatments in psychiatry: the potential value of combining qualitative and quantitative research methods. *International Review of Psychiatry*, 14:6–14.

Creek J (1997) . . . the truth is no longer out there. *British Journal of Occupational Therapy*, 2:50–2.

Cresswell J W (1994) *Research Design* (Newbury Park, CA: Sage).

Denzin W K (1989) *The Research Act: A Theoretical Introduction to Sociological Methods*, 3rd edn (Englewood Cliffs, NJ: Prentice Hall).

Draper J and Draper P (2003) Response to Watson's Guest Editorial, 'Scientific methods are the only credible way forward for nursing research'. *Journal of Advanced Nursing*, 44:546–7.

Greenhalgh T and Taylor, R (1997), Papers that go beyond numbers (qualitative research). *British Medical Journal*, 315:740–3.

Halfpenny, P (1979) The analysis of qualitative data. *Sociological Review*, 27, 4:799–825.

Hammersley M (1992) Deconstructing the qualitative–quantitative divide. In: J Brannen (ed.), *Mixing Methods: Qualitative and Quantitative Research* (Aldershot: Avebury).

Hoque B A, Malhalanbis D, Pelto B and Alam M J (1995) Research methodology for developing efficient handwashing options: an example from Bangladesh. *Journal of Tropical Medicine and Hygiene*, 98:469–75.

Ingleton C (1999) The views of patients and carers on one palliative care service. *International Journal of Palliative Nursing*, 5, 4:187–95.

Kimchi J, Polivka B and Stevenson J S (1991) Triangulation: operation definitions. *Nursing Research*, 40, 6:364–6.

Knafl K A and Breitmayer B J (1991) Triangulation in qualitative research: issues in conceptual clarity and purpose. In: J Morse (ed.), *Qualitative Nursing Research: A Contemporary Dialogue* (Newbury Park, CA: Sage).

Lindsay J (1996) Coupling up: A study of heterosexual cohabitation. Unpublished Ph.D. thesis. La Trobe University, Melbourne.

Maggs-Rapport F (2000) Combining methodological approaches in research: ethnography and interpretive phenomenology. *Journal of Advanced Nursing*, 31, 1:219–25.

Mahoney C A, Thombs D L and Howe C Z (1995) The art and science of scale development in health education research. *Health Education Research*, 10, 1:1–10.

Mariampolski H (1999) The power of ethnography. *Journal of the Market Research Society*, 41, 1:75–86.

McKie L, MacInnes A, Hendry J, Donald S and Peace H (2000) The food consumption patterns and perceptions of dietary advice of older people. *Journal of Human Dietetics*, 13:173–83.

Mechanic D (1989) Medical sociology: Some tensions among theory, method and substance. *Journal of Health and Social Behaviour*, 30:147–60.

Medical Research Council (2000) *A Framework for Development and Evaluation of RCTs for Complex Interventions to Improve Health* (London: Medical Research Council).

Melby V (2004) Personal communication.

Meredith P and Wood C (1996) Aspects of patient satisfaction with communication in surgical care: confirming qualitative feedback through quantitative methods. *International Journal for Quality in Health Care*, 8, 3:253–64.

Morgan D L (1998) Practical strategies for combining qualitative and quantitative methods: applications to health research. *Qualitative Health Research*, 8, 3:362–76.

Myers S T and Haase J E (1989) Guidelines for integration of quantitative and qualitative approaches. *Nursing Research*, 38, 5:299–301.

Paley J (2000) Paradigms and presuppositions: The difference between qualitative and quantitative research. *Scholarly Inquiry for Nursing Practice: An International Journal*, **14**, 2:143–55.

Payne S, Seymour J and Ingleton C (2003) Response to Watson's Guest Editorial, 'Scientific methods are the only credible way forward for nursing research'. *Journal of Advanced Nursing*, **44**:547–8.

Perlesz A and Lindsay J (2003) Methodological triangulation in researching families: making sense of dissonant data. *International Journal of Social Research Methodology*, **6**, 1:25–40.

Risjord M, Moloney M and Dunbar S (2001) Methodological triangulation in nursing research. *Philosophy of the Social Sciences*, **31**, 1:40–59.

Roberts C (2003) Palaeopathologist. In: J Turney (ed.), *Science, Not Art: Ten Scientists' Diaries* (London: Calouste Gulbenkian Foundation).

Rose K E and Webb C (1997) Triangulation of data collection: Practicalities and problems in a study of informal carers of terminally ill cancer patients. *Nursing Times Research*, 2, 2:108–16.

Sale J E M, Lohfeld L H and Brazil K (2002) Revisiting the quantitative–qualitative debate: Implications for mixed-methods research. *Quality and Quantity*, **36**:43–53.

Sandelowski M (1996) Using qualitative methods in intervention studies. *Research in Nursing and Health*, **19**:359–64.

Sandelowski M (2000a) Response to 'Paradigms and presuppositions'. The difference between qualitative and quantitative research. *Scholarly Inquiry for Nursing Practice: An International Journal*, **14**, 2:152–60.

Sandelowski M (2000b) Combining qualitative and quantitative sampling, data collection, and analysis techniques in mixed-method studies. *Research in Nursing and Health*, **23**:246–55.

Smith J K and Heshusius L (1986) Closing down the conversation: the end of the quantitative–qualitative debate among educational inquirers. *Educational Researcher*, **15**, 1:4–12.

Stokes S A and Gordon S E (1998) Development of an instrument to measure stress in the older adult. *Nursing Research*, **37**, 1:16–19.

Strickland O L (1993) Editorial. Qualitative or quantitative: so what is your religion. *Journal of Nursing Measurement*, **1**, 2:103–5.

Tse F Y K and Fok M S M (2003) Development of an instrument to measure the responses and management of Chinese primary caregivers in caring for children with minor upper respiratory disorders. *International Journal of Nursing Studies*, **40**:863–71.

Wakefield J C (1995) When an irresistible epistemology meets an immovable ontology. *Social Work Research*, **19**, 1:9–17.

Watson R (2003) Editorial: Scientific methods are the only credible way forward for nursing research. *Journal of Advanced Nursing*, **43**:219–20.

Webb E J, Campbell D T, Schwartz R D and Sechrest L (1966) *Unobtrusive Measures: Non-Reactive Research on the Social Sciences* (Chicago: Rand McNally).

West C and McDowell J (2002) The distress experienced by people with type 2 diabetes. *British Journal of Community Nursing*, 7, 12:606–13.

Wilde B, Larsson G, Larsson M and Starrin B (1994) Development of a patient-centred questionnaire based on a grounded theory method. *Scandinavian Journal of Caring Sciences*, **8**:39–48.

Wilford H and Hunt J (2003) An overview of sperm cryopreservation services for adolescent cancer patients in the United Kingdom. *European Journal of Oncology Nursing*, 7, 1:24–32.

The Research Process and Ethical Issues

Introduction

One of the first tasks in reading and evaluating a research study is to identify the actions and steps taken by the researcher in order to answer the research question. This chapter describes the research process in quantitative and qualitative research and points out the differences between them. There are ethical implications at every stage of the research process. An outline of the guiding principles to safeguard patients' rights and safety is given.

The meaning of research process

The process of any activity is what happens from its inception to its end. The tasks and actions carried out by the researcher in order to find answers to the research question constitute the research process. Decisions are taken in choosing the tasks and the way in which they are carried out. A number of factors, including the researcher's beliefs and experience, ethical considerations or resources, may influence these decisions. The thinking processes of the researcher, the assumptions made and the theoretical stance are also part of the research process. According to Denzin and Lincoln (1994), there are three inter-related activities which define the research process: the articulation of the researcher's individual world view or basic belief system (in relation to the research domain), decisions on the theoretical perspective and strategies of enquiry, and decisions on methods of data collection and analysis.

Thus, although the research process is often described in terms of the tasks and actions undertaken, it also consists of the decisions and the thinking that underpins these decisions.

Whatever the type of research carried out or the approaches used, the research process invariably consists of four main components:

- the identification of the research question;
- the collection of data;
- the analysis of data;
- the dissemination of findings.

To carry out these tasks, a number of other tasks may be performed. For example, in identifying the research question, a review of the literature and/or discussion with colleagues may be useful. Before data can be collected, a questionnaire or an interview schedule may have to be constructed. The research process, therefore, consists of all these tasks and the decisions made before and during the project.

The research process and the nursing process

A number of authors have compared the research process to the nursing process (Burns and Grove, 1987; Thomas, 1990). They are both problem-solving processes and both consist of a number of steps or stages. However, they differ in the goals they aim to achieve. The main purpose of the nursing process is to provide care to clients. In doing so, nurses gather information in order to assess the nursing problem and to evaluate the care given. The collection of such information is not always as formal as is the case in research. Data for research purposes must be collected more systematically. For example, when assessing clients, nurses can ask questions but do not have to use a tool such as a questionnaire with established validity and reliability in order to do so (although some do). The aim of research, on the other hand, is to find solutions to research questions, which may or may not contribute to better care for clients. Data for research purposes must be collected systematically and rigorously. Table 6.1 shows the main components of the nursing process and the research process.

The process in quantitative research

The research process is often described as having a number of stages and steps. Depending on the type of research, these stages are not necessarily linear (performed one after the other, in one direction only). There are important differences between quantitative and qualitative research in the way in which the research tasks are undertaken.

Table 6.1 Main components of the nursing and research process

Nursing process	Research process
Assessment	Identification of research problem
Planning	Collection of data
Implementation	Analysis of data
Evaluation	

The systematic and inflexible nature of quantitative research means that the research proceeds in a logical and sequential manner. The stages of the process in quantitative research can be broken down into a number of steps. The number of steps varies from author to author (see e.g. Meadows [2003] who lists seven key stages). The difference in the number of steps is not important provided the main tasks are carried out and explained. The main stages of experimental and survey research are described briefly below. The process in quantitative research mirrors the scientific method used in the natural sciences (as described in Chapter 2). The chapters that follow will provide more detail and discussion on these topics.

Stages of the research process

Identification and formulation of the research question

This is the first stage of a research project, when the researcher decides what is to be researched and formulates one or more questions. The next step is for the researcher to define the terms and concepts used in the research questions. A review of the relevant literature helps to clarify issues, informs the researcher of how others have formulated similar research questions and defines concepts. At the end of this stage, the research questions or hypotheses developed must be stated clearly and unambiguously.

Collection of data

A number of tasks will be carried out by the researcher before data are collected. Decisions will be taken in order to choose a design for the study and a conceptual framework (if appropriate), and to select or develop instruments to collect data (for example questionnaires, interviews or observation schedules). This may be followed by the testing (or piloting) of these instruments in order to refine them (sometimes the whole study is piloted on a small scale to find out whether the project is feasible). At this stage of the process, the researcher will define the population from whom the data will be collected. Seeking access to them and obtaining ethical approval from the relevant ethical committees should start well before the project is started. When all these preparations have been completed, data are ready to be collected.

Analysis of data

In the final stage of the process, the researcher analyses, interprets and presents the findings. Prior to data collection, decisions about the type of analysis would have been taken. For example, when questionnaires are constructed, the researcher must decide whether and what statistical test should be carried out and code the questionnaire accordingly.

When the data have been analysed, it is usual for the researcher to interpret the findings, discuss the limitations of the study, make recommendations for practice and further research, and present the study orally and/or in written form.

Conclusions

The stages described above are sometimes listed as a number of steps, as suggested below by Hek (1994):

- Identify the general problem or topic of interest.
- Critically review the relevant literature.
- Develop a theoretical framework.
- Refine the topic into a research question, aim or hypothesis.
- Plan the research design, research approach, population and sample selection, access to sample, ethical considerations, methods of data collection, data collection tool and methods of data analysis.
- Pilot study.
- Collect data for the main study.
- Process and analyse the data.
- Interpret the results.
- Identify the implications and limitations of the study.
- Produce recommendations based on the results.
- Write a report.
- Disseminate the results.

These steps represent the tasks undertaken by the researcher or by others on her behalf. In quantitative research, certain tasks must be carried out before undertaking others. For example, the research question or hypothesis must be clearly formulated before data are collected. The research questions cannot be modified during the data collection phase, and usually analysis starts after the collection of data. According to Arber (1993), 'although the research process can be represented as a series of discrete stages, in practice a number of activities are generally in progress at the same time, for example, you can select a sample while designing the questionnaire and recruiting interviewers'.

The process in qualitative research

The flexible nature of qualitative research is such that the research process takes on different forms. The stages of the research process may also differ from one qualitative study to another. As qualitative research comprises a variety of approaches and techniques, it is difficult to generalise about them.

Researchers using the qualitative approach may or may not define the research question prior to collecting the data. Often, a broad topic is identified and the phenomenon on which the researcher finally focuses is decided during the data collection phase. Sometimes a thorough review of the relevant literature is carried out before the data are collected, and at other times no literature review is conducted as the researcher may not want to be influenced by other people's perspectives. Regarding conceptual or theoretical frameworks, those using a grounded theory approach believe that hypotheses and theories are generated from the data collected. Therefore no attempt is made to use conceptual frameworks, although there are cases where this happens.

Instruments may or may not be constructed in advance of data collection. In qualitative research, although questions can be written and asked of respondents, the researcher is part of the instrument of data collection. Some questions may be thought of and formulated on the spot and new perspectives explored. The researcher is at liberty to alter questions or omit questions asked of previous respondents. The designs of qualitative studies are flexible enough to accommodate these and other changes. The research enterprise is moulded to suit the phenomena being studied.

In qualitative research, the researcher can begin to analyse data as they are collected. Although formal analysis takes place when data collection is completed, the researcher usually processes some of the data mentally or otherwise during fieldwork even before all the data are collected. After data analysis researchers can, and often do, go back to respondents to seek clarification and/or validation.

Do not be disheartened if at this stage you feel confused about some of the terminologies used. This chapter on the research process exposes you to the journeys (Hek, 1994) that researchers undertake. The new terms encountered are like places you will become familiar with on this journey. The rest of the book will clarify the terminologies and topics raised here; in addition, a Glossary has been provided at the end of the book.

Understanding the research process

The research process is presented above as a framework for researchers to present their study and for readers to understand the reasons for the decisions taken and for the main tasks carried out. The research process is more than what is reported. For the purpose of articles or reports, the researcher breaks down the project into a number of parts or steps, which facilitates the reader's understanding of what was done. The final publication is often a sanitised version, purified of the difficulties and frustrations encountered during the process, and almost never gives an insight into the trials and tribulations faced by researchers.

In Buckeldee and MacMahon's (1994) book entitled *The Research Experience in Nursing*, the research process is shown to be 'a messy and, at times, disorganized process, requiring creativity and reflection at all stages and that it is not an ordered linear process implied by many research texts'.

While this applies mostly to quantitative research, Sapsford and Abbott (1992) point out that 'qualitative reports tend to display greater reflexivity: they reflect more on the process of research, on how the participants made sense of it, on their own preconceptions, and on how detailed events may have shaped the nature of the data'.

Publication conventions impose restrictions on how research studies are reported. Although, as pointed out earlier, some qualitative researchers do not consult or review the literature before collecting data, a literature review section invariably appears at the start of an article as if a review were carried out at the start of the research. Journals adopt formats which they believe facilitate the reader's understanding. Invariably, they require research articles to have the following structure or sections: an introduction (which introduces the topic and gives a rationale for the study), a review of selected literature, a description of the design, the main findings and a discussion of them. This extract from the *Journal of Advanced Nursing*'s (www.journalofadvancednursing.com, 2004) 'Guide for Contributors' illustrates this point:

> Papers which are primarily about a research project should be presented with sections as follows:
>
> ● Abstract
> ● Introduction
> ● Background
> ● The study
>   – aims
>   – design/methodology
>   – sample/participants
>   – data collection
>   – validity and reliability/rigour
>   – ethical considerations
>   – data analysis
> ● Results/findings
> ● Discussion
> ● Conclusions

As can be seen, this structure follows closely the stages of the research process in quantitative research. There is a challenge on the part of the author to shift through all the details of the process and to present an account as succinct and brief and yet as comprehensible and complete as possible and in a language that clarifies rather than obfuscates.

Critiquing the research process

One of the first tasks in critiquing a research article is to attempt to describe the actions and tasks undertaken by the researcher. If the process is well described, you will have little difficulty in doing this. However, in some cases, the structure of the article may be such that you will need to 'tease out' what was actually done. It is for the benefit of readers that the research process is reported in a neat version. There is always a desire on the reader's part to know more than what is reported. While it is not possible for the researcher to describe in detail everything that happened, you must not be left with major questions unanswered. For example, if only the size of the sample is given and you are not provided with an explanation of how the sample was chosen, this will limit the extent to which the data can be generalised to other settings (see Chapter 12).

Some details are important in assessing the validity and reliability of data, some are not. For example, there are few implications for the data if the researcher had to make ten telephone calls to a nurse manager in order to gain access to the respondents, but it is vital to know whether the nurse manager 'hand-picked' the respondents, thereby creating the possibility of bias in the sample. When reading a research article or report, it is essential for you to distinguish between information that is and is not relevant.

Ethics and the research process

There are ethical implications at every stage of the research process, including the choice of topic to research, the selection of the design and the publication of the findings. Even the decision to research or not to research has ethical implications. By continuing to base practice solely on customs and traditions, consumers are denied the best possible care (Parahoo, 1991). Therefore, one can ask whether it is unethical not to examine one's practice.

Although this book is not about how to do research, nurses need to know the implications of research to be able to safeguard patients' rights and ensure their safety. These implications are discussed throughout the book. However, there are six ethical principles (ICN, 2003) that health professionals can use to guard their patients or clients from harm. These are:

1 *Beneficence.* The research project should benefit the participating individual and society in general (by contributing to the pool of human knowledge). Sometimes the benefit of participation is access to a new treatment not yet available to others. Participants are also likely to receive more attention and human contact than they might otherwise receive. On the other hand, when this attention is suddenly withdrawn at the end of the study, it can cause a feeling of isolation, which can be potentially harmful.

2 *Non-maleficence.* Research should not cause any harm to participants. While the potential physical harm may be obvious, the psychological effects may not be as transparent.

3 *Fidelity.* This principle is concerned mainly with the building of trust between researchers and participants. For example, if during a study the researcher finds that participants are in some way at risk, they should not put the need to complete the experiment above the participants' safety. Researchers are obligated to safeguard the rights of participants.

4 *Justice.* This involves being fair to participants by not giving preferential treatment to some and depriving others of the care and attention they deserve. Participants' needs must come before the objectives of the study. Researchers must ensure that participants are fairly treated and that the power relation is not unfairly tilted in their (the researcher's) favour.

5 *Veracity.* To build trust between participants and researchers, the latter must tell the truth, even if this may cause participants not to take part or to withdraw during the study. Being 'economical with the truth' can be a form of deception.

6 *Confidentiality.* The confidentiality of the information gathered from and on participants must be respected. Giving consent to participate in a study does not mean giving researchers the right to consult the subject's medical notes as well. Researchers often ask nurses and doctors, but not the participant, for permission. The presentation of the findings can potentially identify participants or participating institutions. Researchers must take care not to inadvertently reveal information that participants may want to remain confidential.

The above six ethical principles have been synthesised into four rights of subjects considering participation in research: the right not to be harmed, the right of full disclosure, the right of self-determination (subjects' right to decide to take part or to withdraw at any time) and the right of privacy, anonymity and confidentiality (ICN, 2003).

Nurses may not always have the necessary knowledge to decide whether a research study can be detrimental to the patients or clients invited to take part. Research ethics committees exist for the purpose of examining the ethical implications of such studies and for granting permission, when appropriate. The panel members should have a range of expertise necessary to carry out this task.

Ethical issues in quantitative and qualitative research

The six ethical principles apply to all types of research. However, each research approach and each study has its own ethical implications. There are some ethical issues which are more prominent in one type of design than in another. For example, in a quantitative study, participants can give informed consent prior to the study (although they have the right to withdraw). The data collection tools are unlikely to change. In qualitative studies often researchers do not know how an interview is likely to unfold. Researchers cannot state in advance all the questions they may ask. Therefore asking for informed consent is a process rather than a one-off event.

The nature of qualitative research can seem harmless but as Alderson (2001) points out:

> qualitative research may seem like only talking to people, or observing them, or using written material they have provided. Surely this can do no harm, and have no side effects . . . Only talking, however, may have strong and possibly distressing effects. The ethics of consent do not simply relate to the legal dangers of being sued for physical harm; people have rights over their lives and beliefs and actions, and the use that is made of information about them.

Richards and Schwartz (2002) listed four potential risks to research participants in qualitative studies. These are: anxiety and distress, exploitation, misrepresentation and identification of the participant in published papers. Distress can be caused to participants in all types of research. Survey items can bring back traumatic memories or cause offence. However, in qualitative studies, the opportunities for sharing 'confidences' are greater than in quantitative research. Strategies such as 'probing' can sometimes put unnecessary pressure on participants to reveal intimate and personal details which they would have preferred to keep to themselves. Balancing 'harm' and 'benefits' in such interactions is not easy, especially when researchers are keen to obtain meaningful insights into peoples' lives.

Seymour and Ingleton (1999) describe the complexity of ethical behaviour as:

> a practical, dynamic and interpersonal activity, and [it] depends on striking a fine balance between the rights of individual participants, the risk of exploitation and the wider purposes of the research.

One must recognise that 'all research is potentially exploitative and researchers' motives can frequently be mixed' (Jones et al., 1995). In health and nursing studies, researchers are often health professionals. This can lead to a 'blurring' of roles, goals and motives. They should ensure that the need to obtain data (compounded by difficulties in recruiting participants) does not take precedence over patients' needs, wishes and rights. Another dilemma frequently faced by nurse researchers is when their participants perceive them as 'nurses' as well as, or instead of, researchers. In such cases participants may disclose information which is not sought by the researcher or the participant may seek advice or help with their problems or conditions. Researchers may also have to intervene when a participant's condition gets worse (see e.g. Fitzsimons and McAloon, 2004). In all these circumstances the rights, well-being and safety of participants should take precedence over research objectives.

Participants' views can be misinterpreted in qualitative research. Some researchers may take transcripts or the findings back to participants for 'validation'. This can potentially cause distress to participants who may feel misrepresented. The small sample size in qualitative studies, and the use of 'quotes' to illustrate participants' views can also potentially lead to the identification of participants in subsequent publications. Such problems of identification are not prominent in quantitative studies, where responses are presented in numerical forms.

To reduce these risks Richards and Schwartz (2002) recommended strategies such as 'ensuring scientific soundness, organising follow-up care where appropriate, considering obtaining consent as a process, ensuring confidentiality and taking a reflexive stance towards analysis'.

Robley (1995) explains how ethics affects all phases of the qualitative research process.

> Decisions about what to study, which persons will be asked to participate, what methodology will be used, how to achieve truly informed consent, when to terminate or interrupt interviews, when to probe deeply, when therapy or nursing care supersedes research, and what and how case studies should be documented in the published results are all matters of ethical deliberation.

Both qualitative and quantitative research have ethical implications, but the differences in process and methods may lead to emphasis on certain issues rather than others.

Research governance

Every society has the responsibility to protect the rights of its citizens and ensure their well-being and safety when they take part in research. This is enshrined in the Declaration of Helsinki on 'ethical principles to provide guidance to physicians and other participants in medical research involving human subjects', including human material or identifiable data (World Medical Association, 2004). The formal and informal regulations may vary from country to country, but ethical principles governing the conduct of research should be the same. The UK government has recently introduced its Research Governance Framework for Health and Social Care (DoH, 2001).

The Research Governance Framework, which became law in May 2004, aims to continually improve standards and reduce unacceptable variations in research practice across health and social care. In particular it

- sets standards;

- defines mechanisms to deliver standards;

- describes monitoring and assessment arrangements;

- improves research quality and safeguards the public (DoH, 2001).

By May 2004, all research-active NHS care organisations in England were expected to comply with the Framework.

Background to Research Governance Framework

There are a number of factors and events which led to the development and implementation of this Framework. The conduct and management of research and its implications have long been a concern to researchers, health professionals and, more importantly, the public. Lapses in ethical behaviour, including misconduct by researchers, have been reported regularly in the press and in the professional literature. In 1998 the editor of the *British Medical Journal* called for the establishment of a national body for research misconduct (Smith, 1998). Many health care organisations were unaware of all research carried out with patients, their relatives and staff on their premises. Not all research in these organisations had formal approval either from the organisation itself or from a research ethics committee (REC). Universities and other organisations employing researchers did not all have policies and codes of practice to ensure that research was carried out properly. The real catalysts, however, seemed, as usual, to be highly publicised cases of malpractice and abuse. In one hospital parents complained that they had not given consent for their babies to be included in research (Ramsey, 2000) and, in another, people discovered that 'whole organ systems had been removed, for research purposes, from their children who died at the hospital, without their knowledge' (Bradbury and Weber, 1999). Other publicised malpractice included a case where the principal investigator did not take adequate steps to ensure that the project ran in accordance with the initial proposal, and another where the scoring or measurement used by the researchers were not peer-reviewed and were 'questionable' (Ramsay, 2000). Other factors which influenced the need for a Research Governance Framework included the Data Protection Act (1998) (United Kingdom Parliament, 1998) and the European Union Directive 2001/20/EC on Good Practice in Clinical Trials (European Union, 2001). Additionally, new scientific knowledge and technological advances in the fields of genetic engineering and embryology focused attention on the need for regulations.

Together all these factors contributed to the development of policies and measures to ensure that research is carried out efficiently, effectively and ethically.

Key responsibilities

Achieving high quality and ethically conducted research depends on cooperation between a number of people and organisations. The Research Governance Framework identifies the following groups and organisations as having key responsibilities: participants, researchers, research funders, research sponsors, universities, organisations providing care, care professionals and research ethics committees.

In health care organisations, it is the responsibility of the Chief Executive to implement the framework. However, everyone in these organisations, no matter how senior or junior, also has a role to play.

Research ethics committees

Prior to Research Governance legislation in the UK there was no consistency in how ethical approval for research with patients and health professionals was applied for or granted. They were not coordinated, used differing application processes and sometimes had different approaches to various research issues (DoH, 2005). The Central Office for Research Ethics Committees (COREC, http://www.corec.org.uk) was set up by the Department of Health (UK) to coordinate 'the development of operational systems for Local and Multi-Centre Research Ethics Committees (RECs), on behalf of the National Health Service (NHS) in England'. COREC works closely with the regional RECs in Scotland, Wales and Northern Ireland.

Anyone undertaking research with patients and staff in the NHS in the UK has to apply for ethical approval from a REC set up as a result of the Research Governance legislation. On-line application forms have been designed for this purpose. There have been a number of complaints about the number of pages that researchers have to complete and the type of information required (DoH, 2005). As a result an Ad Hoc Advisory Group (DoH, 2005) was set up to review these complaints, and the group made a number of recommendations, including the need to review the accessibility and design of the on-line form.

Nurses' role as patients' advocates and as researchers

According to the Royal College of Nursing Research Society Ethics Guidance Group (2004) 'nurses act in a range of roles in research – including carer, student, manager, investigator, research supervisor, sponsor, ethics or governance committee member'. Many of the people in the care of nurses are in vulnerable positions. These include children (see e.g. Allmark, 2002), those who are too ill to take part and those who, because of mental illness or learning disability are not able, temporarily or permanently, to give informed consent. Nurses as gatekeepers have responsibilities towards those in their care and must balance the need to 'protect' their patients with the potential to influence the outcome of research. Redsell and Cheater (2001) explain that using 'intermediaries' to obtain consent from and recruit research participants can increase 'the risk of selection bias, may expose the practitioner to ethical difficulties and may compromise the external validity' of research findings.

'Informed consent', which is the cornerstone of ethically sound research (ICN, 2003), is described as

> a process by which researchers ensure that prospective participants understand the potential risks and benefits of participating in a study, they are informed about their rights not to participate, and they are presented this information in a manner that is free from coercion.

Information should also be presented in a format, language and style that participants can understand. This means that researchers have to be particularly mindful of terminologies and jargons which professionals are acquainted with but which are not familiar to potential participants.

Giving informed consent is a process and not just a one-time event at the start of a project. As participants become more aware of real implications of the study, they may decide that they need more information or decide to withdraw from the study. Their right to do so must take precedence over the need to complete the project. For an excellent example of the on-going process of gaining consent see Seymour and Ingleton (1999).

The RCN 'Guidance for Nurses' (RCN, 2004) recommends that in order to obtain informed consent the following arrangements should be made:

- Provide full information which is easy to understand.
- Ensure the individual's informed consent is given.
- Provide opportunities for participants to withdraw consent.
- Repeat consent procedures in longer studies to ensure consent in continued.

Researchers must be particularly aware of the vulnerability of some participants. Vulnerable populations include those who are physically and/or mentally incapable of giving informed consent. It also includes those 'confined' or 'captive' such as schoolchildren or prisoners who may not feel free to decline if access to them was granted by someone in authority (ICN, 2003). Others can be vulnerable by virtue of experiencing (or having experienced) physical and mental abuse or oppression.

Research ethics committees exist for the purpose of ensuring that the rights of all individuals are respected. However, health professionals, as advocates or researchers, must be sensitive to these issues, and act according to the ethical principles outlined earlier in this chapter.

There is a lot of discussion in the literature about specific issues related to obtaining informed consent from vulnerable people or their guardians (see e.g. Arraf et al. [2004] for ethics in palliative care research; Meaux and Bell [2001] for children as research participants; Schmidt et al. [2004] for patients in emergency departments; and Ferguson [2004] for learning disability research).

For further guidance on ethical issues in research see *Good Research Practice* (Medical Research Council, 2000), the *Code of Ethics for Registered Nurses* (Canadian Nurses Association, 2002), the *Ethical Guidelines for Nursing Research* (ICN, 2003), *Research Ethics* (RCN Research Society, 2004) and the British Sociological Association's 'Statement of Ethical Practice' (2003).

The ethical implications of research are discussed further in relevant parts of the book, more specifically in relation to experiments, questionnaires, interviews and observations.

SUMMARY

Summary and conclusion

The research process constitutes all decisions and actions taken by the researcher. The process is normally reduced to a number of steps for the purpose of reporting. The stages and steps of the research process in quantitative research are more or less linear, while in qualitative research the steps are intertwined and it is possible to revisit previous stages during the project.

Research has many ethical implications, and both researchers and nurses can be guided by the six ethical principles outlined above. Patients' rights, well-being and safety should, at all times, take precedence over research objectives. For the UK, the Research Governance Framework provided guidance and has set up a number of measures designed to ensure that research carried out is of good quality and ethically sound.

References

Alderson P (2001) *On Doing Qualitative Research Linked to Ethical Healthcare* (London: The Wellcome Trust).

Allmark P (2002) The ethics of research with children. *Nurse Researcher*, **10**, 2:7–19.

Arber S (1993) The research process. In: N Gilbert (ed.), *Researching Social Life* (London: Sage).

Arraf K, Cox G and Oberle K (2004) Using the Canadian code of ethics for registered nurses to explore ethics in palliative care. *Nursing Ethics*, **11**, 6:600–9.

Bradbury J and Weber W (1999) Consent requirements for necropsy may change in UK. *The Lancet*, **354**:2055.

British Sociological Association (2003) Statement of ethical practice for the British Sociological Association, http://www.britsoc.co.uk/index.php?link_id=14&area=item1; accessed 1 July 2004.

Buckeldee J and McMahon R (1994) *The Research Experience in Nursing* (London: Chapman & Hall).

Burns N and Grove S K (1987) *The Practice of Nursing Research: Conduct, Critique and Utilization* (Philadelphia, PA: W B Saunders).

Canadian Nurses Association (2002) *Code of Ethics for Registered Nurses* (Ottawa: CAN).

Denzin N K and Lincoln Y S (1994) Introduction: entering the field of qualitative research. In: N K Denzin and Y S Lincoln (eds), *Handbook of Qualitative Research* (Newbury Park, CA: Sage).

DoH (2001) *Research Governance Framework for Health and Social Care* (London: Department of Health).

DoH (2005) *Report of the Ad Hoc Advisory Group on the Operation of NHS Research Ethics Committees* (London: Department of Health).

European Union (2001) Good practice in clinical trials. *Official Journal of the European Communities*, L121:34–44.

Faulkner M (2002) Research notes. *Nursing Standard*, **16**, 17:20.

Ferguson D (2004) Learning disability research: a discussion paper. *Learning Disability Practice*, **7**, 6:17–19.

Fitzsimons D and McAloon T (2004) The ethics of non-intervention in a study of patients awaiting coronary artery bypass. *Journal of Advanced Nursing*, **46**, 4:395–402.

Hek G (1994) The research process. *Journal of Community Nursing*, **8**, 6:4–6.

ICN (International Council of Nurses) (2003) *Ethical Guidelines for Nursing Research* (Geneva: ICN).

Jones R, Murphy E and Crossland A (1995) Primary care research ethics. *British Journal of General Practice*, **45**:623–6.

Meadows K A (2003) So you want to do research? An overview of the research process. *British Journal of Community Nursing*, **8**, 8:369–75.

Meaux J B and Bell P L (2001) Balancing recruitment and protection: children as research subjects. *Issues in Comprehensive Pediatric Nursing*, **24**, 4:214–51.

Medical Research Council (2000) *Good Research Practice: MRC Ethics Series* (London: Medical Research Council).

Parahoo K (1991) Politics and ethics in nursing research. *Nursing Standard*, **6**, 6:36–9.

Ramsey S (2000) UK inquiry highlights urgent need for research governance. *The Lancet*, 355:1706.

RCN Research Society Ethics Guidance Group (2004) *Research Ethics: RCN Guidance for Nurses* (London: Royal College of Nursing).

Redsell S A and Cheater F M (2001) The Data Protection Act (1998): implications for health researchers. *Journal of Advanced Nursing*, **35**, 4:508–13.

Richards H M and Schwartz L J (2002) Ethics of qualitative research: are there special issues for health services research? *Family Practice*, **19**, 2:135–9.

Robley L R (1995) The ethics of qualitative nursing research. *Journal of Professional Nursing*, **11**, 1:45–8.

Sapsford R and Abbott P (1992) *Research Methods for Nurses and the Caring Professions* (Buckingham: Open University Press).

Schmidt T A, Salo D, Hughes J A, Abbott J T, Geiderman J M, Johnson C X, McClure K B, McKay M P, Razzak J A, Schears T M and Solomon R C (2004) Confronting the ethical challenges to informed consent in emergency medicine research. *Academic Emergency Medicine*, **11**, 10:1082–9.

Seymour J E and Ingleton C (1999) Ethical issues in qualitative research at the end of life. *International Journal of Palliative Nursing*, **5**, 2:65–73.

Smith R (1998) The need for a national body for research misconduct. *British Medical Journal*, **316**:1686–7.

Thomas B S (1990) *Nursing Research: An Experiential Approach* (St Louis, MO: C V Mosby).

United Kingdom Parliament (1998) *Data Protection Act* (London: HMSO).

World Medical Association (2004) Declaration of Helsinki: Ethical principles for Medical Research involving human subjects. http//www.wma.net/e/policy/b3.htm; accessed 8 June 2005.

Literature Reviews

We are bombarded with information, but are we better informed?

Anon

Introduction

The purpose of research is to make a contribution, however small, towards understanding the phenomenon being studied and ultimately towards the total body of knowledge. Researchers can benefit from what has been done before and thereafter contribute something in return. The literature review serves to inform the various stages of a project and to put in context what is already known on the subject.

There are different types of literature and different reasons why a literature review is carried out. In this chapter the main purpose of reviewing the literature prior to and during a study will be explored.

The increasing amount of information generated by research studies also needs to be systematically reviewed and summarised to facilitate practitioners in their use of research. The process of systematic reviews will also be outlined and discussed.

The meaning of literature

People are generally familiar with terms such as English or French 'literature'. In research terminology, 'the literature' refers mostly to any published material, although reference is sometimes made to radio, television or other audiovisual media, such as slides, photographs and songs. What normally constitutes literature, however, is mainly books, journals, theses, reports, newspapers, pamphlets and leaflets. Sometimes reference is also made to what was said at a conference or to personal communications (face-to-face or telephone conversations, and letters). Although the value of each of the different types of literature depends on what individuals derive from them, researchers place more value on some than on others. The value of each type of publication varies according to the type and quality of information it contains. The credibility of each type of information itself depends on how objective or subjective it is and whether or not it is verifiable. The nursing and health literature comes mainly in the forms of research papers, descriptions and discussions of practice, policies and issues, conceptual and theoretical papers, opinion articles and anecdotes.

Research information is generated by research studies and systematic reviews. It relates to the topic being researched, the methods of data collection and the findings. This type of information is highly valued by some as it is usually systematically and rigorously collected and analysed, and, in the case of quantitative research, may be verifiable.

Descriptive accounts of nursing practice can be found in nursing journals, especially professional ones. Although they contain valuable information, they tend to be subjective. Nonetheless, where little information is available, descriptive accounts, in particular when the author offers a critical and reflexive perspective, can be useful and informative. More importantly, they are vehicles for sharing experiences of practice between professionals and others.

Conceptual and theoretical discussions are the backbone of all disciplines. They take the form of the intellectual discussion of ideas. Although the views expressed are those of individuals, the arguments put forward must be structured logically and argued coherently for others to understand, contribute to and use.

Nursing and health journals often publish the personal opinions of practitioners and academics. These opinions, based on experience and beliefs, are subjective, although the authors may back their arguments by research and other evidence. The credibility of the information in a personal opinion article depends in part on how the arguments are developed and supported, and on the status of the author. The list of references or the absence of it is an indication of how personal the opinion is or how much effort the author has made to relate her views to available evidence.

There are many areas that remain unresearched or underresearched. Those reviewing the literature on such areas can only rely on anecdotes and personal accounts.

Primary, secondary and tertiary sources

The value of information also depends on whether it is reported first or second hand. Original publications are known as primary sources. Such publications as the Briggs Report (Briggs, 1972) and *Introduction to Nursing: An Adaptation Model* (Roy, 1976) are primary sources. Secondary sources are publications that report on the original work. *Callista Roy: An Adaptation Model* (Lutjens, 1991) is a secondary source because Lutjens reports on Roy's original work published in 1976. Besides reporting on the original work, the authors may explain, comment or discuss the original ideas. By doing so, secondary sources are sometimes useful in that they simplify, discuss and summarise the primary material. However, there is the possibility that the original work may be distorted, misinterpreted and selectively reported as the information is first filtered through the mind of someone else. Therefore, when reading secondary sources the reader depends on a 'middle person' to accurately report what the original author(s) wrote.

It is not always possible to review primary sources because some of these are out of print or not easily accessible, or the material is too 'hefty' and time-consuming to read. Although a secondary source may shed some light on the original material, it conveys the essence of the work and is not the work itself. When research projects are reported second hand, they can lack the details necessary to fully understand how the study was carried out. As far as possible, primary sources must be consulted. The reviewer has to make a judgement on how and when to use either of the sources. It is sometimes easier to quote Roy or the Briggs Report, for example, from a secondary source near at hand than to search for these quotes in the original works. However, if Roy's model is used as a conceptual framework in a study, it is inadmissible not to use the primary source. Reading the list of references at the end of a chapter or article will give you an idea of whether there is a reliance on secondary rather than primary sources.

Tertiary sources are databases and bibliographies. Databases in electronic versions are increasingly being used, especially as they provide instant access to large amounts of literature. This is further discussed later on in this chapter.

Assessing the value of publications

Let us now evaluate each type of publication according to the type of information it contains and assess its value as a source of material for a literature review.

Books

There are different types of nursing books, such as, among others, general textbooks, books that contain a number of research projects and specialist books (for example on stress or models of nursing). Books are good sources of material that can be used in a literature review. Textbooks provide some understanding of concepts and issues but are limited in that they may cover a wide range of topics. Some textbooks make extensive reference to research, while others do so sparingly. There are also books that report exclusively on one research project or a number of projects. They provide useful information that can be used in literature reviews. It is worth noting, however, that by the time books are written, published and read, the research and statistical information they contain is already dated. Heavy reliance on books as sources of material for a review is a sign that the reviewer has missed what has recently been researched and written. Books are reviewed by 'experts' on the topic before publication. As such, they would be credible sources of information. Their value also depends on how well researched they are and on their academic status.

Journals

The main sources of literature for researchers are journal articles, which are self-contained entities. This means that, unlike a chapter in a book, which should be read in relation to previous and later chapters, an article contains, in a few pages, all the messages the author wants to convey. Another advantage of articles over books is that they can be read quickly. Although on average it may take over a year from acceptance to publication, they are more 'fresh' than any other sources of information on research and other issues, excluding perhaps conference papers and personal communications.

A distinction is sometimes made between scholarly/academic and professional journals. Academic journals (for example the *Journal of Advanced Nursing*) contain articles of high intellectual quality. These are written in a language and style that tend to appeal more to academics than practitioners. Professional or popular journals (for example, *Nursing Times, Nursing Standard* and *British Journal of Community Nursing*) are written mainly for practitioners although they contain research papers as well. They tend to be more descriptive, seeking to identify practice implications, while academic ones are more abstract and put more emphasis on theory and research. The popular journals have a useful contribution to make, as Smith (1996) explains:

> The popular nursing journals aim to keep their readers regularly informed about up-to-date and topical professional developments, trends in nursing care and practice, news about individuals and the profession, and by providing conference reports. They also provide a marvellous forum for novice writers to air their views and to develop their writing and critical abilities in the correspondence columns and book reviews sections.

Journal articles submitted for publication are normally refereed; that is, they are sent to 'experts' who advise the journal on the feasibility of publication. The 'experts' are normally other authors, which is why this practice is referred to as 'peer review'. It helps to maintain standards in publishing and gives credibility and value to the published material as unsuitable articles are either rejected or sent back to the author for revision. On average, an article is sent by the journal editor to two referees, although some journals may require only one, and others three or more. Referees are not normally made aware of who the author is. Thus a 'double-blind peer review' means that referees do not know who the author is nor does the author know who the referees are.

Theses

Doctoral and other postgraduate theses are useful and credible sources of information. They should contain not only a thorough review of concepts, theories and research studies, but also details of the research process and findings. Some doctoral theses are published as books (for example McKenna [1994], *Nursing Theories and Quality of Care*) or monographs (for example Gott [1984], *Learning Nursing*). Unfortunately, many theses remain unpublished, but they can be obtained through inter-library loan from the particular libraries where they are kept. Theses are examined and the status of the information they contain is enhanced by this process.

Research reports

Although doctoral theses follow a more or less prescribed format, research reports come in different sizes and forms of presentation. They tend to have less literature review but focus instead on the data collection, findings, conclusions and recommendations. This is, perhaps, because sponsors, for whom research reports are primarily written, are more interested in the findings and their implications for policy and practice than they are in the literature review. Many of these research reports are also published in their original forms or as research articles. Research reports do not as a rule undergo a peer review process before publication, although they are subsequently scrutinised by researchers, clinicians and others. These projects are normally carried out by experienced researchers. An example of a research report is *Exploring Staff Views of Old Age and Health Care* by Davey and Ross (2003).

Conference proceedings

The main reason to refer to, and review, conference proceedings is because the information is not available elsewhere in print. Conference proceedings are in fact abstracts or summaries of papers submitted to conferences, and, as such, they contain only brief information. Their value is mainly in being 'hot off the press'. They are limited in that not enough details are available for the reader to evaluate the project. For example, the Royal College of Nursing Research Society organises annual research conferences and publishes summaries of all papers presented at these conferences. Some presenters make copies of their talk available to conference attendees.

Other forms of information

The value of newsletters, pamphlets and leaflets as sources of information is limited in that they are brief communiqués of news and comments. They only present information with few opportunities for discussion and explanation. They also report much of their information second hand, although they have an advantage because they deal with topical issues. Leaflets and pamphlets from drug companies do contain useful information, but they can also be selective in their evidence, which they may produce in order to sell their products.

Editorials and letters written to professional journals reflect the topical interests and concerns of practitioners and others, and express the views of the authors on topics they want to draw attention to. Their value lies in the fact that they are often the expressions of practitioners who are working 'on the ground'. Newspapers and popular magazines also publish material related to health and nursing. They are interested in topical and sometimes 'sensational' issues and report the latest news on selected issues. The quality and credibility of the information depend on the author of the article and the type of newspaper or magazine.

Accessing information sources

All these sources of information can form part of a literature review. The researcher should cast her net wide in order to 'feel the pulse' of the phenomenon she is studying. The uses to which different types of information are put depends on what the reviewer wants to achieve. For example, if the reviewer wants to show that there is controversy over the benefits of Roy's model for the care of older people, she may refer to letters in the *Nursing Times* or the *Nursing Standard* to illustrate the point. However, she would have to look for discussions of models, in particular Roy's model, in academic books and journals. She would also need to search and review previous research on this issue, information that can be found mostly in academic journals and possibly in postgraduate theses.

Researchers must look for the most up-to-date, relevant and credible information they can find. In practice, this usually means relying more on academic/scholarly journals and books, research reports and theses than on professional journals, newspapers, leaflets and anecdotes.

Purpose of literature reviews

There are four common reasons why a literature review is carried out. These are:

● to prepare for an essay or assignment;

● to increase understanding of a topic or issue;

● to inform a research project;

● for a systematic review.

To prepare for an essay or assignment

For students writing an essay or undertaking an assignment, the literature provides useful information which they can use for describing and discussing relevant issues. In this case the essay or assignment is the outcome and the literature only serves to illustrate and discuss some of the ideas put forward. Sometimes the literature review is itself the assignment.

To increase understanding of a topic or issue

A literature review can also explore aspects of a phenomenon with the aim of increasing our understanding of it. For example, Davies (2004) carried out a literature review of 'parental grief'. As she explained:

> the aim of this review was to trace how theoretical perspectives on parental grief have changed over the last century and show how these influence therapeutic interventions with bereaved parents.

To inform a research project

Most researchers turn to the literature for ideas before or during a study. Many of those who start constructing a questionnaire find that they very quickly run out of questions to ask. Some learn later, to their cost, that they have omitted asking relevant and pertinent questions. The greatest feeling of frustration is to discover afterwards that the same research has already been carried out, and that, had this been known, 're-inventing the wheel' would have been unnecessary. More importantly, researchers find that they could have benefited from reading other similar studies, had they known about them prior to starting their own. There seems to be a natural tendency to get on with the project and start collecting data instead of (what could be seen as) 'wasting time reading the literature'.

A literature search and review serves to put the current study into the context of what is known already on the phenomenon. It should stimulate the researcher's thinking and can provide a wealth of ideas and perspectives. This is useful in helping to identify, refine and formulate questions. Research on the same or similar topics can, in many ways, be very informative and useful. Two questions researchers should ask are:

● What can the current literature contribute to their research?

● What can their research contribute, in particular, to the understanding of the phenomenon under investigation, and to knowledge in general?

In order to review the literature, a search must first be carried out. A literature search simply means locating and identifying the most up-to-date and relevant material. A literature review involves the critical reading of the selected literature to find out how it can be useful to the current research. From the review, a case can be made for the importance of the current research (in particular how it builds on current knowledge or what gaps it fills) and for justifying the design of the study. The scene is also set for comparing the current findings with those of similar studies. The review carried out by the researcher is much more than the written summary that appears in articles or what is reported in theses and research reports. Much more literature is read and analysed than is discussed and presented.

The literature review, as part of a research project, should perform the following functions:

- provide a rationale for the current study;
- put the current study into the context of what is known about the topic;
- review the relevant research carried out on the same or similar topics;
- discuss the conceptual/theoretical basis for the current study.

Providing a rationale for the current study

Researchers need to provide reasons for their study. In doing so, they can try to convince readers that the study is of sufficient importance. Some give as many reasons as possible, perhaps in an attempt to convince the journal's editor and referees that the current research is important. Sometimes the real reason for doing research is because of the requirement of a course or because of the pressure on academics and others to publish. Ideas for research projects come mainly from one's observation of practice and/or from the literature.

The most frequently cited reason for doing a study is the lack of research on the particular aspect of the topic being researched. For example, While and Biggs (2004), reviewing the literature for a study on 'benefits and challenges of nurse prescribing', noted that while there were more than 20,000 qualified nurse prescribers working in primary and community care, 'little has been published regarding the views of practicing health visitors and district nurses who could have been prescribing since national training was implemented in 1998', in England.

The reduction of morbidity and mortality, the prevention of illness and the economic and social costs of a particular illness or treatment are often cited as arguments for conducting a study. Abayomi and Hackett (2004), in their rationale for a study on the 'assessment of malnutrition in mental health clients: nurses' judgement vs. a nutrition risk tool', gave a number of reasons including the fact that 'malnutrition has a disabling effect on the NHS', and that 'up to 50% of hospital food in the UK is wasted, at a cost of £45 million a year'. They pointed out that previous studies evaluating the effectiveness of nutrition assessment tools have focused on physically ill people and not on those with mental illness. Using findings of previous studies they explained that nutritional status affects recovery and that poor nutrition 'can lead to increased risk of morbidity and death, impaired mental and physical function, apathy, depression, self-neglect, increased risk of complications, increased risk of pressure ulcers, reduced immune response, delayed wound healing, longer hospital stay and reduced quality of life'.

Statistical data and research findings can provide valuable back-up for the arguments put forward by researchers for their studies. Another reason often given as rationale for a study is to inform the debate on controversial issues. For example, while there is demand among women for greater choice in the type of maternity care they receive, there is also opposition to home births on the grounds of safety (Woodcock et al., 1994). To make a research contribution to this debate, Woodcock et al. (1994) carried out 'a matched study of planned home and hospital births in Western Australia'.

The ultimate goal of nursing research is to improve clinical practice. It is therefore expected that the rationale for research projects often includes the need to evaluate the effectiveness of a particular practice or compare one nursing intervention with another. Questioning practice often provides ideas for research. For example, Fader et al. (2003) questioned the effects of prolonged wearing of incontinence pads by older people on skin care. As they explained:

> based on current evidence, we cannot be confident that *less frequent* pad changing (resulting in *prolonged* skin contact with urine) does not compromise skin health, and there is a need to establish whether or not the nighttime management of incontinence involving less *frequent* pad changing is justifiable.

Policy-related reasons are often cited as a rationale for research studies. Researchers may set out to investigate professionals' reactions to policies or recommendations. The need to evaluate the effects of particular aspects of policies, old and new, is frequently given as part of the reason for research being carried out.

In addition, researchers may simply want to replicate or follow up other studies. Whatever the reasons, the rationale for a study must be relevant, clear and convincing. It must be supported, where appropriate and possible, by research findings, statistical data and, in some cases, expert opinion.

Putting the current study in context

The literature review must place the present study in the context of what is already known about the topic. It should also, where appropriate, explain or discuss the concepts, variables and issues relevant to the research problem being investigated. In a study of factors influencing the job satisfaction of hospital nurses, the researcher should discuss the concept of job satisfaction. It is likely that she will compare and contrast various definitions and descriptions offered by others who have grappled with the concept, and choose the meaning she will give to job satisfaction in her study. She will also look for previous research findings and other conceptual/theoretical literature relating to factors affecting job satisfaction. If there is little or no literature relating to hospital nurses, the researcher will draw on literature on community nurses. Failing this, she could consult relevant research and non-research material relating to job satisfaction from other professions.

In reviewing the literature, the researcher will shed some light on what is known already about variables such as gender, expectation, the nature of the job or pay, which may influence job satisfaction. Although different researchers may approach this exercise in different ways, the key concepts, variables and issues must be explained, if not discussed.

Researchers have to be selective about what they present to readers. They cannot possibly write about everything known about the topic. They can only discuss material relevant to the case they want to make, but in doing so they must back up their arguments with evidence and also present a balanced view in their discussions. Biases will be obvious when one-sided arguments are put forward, especially when readers are aware of counter-arguments.

Among the issues discussed in the study by Duxbury (1994) on primary nursing and night medication are: sleep requirements and sleeplessness as a common problem for hospital patients; factors that affect sleep (such as noise, pain, temperature, discomfort and anxiety); the relationship between work organisation and disturbance; night nurses' role and attitudes in general; night nurses' role, relating to sleep and sleep problems, in particular; and primary nursing's effect on care at night. While putting her case for carrying out the study, the author presents a summary of what is known on relevant aspects of the topic and does so by referring to research and non-research literature.

Reviewing relevant research

In reviewing the literature, the researcher tries to identify research previously carried out on the topic. By comparing, analysing and summarising their focus, methodologies and findings, she can come to some conclusions as to the state of research in this particular area. For example, Patterson (1994), studying 'perspectives of clinical teaching', found that 'much of the research pertaining to the thinking of clinical teachers has occurred in disciplines other than nursing'. She also observed that 'a great deal of the research in teacher thinking has focused on identifying the impact of teacher perspectives on students' learning'. This exercise informs the researcher of the main focus of similar studies and of aspects of the topic that have been over researched or still remain to be investigated.

In the above study, Patterson's (1994) review also revealed that methodologies that have been used included 'ethnomethodology, phenomenology, case study, interview and participant observation'. Researchers can build on the strengths of previous methodologies or adopt other strategies. The pitfalls of previous research can also be avoided. Perhaps one of the major benefits is to be able to make use of other researchers' tools, such as questionnaires or other measuring instruments.

Comparing the findings of similar studies is an important exercise in understanding the phenomenon being studied. Similar results may reinforce their validity, while contradictory ones may raise questions about, among others, the data collection and analysis methods.

It is not important or necessary to discuss every previous research study in detail. How much the reviewer reports on or discusses depends on the particular points she wants to make. In literature reviews, the most common aspect of previous research reported is the findings. When the findings from different studies are contradictory, a good reviewer should attempt to speculate on why this may be so. A close look at their methods, samples or data analysis would probably be required to explain the differences. For example, one study looking at the health of carers of spouses with cancer found that only 10 per cent of carers consulted a general practitioner about their own health. Another similar study found that general practitioner consultation was 23 per cent. There may be good reasons why these findings are different. It could be that these studies were carried out in different populations with different types of cancer. Cultural differences as well as different health-care systems may explain why consultation patterns vary. Alternatively, the explanation may also be found in the methods, response rates or data analysis. Whatever the reasons, the reviewer should not leave the reader to speculate on contradictory findings but must try to offer explanations, as it is the reviewer who has read these studies in detail. By reviewing previous studies, the researcher can explain what has been achieved so far and what contribution her study proposes to make, and also learn from the achievements and mistakes of other researchers.

Discussing the conceptual/theoretical basis for the current study

The purpose of research is to contribute to the pool of knowledge, and, as we found in Chapter 2, knowledge is organised, among other ways, in the form of theories. The use of conceptual frameworks is a step towards this contribution. Not all research uses a framework. However, a review of the literature will inform the researcher of what frameworks are available and how others have used them. The use of conceptual frameworks in nursing research is the subject of Chapter 8.

These functions of a literature review apply mainly to quantitative research. What is already known is then tested and built upon, which is why quantitative researchers, prior to starting their own research, need to know what has previously been done. In qualitative study, the researcher does not want to be influenced by previous knowledge but she needs to know what contribution to knowledge she wants to make. She also needs to know enough about the subject she is researching. For example, if an ethnographic study of the use of nursing models is carried out in a medical ward, the researcher must at least know what models are. She may not be interested, at the initial stage, in the findings of other studies, but may later want to compare hers with others.

In practice, it is unlikely that qualitative researchers do not read the literature. They may have to be selective and read enough to enable them to carry out the study without being unduly influenced by previous research. Qualitative researchers do not normally use existing conceptual frameworks or theories but instead try to formulate their own from the data they collect. Finally, in quantitative research, the literature is reviewed and completed prior to data collection, whereas in qualitative research there is more flexibility. In practice, many quantitative and qualitative researchers continue to read and review the literature at any time in the research process, right up to the completion of the report or thesis.

Critiquing the literature review

While a literature review primarily benefits those conducting the study, you as a reader may want to know why the current study is important, what research, if any, has been carried out previously and what the researcher proposes to contribute. Books, theses and research reports give the authors ample scope to present extended literature reviews, while journal articles restrict them to a summary of the main arguments. The word-limit restriction should not, however, be used as an excuse for poor and inadequate reviews. The ability to present up-to-date, relevant information clearly, concisely and logically is crucial. The review should not be a collection of disparate, unconnected views or a series of quotes.

In critiquing a literature review, you may want to use the four functions described above as a framework to assess whether these four areas are covered. Is a rationale provided? If so, what is it? Sometimes more than one reason for the study can be given. How convincing are these reasons? For example, in a study of 'attitudes of undergraduate nurses towards mental illness', the author stated that nurses' attitudes and values are of considerable importance. However, the only reason put forward for this was that 'they will be the leaders of tomorrow', undoubtedly a poor reason. Not only is the author making an assumption about 'undergraduates and leadership', but, more importantly, the relationship between 'attitudes and practice', which is more relevant, is not mentioned, let alone discussed.

Even when the rationale is convincing, the author needs to support it with such evidence as research findings, statistical data and, to a lesser extent, expert opinion. References to this evidence need to be relevant and up to date. Although statistical data take time to collect, analyse and publish, you must watch out for outdated figures. For example, in one study it was stated that 'there is a high incidence of incontinence in residential homes'. This was backed up by a reference dated 1992, while the article was written in 2004. The incidence rate could have changed since the data were collected.

Does the author inform you of similar research carried out? You should not assume that no previous research exists when the author does not mention it. It is incumbent on the researcher to provide a brief critical overview of previous research. Making selective references to one or more studies whose findings may be favourable to her cause can only bring charges of bias against the author. Readers may be aware of the existence of contradictory findings or counter-arguments.

A detailed critical review of all previous research may be boring and irrelevant. The author should guide you to make sense of the focus, methodologies and findings of other studies, rather than just describe them. Where necessary, inconsistent or contradictory findings must be explained. Prior to writing the review, it is the task of the reviewer to read, digest, compare and analyse most of the relevant material, and draw general conclusions.

If the current research study proposes to adopt approaches and methods different from those of previous research, you will be left wondering, if you are not told, which approaches and methods were previously used and why they have been discarded. When critiquing a literature review, you must identify information that is often omitted yet is crucial to your understanding of the review.

You must also find out whether important issues and concepts are dealt with adequately. It is unfair to expect the author to present a discussion of everything related to the topic. However, if, for example, in a study investigating 'health promotion strategies of health visitors', the concept of 'health promotion' is not explored, you may find it difficult to understand what constitutes health promotion for the author. You would also like to know what health promotion strategies are and, briefly, what the state of knowledge on them is.

As explained earlier, it is important to pay attention to the publication dates of the literature referred to in the review. It is difficult to generalise about what constitutes a 'dated' reference. If you read the nursing literature frequently, you will be aware of areas that are well researched. If you find that references are more than five years old, you can ask yourself whether there is more recent literature on the topic. It is up to the author to mention why the literature she refers to is 'dated'. You must also take into account that it can take time for an article, once accepted for publication, to be published. You should also question the author's reliance on secondary sources if this is the case.

Not every literature review fulfils the four functions mentioned above. In practice, the author focuses on one or more of these and pays little attention to the others. This choice depends on the case she wants to put across. Provided crucial information – such as a discussion of concepts relevant to the study and information about previous studies – is not omitted, the review may be adequate. You must also look out for assumptions and generalisations. In a study of 'psychiatric nurses' attitudes and behaviours towards patients in acute wards', the authors make the assumptions in the literature review that 'the management approach in acute psychiatric care needed to be changed' and that 'nurses working in these settings needed to have greater skills in rehabilitation and health promotion'. No evidence was offered to support either of these two statements. The study itself did not set out to investigate management approaches or the skills of psychiatric nurses.

It is unfair to be overcritical of literature reviews, especially in journal articles where the authors are limited for space. Not every issue, concept or research study can be discussed in depth. If the information is not there, you can ask yourself whether the lack of it affects your understanding of the study. If it does, this is a good indication that this information should have been included in the review. A good literature review provides you with essential, relevant information to put the current study in the context of present knowledge and research available on the topic.

Systematic reviews

The current emphasis on evidence-based practice has focused attention on the 'systematic review' which aims to search, appraise and summarise available evidence for practice. The glut of information, coupled with competing demands on practitioners' time mean that it is difficult for them to keep abreast of the knowledge that surrounds them. We continue to produce knowledge, much of which gets lost in the sea of information. Like the sea, information is a valuable resource, and unless we learn how to harness it and make use of it, we can drown in it.

Evans and Pearson (2001) explain that the findings of the systematic review 'frees the decision maker from reliance on the mass of published primary research'. In any case most practitioners do not have the resources and expertise to search and appraise the large number of studies that are relevant to their practice.

A systematic review can be defined as the rigorous search, selection, appraisal, synthesis and summary of the findings of primary research in order to answer a specific question. The process of systematic reviews from question formulation to the summary of evidence should be transparent and, therefore, potentially replicable. The rationale and actions of the systematic reviewer should be clear for readers to assess the reliability, validity and relevance of the review for their practice. The word 'systematic' refers to the system adopted by the reviewer, which details the parameters set (e.g. the time-frame from which studies are selected), the method of appraisal (e.g. tools used to evaluate the quality of the studies) and the method of synthesis (e.g. qualitative summaries or statistical calculations).

Systematic reviews can be broadly termed as 'research on research'. It is sometimes called secondary research because it does not collect new information (primary research) but makes use of the findings of previous research. Table 7.1 makes a comparison between primary research and systematic reviews.

In contrast, a non-systematic literature review is normally broad. The questions for which evidence are sought may not be stated or may be unclear. The method of selecting items for review is not always transparent, nor is the method of appraisal. Readers are unsure how the review was carried out. A

Table 7.1 Comparison of primary research and systematic reviews

Primary research	Systematic reviews
Choose a topic and formulate a question, objectives or hypothesis for which data are to be collected	Choose a topic and formulate a question, objectives or hypothesis in order to begin a systematic search
Select a sample or population and study site/s	Select databases and set inclusion/ exclusion criteria for selection of studies/other evidence
Choose data collection methods (e.g. questionnaires, interviews or observations) and collect data	Search the literature and extract relevant, valid and reliable information from articles (through critical appraisal) with the use of a checklist of questions
Analyse data collected	Analyse and synthesise the findings of the selected (methodologically sound) studies
Draw conclusions from the analysis of data	Draw conclusions from the findings of the review

non-systematic review, often called a 'narrative' or 'descriptive' review, is often 'haphazard and biased, subject to the idiosyncratic impressions of the individual reviewer' (Mulrow, 1994).

Systematic reviews can be used to answer specific and focused questions relating to clinical practice, policy, education or methodologies. Below are some examples:

Clinical   To identify differences between gauze and tape and/or transparent polyurethane film dressings in the incidence of central venous catheter-related infection and in a number of other outcomes (Gillies et al., 2003).

Policy   To assess the effectiveness of home-based support for older people (Elkan et al., 2001).

Education   To assess whether self-management educational intervention improves lung function and decreases morbidity and health care use in children and adolescents with asthma (Cicutto, 2003).

Methodology   To assess the quality of quantitative psychiatric/mental health nursing research articles published in English between 1982 and 1992 (Yonge et al., 1997).

The terms 'systematic reviews' and 'meta-analysis' are sometimes used interchangeably. However, meta-analysis is one form of systematic review. Meta-analysis has been defined as 'a mathematical synthesis of the results of two or more primary studies that addressed the same hypothesis in the same way' (Greenhalgh, 1997b). Meta-analysis is a term normally used to describe a process of combining and summarising the findings of a number of clinical trials.

The association of systematic reviews with randomised controlled trials (RCTs) comes mainly from those who believe that there is a hierarchy of study designs for studies of effectiveness (National Health Service Centre for Reviews and Dissemination [CRD], 2001) in which systematic reviews of RCTs provide the best evidence. In this hierarchy, evidence from other research approaches and designs, including qualitative ones, is not highly regarded. This view, however, is not shared by all and is indeed contested (see Chapter 19). Recently there have been indications that qualitative evidence is becoming more valued. Dixon-Woods and Fitzpatrick (2001) noted that the recent publication of the NHS Centre for Reviews and Dissemination (NHS CRD, 2001) on the guidance of undertaking systematic reviews shows increased recognition of the diverse types of evidence. They believe that 'this suggests that the rigid insistence on controlled trials as the sole source of evidence on effectiveness that characterised the beginnings of the evidence-based healthcare movement is fading'. Pearson (2004) also points out that 'the Evidence-Based Practice movement' is beginning to adopt a more comprehensive view of what counts as evidence. For a useful discussion of the practical issues in conducting systematic reviews of qualitative studies, see Lloyd Jones (2004).

Meta-synthesis (Jensen and Allen 1994; Sandelowski et al., 1997), another form of systematic review, is the term that has been used to describe the technique or method to search, appraise and synthesise (combine) the findings of qualitative studies. For examples of systematic reviews of qualitative studies see Evans and Fitzgerald (2002), Beck (2002) and Sandelowski and Barroso (2003). According to Evans and Pearson (2001), methods for reviewing, summarising and synthesising qualitative research are still evolving. The task of appraising and synthesising qualitative studies is made more difficult because of the 'widely varying theoretical perspectives and diverse analytical approaches' used in these studies (Dixon-Woods and Fitzpatrick, 2001). A number of papers, including Sleep and Clarke (1999), Evans and Pearson (2001) and Sandelowski et al. (1997), provide useful discussions on this issue.

The systematic review process

As with primary research, there are a number of key steps which have to be followed when undertaking a systematic review. These are:

- Formulate/select question, aim, objectives, or hypotheses

- Define terms or concepts

- Set inclusion/exclusion criteria

- Search the evidence

- Select items to review

- Appraise the evidence

- Synthesise the evidence

- Conclude and make recommendations.

Formulating questions for a systematic review

No systematic review can take place without a question, an aim or a hypothesis. According to Pearson (2004) 'a sound, systematic review rests on a well defined review question'. These have to be clear and unambiguous. Questions for reviews can come from one's practice or professional interest. Systematic reviews are associated with clinical practice, mainly because they are an integral component of evidence-based practice. However, a systematic review is a technique or design to answer a range of questions, including non-clinical ones. Below are examples of questions for which systematic reviews have been carried out. They show that more than one question can be formulated and that they have to be focused and realistic as well. The broader the review question the more difficult it can be to conduct the review and reach conclusions.

- From Shade (1992) 'Patient-controlled analgesia: can education improve outcomes?'
  Would specific, structured pre-operative instruction by nurses with patients, concerning the use and purpose of the PCA (patient-controlled analgesia) device: (a) reduce the amount of analgesic that the patient uses from the pump postoperatively; and (b) reduce the patient's perception and experience of pain, as measured on a validated measuring tool?

- From Yonge et al. (1997) 'A systematic review of psychiatric/mental health nursing research literature 1982–1992'
  They asked the following questions:

  1 What is the quality of the existing literature?
  2 In which country is the research being done?
  3 What is the academic preparation of the researcher(s)?
  4 Was the research project funded?

Defining terms or concepts

When terms such as 'pain', 'effectiveness', 'mobility' or 'therapeutic interventions' are used in the question/s, they have to be operationally defined. In particular the outcome measures of 'effectiveness' have to be clearly stated. For example, in a review on the effectiveness of nicotine replacement therapy in helping people to stop smoking (Tang et al., 1994), 'effectiveness' was defined as 'the difference between percentages of treated and control subjects who had stopped smoking at one year'.

Setting inclusion/exclusion criteria

The questions and the available resources determine to a great extent the scope of the review. Therefore inclusion and exclusion criteria are set to define the boundaries of the review. These criteria must be justified, and their implications for the validity of the review must be recognised. For example, if the evidence is searched manually from selected journals, or if only English-language publications are considered, the findings will have limitations as it is possible that significant evidence may be missed. The generalisability of the findings depends on how inclusive or exclusive the review is in its identification and selection of evidence. For example, one of the exclusion criteria in Brooker et al.'s (1996) review of the 'effectiveness of community mental health nursing' (CMHNs) was 'interventions carried out by multi-disciplinary teams in which CMHNs work'. Therefore the findings are not generalisable to interventions used by nurses working in these teams. Setting this exclusion criterion was deliberate on the part of the reviewers as they wanted to focus on interventions carried out by nurses only.

Setting inclusion/exclusion criteria can depend on reviewers' definition of evidence. It is not unusual to find that some would include RCTs only. The lack of studies on a particular topic can also influence the decision of the reviewer to be less 'choosy' and more inclusive.

For an example of inclusion criteria for a systematic review see Cheater and Closs (1997) who reviewed 'the effectiveness of methods of dissemination and implementation of clinical guidelines for nursing practice'.

Searching the evidence

The aim of a systematic review is to answer the review question. For this answer to be credible every effort to locate all relevant studies must be made. The resources and skills to do so often determine how successful reviewers will be in identifying all relevant literature.

The most common format in which research findings are presented is the journal article. Abstracts (a brief summary outlining relevant information) of these articles are compiled in registers, known as databases, which are available on-line or as CD-ROMS. Three of the most relevant and useful databases for nurses are the Cumulative Index to Nursing and Allied Health (CINAHL), MEDLINE, and Allied and Complementary Medicine (AMED).

MEDLINE is widely recognised as 'the premier source for bibliographic and abstract coverage of the biomedical literature' (MEDLINE, 2003). It also covers other areas including medicine, health, nursing, dentistry and the health care system. MEDLINE contains over 11 million citations from more than 4600 journals dating back to the mid-1960s.

The CINAHL database provides coverage of the literature related to nursing and allied health from over 1200 journals. This database 'also provides access to healthcare books, nursing dissertations, selected conference proceedings, standards of professional practice, educational software and audiovisual materials in nursing (CINAHL, 2003). Approximately 70 per cent of CINAHL headings also appear in MEDLINE (CINAHL, 2003). Subirana et al. (2002), who compared the efficiency of MEDLINE and CINAHL in identifying references, concluded that searches on nursing-related subjects should combine CINAHL and MEDLINE in order to obtain the best results. There are other databases relevant to nurses including CANCERLIT which is produced by the US National Cancer Institute and which covers all aspects of cancer therapy. PsycInfo is another database which contains citations and summaries in the field of psychology with particular reference to medicine, psychiatry, nursing and other related disciplines.

Reviewers rely mainly on databases. However, depending on a number of factors, including which journals are included in the database and how articles are indexed, it may not be possible to identify all relevant literature. Some literature are published in-house and some researchers do not publish their projects. These studies are known as the 'grey literature'. They are important to include in the review. Hopewell et al. (2003) reviewed research studies that have investigated the impact of the grey literature in meta-analysis of randomised trials of health care interventions. They concluded that 'published trials are generally larger, and may show an overall greater treatment effect than grey trials'. According to them 'reviewers need to ensure they identify grey trials in order to minimise the risk of introducing bias into their review' (Hopewell et al., 2003).

Reference lists of published papers and manual searches of relevant journals can also be useful. Databases, the grey literature, reference lists and manual searches are all important sources of literature which should be accessed, where possibly, in the process of a systematic review.

Searching computerised databases successfully is a skill which requires training and experience. The use of appropriate search terms is the key to the successful identification of relevant material. Each database has information on how to search the literature. Librarians can also be helpful in advising how to access them or what courses are available for training. There are a number of useful resources to help you in this process (see for e.g. Greenhalgh, 1997a). *Undertaking Systematic Reviews of Research on Effectiveness* (NHS CRD, 2001) describes all the stages of the review process.

In the extract below, Petticrew et al. (2002) described how they searched and identified the literature for their review of the 'influence of psychological coping on survival and recurrence in people with cancer'.

Search strategy – Following systematic review guidelines we searched several databases for published and unpublished studies (in any language) on the association between progression of cancer, recurrence or survival, and psychological coping: Medline 1966–June 2002, PsycINFO 1887–June 2002, ASSIA 1987–June 2002, Embase 1980–June 2002, Cancerlit 1966–June 2002, Dissertation Abstracts 1975–June 2002, the NLM gateway (accessed 21 June 2002), and CINAHL 1982–June 2002. We searched bibliographies and reviews and contacted key individuals and authors for additional unpublished information when necessary.

Knowing what sources of information to access and how to access them are key requisites for locating the evidence.

Selecting items to review

The search for literature will identify relevant and non-relevant items. The next task of the reviewer is to select only those that meet the inclusion criteria. Reading the abstracts or summaries of the selected items will quickly determine which items should be included. Sometimes, however, abstracts may not be clear or may not provide adequate or relevant information for the reviewer to make a decision. This can be done when the full article is accessed.

Appraising the evidence

Before synthesising the findings of the selected items, the quality of these studies must be appraised since not all studies are valid and reliable. There are a number of tools or checklists available to help in this process. CASP (Critical Appraisal Skills Programme) has developed a number of tools which are available and free for personal use at http://www.phru.nhs.uk/casp/appraisa.htm. Other references for checklists include Treloar et al. (2000) and Greenhalgh (1997a). The Cochrane Reviewers' handbook (http://www.cochrane.org/resources/handbook/index.htm) can also be useful. The appraisal of research studies is explained further in Chapter 17.

To avoid subjectivity in the use of these tools it is usual for two or more reviewers to carry out the appraisal independently and to compare the results. Differences can be ironed out and a consensus can be reached. Only items that meet the quality criteria set by reviewers are included in the next stage of the review.

Synthesising the findings from selected studies

The aim of data synthesis is to collate and summarise the data extracted from primary studies selected in the review (NHS CRD, 2001). There are different ways in which these findings can be synthesised (combined) depending on whether the reviewed studies are RCTs, non-RCTs, quantitative studies, qualitative studies or those combining qualitative and quantitative studies.

For meta-analysis of RCTs, the aim of the synthesis is to find out if there is a difference between the intervention groups and the control groups in terms of the pre-selected outcome measures. These could be 'the difference in number of days in which a condition is treated with a new drug when compared to a placebo', 'the risk of developing infection (in the two groups) following two types of wound care' or 'the incidence of relapse between two different treatments'. These are normally expressed in terms of odds ratio (the ratio of the odds of an event in the intervention group to the odds of an event in the control group), the relative risk (the ratio of risk in the intervention group to the risk in the control group) or the mean difference (the difference between the mean scores (e.g. quality of life) of the two groups. These are only some of the measures in which the synthesised data can be presented.

The findings of the selected studies are not just added up and averaged. Weightings can be given according to the size and the quality of individual studies. Larger studies and those judged to be of higher quality can be given more 'weight'.

The heterogeneity (variability in the characteristics of the sample of individual studies) and 'publication bias' (the likelihood that RCTs which show that the interventions had little or no effects were not published) are two of the other factors that can be taken into account when the results of the studies are combined. Statistical techniques to carry out these calculations and test the accuracy of the results are well developed (for more details see NHS CRD, 2001). Most people may find it difficult to interpret data on 'odds ratio' or 'relative risk' or 'number needed to treat'. Therefore the findings are also summarised and presented in a prose form that is easier to understand.

The synthesis of qualitative studies requires a more descriptive and narrative approach since the findings are normally presented in the form of themes. The process is similar to the analysis of data from a number of interview scripts. However, when the populations in these studies are not similar and the approaches are diverse, the reviewer may be faced with difficult decisions especially if the findings are divergent too.

According to NHS CRD (2001) 'there are no formal procedures available to aid narrative synthesis of findings from qualitative studies within the context of a systematic review'. The synthesis is likely to be a subjective interpretation of these findings. However, as with meta-analysis, the process of synthesis should be made transparent.

Evans and Fitzgerald's (2002) review of the 'experience of physical restraint' and Sandelowski and Barroso's (2003) 'metasynthesis of qualitative findings on motherhood in HIV-positive women' are useful examples of qualitative systematic reviews.

Concluding and making recommendations

Systematic reviews are carried out in order to appraise and synthesise the available evidence in answer to a specific question. Readers are eager to know what the conclusions are and how they can use the findings in their practice. Reviewers, by virtue of appraising a number of studies, can also comment on the quality of the evidence and make recommendations for future research. For example, after reviewing seven randomised trials on acupuncture for depression, Mukaino et al. (2005) concluded that 'the evidence from controlled trials is insufficient to conclude whether acupuncture is an effective treatment for depression, but justifies further trials of electroacupuncture'.

Conclusions and recommendations in systematic reviews should be based on the findings and should be made with care as they may subsequently influence practice.

Systematic and exploratory reviews

The increasing emphasis on the need for literature reviews to be systematic and rigorous has raised concerns about other types of reviews which do not follow rigorously the process of systematic reviews. Does every literature review have to be systematic? If you want to know if there is evidence that 'discharge preparation' reduces anxiety among older patients in hospitals, then the review has to be valid and reliable, otherwise the results will be contested. Duley (1996) points out that different reviewers have reported conflicting conclusions to the same question and therefore have added confusion about what clinicians should do. To avoid this, every step of the review, from question formulation to conclusions, has to be explained and justified. Readers can thus judge the rigour with which the review was carried out and decide whether the conclusions are credible or not.

On the other hand, if you want to use the literature to explore and discuss a particular concept such as 'discharge anxiety', you have the freedom to use the literature to explain your perspective on the topic. It is no more than a 'well-researched' essay, but it serves the purpose of giving readers an insight into 'discharge anxiety', and, as such, has a valuable contribution to make to practitioners' knowledge. The quality of the review depends on how you draw from the existing literature, and on the strength and nature of your arguments. It is not possible or even desirable that every bit of literature on 'discharge anxiety' is searched and reviewed. You must, however, demonstrate adequate awareness of the relevant literature on the subject, and not be biased in selecting only literature that supports your views.

Williams (2001) wrote a literature review on the concept of intimacy in nursing. The areas selected for discussion reflect what she perceived as important when discussing the concept. These areas were 'historical background of the nurse–patient relationship and intimacy', the 'nature of intimacy', 'research on intimacy in nursing' and 'the implications of intimacy'. Someone else reviewing this topic may have selected some similar and some different aspects to write about. No indication of how the literature was searched or appraised was given nor is this necessary for this type of review. Although it is a subjective exploration, its credibility depends on how comprehensively the author deals with the concept of intimacy, how critical she is of the literature, how she uses it in her exploration and what contribution she makes to existing knowledge. This type of review serves to clarify concepts or issues. It also offers various ways in which they can be viewed and identifies areas for future investigation. It is not to be compared with, or judged by, the standards of a systematic review. The problem often lies with reviews of evidence which claim to be systematic but often are not.

Relying on systematic reviews

Evidence-based practice is expected to reduce practitioners' reliance on expert opinion by providing them with 'objective evidence' on which to base their decisions. Practitioners, in general, do not have the time nor the skills necessary to search and review large amounts of literature. The summaries of systematic reviews present evidence in a form that can be easily accessed and read. As Evans and Pearson (2001) explain:

> The single document of the review replaces many individual study reports, and as such, frees the decision maker from reliance on the mass of published primary research. This research summary aids the translation of research evidence into practice because the identification, selection, appraisal and summary does not have to be performed by the end-user of the research.

At the same time practitioners rely on these summaries to provide valid and reliable evidence. They are at the mercy of reviewers except if they have access to all the details of the review and are able to critically appraise it. Such a task can be expected to be beyond the role of individual practitioners. There are, however, some built-in safeguards which could, to some extent, reassure practitioners that they can rely on systematic reviews. For example, the Cochrane Collaboration and the Centre for Research and Dissemination based at York University are dedicated to achieving the highest standards in systematic reviews and they allocate 'Kite Marks' to the reviews which they endorse. Yet a systematic review (Olsen et al., 2001) of the quality of 53 Cochrane reviews first published in issue 4 of the *Cochrane Library* in 1998, found:

No problems or only minor ones were found in most reviews. Major problems were identified in 15 reviews (29%). The evidence did not fully support the conclusion in nine reviews (17%), the conduct or reporting was unsatisfactory in 12 reviews (23%), and stylistic problems were identified in 12 reviews (23%). The problematic conclusions all gave too favourable a picture of experimental intervention.

They concluded that while the *Cochrane Library* remains a key source of evidence about the effects of health care practice, there is always room for improvement. Olsen et al. (2001) suggest that 'users should interpret reviews cautiously, particularly those with conclusions favouring experimental interventions'. Practitioners do not normally have the skills and experience of these reviewers to begin to cast doubt on the results (often couched in statistical terms) and the conclusions of systematic reviews. They are dependent on reviewers (another set of experts!) to provide them with valid and reliable evidence.

Systematic reviewing has experienced a great deal of development in the last decade. Methods to access, search, appraise and synthesise evidence have been developed at a level of sophistication which could have hardly been expected within such a short time. Yet despite being referred to as a 'science' it is still subject to a number of validity and reliability threats. Bias related to publication, searching, appraising, synthesising and concluding can all affect the final product. Jadad and McQuay (1996) found that 90 per cent of meta-analysis of studies which evaluated analgesic interventions had methodological flaws that could limit their validity. And when one considers that there is rarely a systematic review that does not conclude that many of the primary studies which they reviewed were flawed, one can begin to understand why the results of systematic reviews should be treated with caution. However, according to Crombie and McQuay (1998) 'they may not be correct all the time but they give a good guide most of the time'.

Appraisal of systematic reviews

Although most nurses and other health professionals cannot be expected to carry out systematic reviews, they should be able to appraise or evaluate these reviews. Not all reviews are prepared by, or in collaboration with, the Cochrane Review Groups or the NHS Centre for Reviews and Dissemination. Both these and other reviews have to be appraised before their recommendations could be applied to practice. The following checklist is offered as a framework for appraising systematic reviews. It is based on the steps of systematic reviews outlined earlier in this chapter.

1   Are the questions for the review clearly stated?
2   Are the terms or concepts operationally defined? This will help you decide whether you understand the terms used in the review question in the same way as the reviewers.

3   What are the inclusion and exclusion criteria? This has implications for the generalisability of the findings.

4   What databases and other sources were accessed? This will inform you of the extensiveness of the search.

5   What terms and combination of terms were used in the search?

6   How were the items (studies) in the review appraised? If a checklist was used, is it rigorous?

7   How was the evidence combined or summarised?

8   What were the conclusions?

9   What were the limitations of the review?

10 Overall, do the findings of the review help or confuse you?

A clear and unambiguous question, transparency in how the search was carried out, how the selected studies were appraised and how the conclusions were reached are all crucial for readers to assess the validity, reliability of the findings, their relevance to, and usefulness in their particular practice.

SUMMARY

Summary and conclusion

The main purpose of a literature review is to show why the current study is needed and where it fits into the overall body of knowledge on the phenomenon being researched. Additionally, the review sets the scene by discussing the relevant issues and concepts in, and related to, the research question, objectives or hypotheses. In designing their studies, researchers can draw upon the theoretical and research literature available. There are different types of literature, and the information they contain varies according to the type of publication. Researchers must as far as possible consult, and refer to, reliable and credible sources. This invariably means research-based literature, although there is other valuable information in the non-research literature as well. Primary sources should be consulted and reported where possible. A literature review, as part of a research study, can have four functions and they can be used as a framework for critiquing reviews.

In this chapter the purpose and process of systematic reviews were discussed. The process consists of formulating clear questions, searching relevant databases, appraising the quality of relevant studies and summarising their findings. Finally, a checklist to evaluate systematic reviews was provided.

References

Abayomi J and Hackett A (2004) Assessment of malnutrition in mental health clients: nurses' judgement vs nutrition risk tool. *Journal of Advanced Nursing*, **45**, 4:430–7.

Beck C T (2002) Postpartum depression: a metasynthesis. *Qualitative Health Research*, **12**, 4:453–72.

Briggs A (1972) *Report of the Committee on Nursing* (London: DHSS).

Brooker C, Repper J M and Booth A (1996) The effectiveness of community mental health nursing: a review. *Journal of Clinical Effectiveness*, **1**, 2:44–50.

Cheater F M and Closs S J (1997) The effectiveness of methods of dissemination and implementation of clinical guidelines for nursing practice: a selective review. *Clinical Effectiveness in Nursing*, **1**:4–15.

Cicutto L (2003) Review: self management education improves outcomes in children and adolescents with asthma. *Evidence-Based Nursing*, **6**, 4:106–7.

CINAHL (2003) http://gateway.uk.ovid.com/re1600/server1/fldguide/nursing/htm

Crombie I K and McQuay H J (1998) The systematic review: a good guide rather than a guarantee. *Pain*, **76** :1–2.

Davey B and Ross F (2003) *Exploring Staff Views of Old Age and Health Care* (London: Nursing Research Unit, King's College).

Davies R (2004) New understandings of parental grief: literature review. *Journal of Advanced Nursing*, **46**, 5:506–13.

Dixon-Woods M and Fitzpatrick R (2001) Qualitative research in systematic reviews. *British Medical Journal*, **323**, 7316:765–6.

Duley L (1996) Systematic reviews: what can they do for you? *Journal of the Royal Society of Medicine*, **89**:242–4.

Duxbury J (1994) An investigation into primary nursing and its effect upon the nursing attitudes about and administration of prn night medication. *Journal of Advanced Nursing*, **19**:923–31.

Elkan R, Kendrick D, Dewey M and Hewitt M (2001) Effectiveness of home-based support for older people. A systematic review and meta-analysis. *British Medical Journal*, **323**:719.

Evans D and Fitzgerald M (2002) The experience of physical restraint: A systematic review of qualitative research. *Contemporary Nurse*, **13**:126–35.

Evans D and Pearson A (2001) Systematic reviews of qualitative research. *Clinical Effectiveness in Nursing*, **5**:111–19.

Fader M, Clarke-O'Neill S, Cook D, Dean G, Brooks R, Cottenden A and Malone-Lee J (2003) Management of night-time urinary incontinence in residential settings for older people: an investigation into the effects of different pad changing regimes on skin health. *Journal of Clinical Nursing*, **12**, 3:374–86.

Gillies D, O'Riordan E, Carr D, O'Brien I, Frost J and Gunning R (2003) Central venous catheter dressings: a systematic review. *Journal of Advanced Nursing*, **44**, 6:623–32.

Gott M (1984) *Learning Nursing* (London: Royal College of Nursing).

Greenhalgh T (1997a) *How to Read a Paper* (London: BMJ Publishing Group).

Greenhalgh T (1997b) Papers that summarise other papers (systematic reviews and meta-analysis). *British Medical Journal*, **315**:672–5.

Hopewell S, MacDonal S, Clarke M and Egger M (2003) Grey literature in meta-analyses of randomised trials of health care interventions. *The Cochrane Library*, **1**:1.

Jadad A R and McQuay H J (1996) Meta-analyses to evaluate analgesic interventions: a systematic qualitative review of their methodology. *Journal of Clinical Epidemiology*, **49**: 235–43.

Jensen L A and Allen M N (1994) A synthesis of qualitative research on wellness–illness. *Qualitative Health Research*, **4**, 4:349–69.

Lloyd Jones M (2004) Application of systematic review methods to qualitative research: practical issues. *Journal of Advanced Nursing*, 48, 3:271–8.

Lutjens L R J (1991) *Callista Roy: An Adaptation Model* (Newbury Park, CA: Sage).

McKenna H P (1994) *Nursing Theories and Quality of Care* (Aldershot: Avebury).

MEDLINE (2003) http://gateway.uk.ovid.com/rel600/server1/fldguide/medline.htm; accessed 7 April 2003.

Mukaino Y, Park J, White A and Ernst E (2005) The effectiveness of acupuncture for depression – a systematic review of randomised controlled trials. *Acupuncture in Medicine*, 23, 2:70–6.

Mulrow C (1994) Rational for systematic reviews. *British Medical Journal*, 309:597–9.

National Health Service Centre for Reviews and Dissemination (2001) *Undertaking Systematic Reviews of Research on Effectiveness*, 2nd edn (York: University of York).

Olsen O, Middleton P, Ezzo J, Gotzsche P C, Hadhazy V, Herxheimer A, Kleijnen J and McIntosh H (2001) Quality of Cochrane reviews: assessment of sample from 1998. *British Medical Journal*, 323:829–32.

Patterson B (1994) The view from within: perspectives of clinical teaching. *International Journal of Nursing Studies*, 31, 4:349–60.

Pearson A (2004) A response to 'the effectiveness of public health nursing: the problems and solutions in carrying out a review of systematic reviews'. *Journal of Advanced Nursing*, 47, 1:109–10.

Petticrew M, Bell R and Hunter D (2002) Influence of psychological coping on survival and recurrence in people with cancer: a systematic review. *British Medical Journal*, 325:1066.

Roy C (1976) *Introduction to Nursing: An Adaptation Model* (Engelwood Cliffs, NJ: Prentice Hall).

Sandelowski M and Barroso J (2003) Towards a metasynthesis of qualitative findings on motherhood in HIV-positive women. *Research in Nursing and Health*, 26:153–70.

Sandelowski M, Docherty S and Emden C (1997) Qualitative metasynthesis: issues and techniques. *Research in Nursing and Health*, 20:365–71.

Shade P (1992) Patient-controlled analgesia: can client education improve outcomes? *Journal of Advanced Nursing*, 17, 4:408–13.

Sleep J and Clark E (1999) Weighing up the evidence: the contribution of critical literature reviews to the development of practice. *Nursing Times Research*, 4, 1:306–13.

Smith J P (1996) Editorial: The value of nursing journals. *Journal of Advanced Nursing*, 24:1–2.

Subirana M, Sola I, Garcia J M, Guillawet A, Paz E, Gich J and Urrutia G (2002) Importance of the database in the literature research: the first step in a systematic review (in Spanish). *Enfermeria Clinica*, 12, 6 :296–300.

Tang J L, Law M and Wald N (1994) How effective is nicotine replacement therapy in helping people to stop smoking. *British Medical Journal*, 308:21–6.

Treloar C, Champness S, Simpson P L and Higginbotham N (2000) Critical appraisal checklist for qualitative research studies. *Indian Journal of Pediatrics*, 67, 5:347–51.

While A E and Biggs K S M (2004) Benefits and challenges of nurse prescribing. *Journal of Advanced Nursing*, 45, 6:559–67.

Williams A (2001) A study of practising nurses' perceptions and experiences of intimacy within the nurse–patient relationship. *Journal of Advanced Nursing*, 35, 2:188–96.

Woodcock H C, Read A W, Bower C, Stanley F J and Moore D J (1994) A matched cohort study of planned home and hospital births in Western Australia 1981–1987. *Midwifery*, 10:125–35.

Yonge O, Austin W, Quiping P Z, Wacko M, Wilson S and Zaleski J (1997) A systematic review of the psychiatric mental health nursing literature 1982–1992. *Journal of Psychiatric and Mental Health Nursing*, 43, 3:171–7.

Research and Theory

Science is built up of facts, as a house is built up of stones; but an accumulation of facts is no more a science than a heap of stones is a house.

Henri Poincaré

Introduction

In science, research is one of the main processes by which data are collected to support, reject or modify theories, or to develop new ones. Researchers often use theories implicitly or explicitly to underpin their studies. Others formulate their own hypotheses and theories from observations.

The development of any profession or discipline depends on the accumulation of a body of knowledge. Theories play an important part in this process by making the link between knowledge and practice. In this chapter, we will explore the meaning of theory and examine its relationship to knowledge, research and practice.

What is a theory?

The term 'theory' is often defined in relation to 'practice', as when, for example, a teacher describes in the classroom the process of giving an injection, as opposed to students actually giving injections to patients. Theory, in this sense, means dealing with a topic (in this case the administration of an injection) in an abstract form. Everyday conversations are full of theories. For example, people have their own theories as to why working-class children are poor achievers at school or why there is an increase in crime. These lay theories (from non-experts) differ from scientific theories because the latter must go through a process of falsification of verification before they are accepted, at least for a while, before new data come to light to modify or replace them with new theories. The theory that the earth was flat was replaced when new observations caused scientists to think again. Many scientific theories began life as speculations (see Chapter 2). In the absence of empirical evidence (as observed by the human senses), the best that people could offer was speculation. Even today, many of the theories about 'space' and 'black holes' are speculations, even though great strides have been made in astronomy.

Theories are merely interpretation of phenomena. They are not the definitive explanation as they may in time be rejected or modified. There may also be competing theories to explain the same phenomenon. For example, the theory about the origin of man in the Bible's book of Genesis is different from Darwin's theory of human evolution.

Morse (1992) sums up the nature of theories thus:

> theories are not fact. They are not the truth. They are tools. They are merely abstractions, conjectures, and organizations of reality, and as such, are malleable, changeable, and modifiable. There are historical examples of theory adopted as doctrine that with the benefit of hindsight look ridiculous and even silly to our sophisticated eyes. As a theory is changeable, anyone has the privilege of making modifications, for on the day that theory is believed and accepted as fact, science will cease to advance.

Defining a theory

There are a number of definitions of a theory. At its most basic, theory explains the occurrence of phenomena. To do this, it has to explain the relationship between variables or concepts. To borrow an example from the field of physics, 'an expansion in a bar of metal occurs when it is heated'. The phenomenon of expansion is therefore explained by the relationship between 'metal' (one variable) and heat (another variable). After a number of observations, it can be deduced that when heat is applied to a bar of metal it will cause the latter to expand.

In offering an explanation of why a phenomenon occurs, a theory must also predict that each time the variables happen to be in the same relationship, the same results will be obtained. In other words, the theory of metal expansion predicts that each time heat is applied to metal, the latter will expand. These explanatory and predictive functions of a theory are expressed in Kerlinger's (1986) definition:

> A theory is a set of interrelated constructs (concepts), definitions and propositions that present a systematic view of phenomena by specifying relations among variables, with the purpose of explaining and predicting the phenomena.

From these two definitions, it is clear that a theory is made up of a number of concepts which form not one but a set of interrelated propositions or hypotheses. Thus, from the above example, the theory of metal expansion comprises a number of propositions, mainly:

- Metals are made up of atoms.

- The structure of atoms is changed by heat.

- Heat causes atoms to expand.

In each of these propositions or hypotheses, there are a number of concepts (metals, atoms, heat and expansion). A concept is a word or phrase that summarises the essential characteristics or attributes of a phenomenon (Fawcett, 1999). The relationship between concepts, propositions and theory can be explained in a simplified way by stating that a theory is made up a set of propositions, and each proposition is made up of concepts. Without concepts, there are no theories; this is why concepts are referred to as the 'building blocks' of theories (Waltz et al., 1991). Therefore, the importance of operationalising concepts (see Chapter 9) for the development or testing of theories cannot be overemphasised.

Fawcett (1999) finds that definitions that emphasise that a theory must state relationships between variables are too restrictive, as they exclude descriptive themes. She defines theory as 'a set of relatively concrete and specific concepts and the propositions that describe or link those concepts'.

Types of theory

Moody (1990) identifies three types of theory: descriptive, explanatory and predictive. She refers to 'descriptive theories' as the most basic type of theory. According to her:

> They describe or classify specific dimensions or characteristics of individuals, groups, situations, or events by summarizing the commonalities found in discrete observations. They state 'what is'. Descriptive theories are needed when nothing or very little is known about the phenomenon in question.

While description and classification are important parts of the scientific process (as described in Chapter 2), they would not, according to positivists, constitute theories in themselves, because they do not seek to explain the causes of phenomena. On the other hand, qualitative researchers do not see theories in the social sciences as necessarily having explanatory and predictive functions. They believe in the uniqueness of individuals and situations, and while they seek to find commonalties between different and similar situations, some are concerned not with explaining why things happen but what actually happens, from the respondents' perspectives.

Explanatory theory is described by Moody (1990) as one which specifies:

> relations between dimensions or characteristics of individuals, groups, situations, or events. These theories explain how the phenomenon is related to

another. They can be developed only after the phenomenon has been explored and described, that is, only after descriptive theories have been developed or validated.

It is clear that explanatory theories are seen as a 'step up' from descriptive theories in the scientific process of theory development. Few researchers would be content to know only what happens; most would probably want to know why these things happen, without necessarily seeking to find general laws to explain human behaviour.

Predictive theories, according to Moody (1990):

> move beyond explanation to the prediction of precise relationships between dimensions or characteristics of a phenomenon or differences between groups. This type of theory addresses cause and effect, and 'why' changes occur in a phenomenon. Predictive theories may be developed after explanatory theories have been formulated.

This type of theory is normally developed in the natural sciences (where 'cause and effect', as for example between chemicals, is more easily established) and aspired to by positivists, in the social sciences. It is likely, however, that most research in the social sciences falls within the first two categories: descriptive and explanatory.

Levels of theory

Another way of describing and classifying theories is in terms of levels. Three levels – grand theory, middle-range theory and laws – will be described here.

Grand theory

These are broad and abstract ideas put together to give a vision of a phenomenon. Examples of 'grand theories' include Darwin's theory of evolution, Marx's theory of social structure and Freud's theory of human motivation. These theories are based on the synthesis of the theorist's own ideas and those obtained from other sources. They are examples of 'armchair' theorising, although, as in the case of Darwin and Freud, some experiments were carried out. Philosophers have for centuries formulated grand theories describing and explaining such phenomena as morality or human nature.

Grand theories tend to be all-encompassing of the phenomenon they describe. The Marxist theory of social structure comprises ideas, among others, about the relationship between those who produce (workers) and those who own the means of production (capitalists), the evolution and existence of social classes historically and cross-culturally, and ideology and its role in maintaining the *status quo*. Marx's theory is contained in many books and cannot be adequately described here. As can be seen, this type of theory comprises a multitude of other theories. Because they are broad conceptualisations, they have also been termed 'conceptual frameworks'.

Nursing theories tend to fall in the category of grand theories. Most of them offer broad conceptualisations of nursing. Fawcett (1999) describes nursing as having at least seven major conceptual models, including Johnson's Behavioural System Model, King's Interacting Systems Framework, Levine's Conservation Model, Neuman's Systems Model, Orem's Self Care Framework, Rogers' Science of Unitary Beings, and Roy's Adaptation Model. Walker and Avant (1988) believe that the grand theories of nursing 'have made an important contribution in conceptually sorting out nursing from the practice of medicine by demonstrating the presence of distinct nursing perspectives'.

Middle-range theories

Grand theories themselves cannot be empirically tested as they contain too many theories and propositions. Other researchers can take some of these propositions and develop smaller, more manageable theories with fewer concepts, and can be more specific about the relationship between them. These middle-range theories (Merton, 1967) fit the definition of scientific theories, as discussed in Kerlinger's definition given earlier. Layder (1993) explains that 'middle range theories describe the relations between empirically measurable variables . . . which can therefore be "tested" against empirically observed evidence'.

Examples of middle-range theories which are frequently used in nursing research include the Health Belief Model (Rosenstock, 1974) and the Theory of Planned Behaviour (Ajzen, 2001).

Laws

Laws are the definitive type of theory to which scientists in the natural sciences aspire. As George (1985) explains:

> In other fields, especially the biological sciences, there are laws as well as theories. Laws are truly predictable and can be utilised with assurance because they provide a sound body of knowledge in which to function. For example, in chemistry, if one correctly places a salt and an acid in the same vehicle, one can predict the results.

As explained earlier, the purpose of theory in the view of positivists is not only to explain, but also to predict and control phenomena. Since nursing deals with human beings in a social and cultural context, it is unlikely that laws, in the way described above, can be developed. Instead, middle-range theories, clearly defined and tested, comprehensive and of value to practitioners, remain the goal to be aspired to, at least for the near future.

Practice, research and theory

You may think at this point that all this is too 'theoretical' (i.e. abstract) or that theories are of interest and use only to academics. You may also wonder how theories in fact contribute to the accumulation of knowledge. Consider the following example. Suppose nurses in one hospital observe that patients rarely follow their advice on healthy eating. They may speculate or find out by reading the research literature that the following factors are associated with this type of behaviour: lack of motivation, lack of incentive and poor nutritional knowledge. Nurses in other hospitals, clinics or nursing homes may also have similar problems. They may find that this type of non-compliant behaviour is associated not only with lack of motivation, but also with the patients' age, social class or personality. Non-compliance with dietary advice is not restricted to one country or culture. Nurses in African or Asian hospitals may face similar problems. For them, a lack of nutritional knowledge, the influence of the family and local food customs may stand in the way of the implementation of a healthy diet.

Thus, casual observations, speculations and research findings together point to a multitude of factors that may be associated with non-compliance with dietary advice. These factors together constitute what can be called an accumulation of facts. A researcher may try to make sense of all these data by describing the non-compliant behaviour and by classifying these factors into, for example, individual factors (age, gender), psychological factors (motivation, incentive, personality), social factors (family influence, social class background, local customs) and economic factors (earnings, cost of food). Additionally, the researcher may compare this type of non-compliant behaviour with others, such as failure to act on advice on smoking, breast self-examination or the wearing of seat belts. The outcome of this process may be a descriptive theory describing and classifying non-compliant behaviours and the factors associated with them.

Researchers can also contribute by investigating more closely the relationship between some of these factors and non-compliant behaviour. Thus, not only has a large amount of knowledge been accumulated on non-compliant behaviours, but also attempts have been made to make sense of it. The researcher processes the mass of information available from various groups of people in different situations who experience the same phenomena. However, she may not be content with explaining specific situations but is rather more ambitious and may seek to explain non-compliant behaviours in general. By moving from the specific to the general, the researcher becomes the theorist.

Having identified the problem in the first place, nurses all over the world can thereafter benefit from such a theory to guide their practice. Many nursing practices, such as choosing an injection site, rehydrating a patient, giving information to patients prior to surgery and helping people to quit smoking, are based on physiological, sociological or psychological theories.

Theories are not always invented in ivory towers. It is true that they can be formulated through the process of speculation, but most theories are based on observations by people in various situations and settings. The relationship between practice and theory is symbiotic, in that each one feeds on the other to their mutual advantage. The practice setting presents problems, while observations and theories help to make sense of these. Practitioners can thereafter apply them to their practice and, in so doing, help to provide information that can be used to support, reject or modify them; and so the process continues. Moody (1990) explains the relationship between theory and practice:

> Theorizing is not reserved for academicians – good practitioners are often some of the best theorists in that their hunches provide the basis for developing propositions that can be empirically tested.

Billings (1995), referring to Klaus and Kennell's (1976) bonding theory, explained that it would appear to be that 'it has several fundamental shortcomings that potentially limit the usefulness of the practical application of the theory to nursing'. Billings (1995) went on to say:

> Evaluative research and debate following in the wake of bonding theory has highlighted the following points: (i) that the theory appears to be insufficiently validated in research terms; (ii) that its narrow view fails to explain attachment behaviour in situations other than the immediate post-delivery period; and (iii) that its practical application has been shown conversely to be of detriment to the mother–child relationship.

This is an example of how a theory has been used to inform nursing and midwifery practice and how, in return, nursing and midwifery practice have questioned the value of the theory.

Some theorists may try to draw general principles from observations of non-compliant behaviours in order to predict and prevent such behaviours in the future. Others may see theories only as showing a range of possible factors associated with this type of behaviour, thereby increasing their understanding of this particular problem. Theories, in this case, are expected to guide nurses' actions rather than to prescribe them.

One theory which has been used to study behavioural intention is the Theory of Planned Behaviour (Ajzen, 2001). According to this theory behaviour is determined by intention which in turn is determined by attitude, subjective norm and perceived control. Dodgson et al. (2003) used the Theory of Planned Behaviour (TPB) to study breastfeeding duration among mothers in Hong Kong. They found that the average duration of breastfeeding was short and that the TPB variables predicted duration of breastfeeding in first-time mothers in Hong Kong.

Theory and research

Research is the process by which evidence is provided in order to support, reject or modify theories and develop new ones. Thus research has theory-testing and theory-generating potential. Science needs research (the process) to achieve its outcome – the production of theories. As explained in Chapter 2, there are two main routes by which research can make this contribution: deduction and induction. Theory-testing research adopts the deductive approach, while theory-generating research uses the inductive one.

Theory-testing research

Theory-testing research is mainly in the positivist tradition and is characteristic of middle-range theories. Layder (1993) explains how theory is tested in research through the deductive process:

> a testable hypothesis or proposition is logically deduced from an existing set of assumptions. The empirical data that is then collected either confirms or disconfirms the original hypothesis or propositions.

Only hypotheses or propositions drawn from a theory, and not the theory itself, can be empirically tested through research. For example, Skinner's theory (Skinner, 1938) of positive reinforcement (which occurs when a pleasant consequence follows a particular response, strengthening that response and therefore making it more likely to happen), is stated in an abstract form and has to be translated into real-life situations for it to be tested. An example of a proposition or hypothesis that can be derived from nursing practice based on Skinner's theory (Skinner, 1938) is: 'there are fewer drop-outs among patients who are praised about their weight loss in the early sessions of a weight loss programme than among those who are not'. By collecting and analysing data to support or reject this hypothesis, a researcher is at the same time putting Skinner's theory to the test.

One proposition or hypothesis is hardly enough to test a theory. Many more from different situations would have to be drawn and tested. The Theory of Planned Behaviour, as mentioned above, is an example of a theory from which many hypotheses have been developed and tested, relating to such phenomena as 'exercise among blue collar workers' (Blue et al., 2001), 'health care workers' glove use' (Levin, 1999) and 'breastfeeding' (Dodgson et al., 2003).

Theory-generating research

Much credit for pioneering the theory-generating role of research in the social sciences is given to Glaser and Strauss (1967). They pointed out that theory generation had been hampered by an overemphasis on the testing of existing theories, which were often limited in explaining reality as they were based not on observation but on speculation.

Glaser and Strauss (1967) saw the generation of theories from observation as a preliminary stage before they can be tested by quantitative methods later, thus acknowledging the dual functions of research as theory generating and theory testing. They, however, put more emphasis on the role of research in generating theories since, according to them, the inductive process is capable of producing more relevant theories. Glaser and Strauss (1967) also agreed with positivists that the role of research 'is to enable explanation of behaviour, prediction and control'. This view is not shared by all qualitative researchers, many of whom believe that the aim of research is to describe how phenomena are perceived, rather than to explain, predict and control phenomena. Layder (1993) believes that there is a place, in qualitative research, for theory generation and for approaches that 'seek to develop theory' and 'employ systematic methods of study'. According to him, 'there is no reason for the two to be seen as competing approaches'.

Since it is believed that theories can be generated by the collection of data, many researchers feel the pressure to invent or discover a theory each time they carry out a qualitative study. Theories do not grow on trees. They are the result of much intellectual and physical labour and patience. What most small research projects can hope to achieve is to describe and clarify concepts. This in itself contributes to knowledge and practice and is a worthwhile enterprise that can thereafter be built upon.

Finally, as explained in Chapter 2, few theories are formulated without some prior observations, conscious or unconscious, systematic or informal, made by the theorists or derived from the observations of others. Similarly, theories derived from qualitative data could somehow be influenced by the researcher's knowledge (of existing theories among others) and experience, despite the conscious effort not to allow these to influence the research process. As Morse (1992) aptly puts it:

> Although most researchers agree that a conceptual framework should not be used in qualitative research and that prior knowledge of the topic should be 'bracketed', we would be fooling ourselves if we thought that qualitative enquiry was divorced from established knowledge.

Conceptual definition and conceptual framework

These terms are sometimes used interchangeably in clinical practice and nursing research. They provide a framework within which practice and research are sometimes conducted. The term 'theoretical framework' is perhaps more appropriate for research underpinned by one identified theory.

A conceptual framework draws on concepts from various theories and research findings to guide the study. The conceptual framework may or may not be stated. For example, in a study of the 'effects of dynamic exercise on subcutaneous oxygen tension and temperature', Whitney et al. (1995) do not mention the use of any particular theory, but make reference to physiological theories.

Conceptual models are the diagrammatic representation of concepts or theories, the purpose of which is to minimise the use of words. An example of a conceptual model is Braden's 'Self-help Model: Learned Response to Chronic Illness Experience' (Braden, 1990). Le Fort (2000) used this model to study adults with chronic pain.

Fawcett and Gigliotti (2001) emphasise that it is not sufficient to state that a study is guided by a particular conceptual model but that researchers should specify how the model or framework is integrated in all aspects of a study. They gave an example of how a conceptual model can be used to guide nursing research (Fawcett and Gigliotti, 2001).

Although a distinction has been made between these three terms (theoretical framework, conceptual framework and conceptual model), researchers do not always differentiate between them in practice. For the purpose of this chapter, 'theoretical framework' will be used interchangeably with 'conceptual framework' and 'conceptual model', in the sense that they are 'abstractions that may shape perception, reality, and inquiry' (Morse, 1992). Instead of engaging in the exercise of finding out whether researchers have used the correct terminology, our effort can be better spent in identifying if and how concepts and theories have been used to underpin these studies.

The importance of the relationship between theory and research is stressed by Moody (1990), who states that, 'progress in nursing science is best advanced when the researcher identifies the theoretical notions underpinning the research and attempts to formalise the link between theory and all phases of the research'.

In many research reports, there is no mention of theoretical frameworks, and in some cases where one is mentioned, there is little explanation of how it guides the study design and how the data relate back to the theory or theories discussed earlier in the article. Downs (1994), in an editorial in the journal *Nursing Research*, makes the following comments:

> research without theory really does little to advance knowledge . . . The study that lacks a theoretical rationale lacks substance and fails to answer the 'so what' question. The findings just sit there, begging to be hitched to something. They are wagons stalled for lack of a horse. Perhaps the saddest thing about atheoretical studies is that they describe events in isolation from a context that allows the results to be generalized.

Although some researchers may not consciously use a theoretical framework to guide their studies, the decisions they take are influenced by the beliefs they hold. These beliefs represent the world view of researchers. For example, in deciding to carry out qualitative interviews, the researcher holds the belief that it is important to listen to respondents rather than to ask them to place 'ticks' on a questionnaire to response categories framed by the researcher. It signifies the value that the researcher places on the rights of respondents to formulate their own responses. Morse (1992) states that the choice of phenomenology, ethnography or grounded theory approach is itself influenced by the theories of Husserl and others (phenomenology), cultural theories (ethnography) and symbolic interactionism (grounded theory).

Similarly, those who decide to use structured observation (see Chapter 15) as a method of data collection are making the statement that it is possible to obtain valuable data using the positivist approach. Some researchers do not specify how they come to select items for inclusion in a questionnaire. However, their choice reflects their beliefs that these items are more important than others. We are not neutral beings. Our beliefs and knowledge are made up of assumptions about the world.

Conceptual frameworks in quantitative research

Not all quantitative research is theory testing. Often the purpose is to find answers to particular localised problems. For example, a survey of newly qualified midwives' knowledge of breastfeeding can be carried out to identify gaps in their knowledge, with a view to improving midwifery education in their school. Or patients can be interviewed to discover their views about the care they receive in a particular hospital. In both cases, researchers may only be interested in finding answers to their specific research questions. However, the link with previous knowledge (which includes theories, research findings, expert opinions and descriptive accounts of practice) is important because researchers can learn from it and, in return, contribute to it. Without reference to existing knowledge, the study and its findings will exist in isolation from other similar work or studies. To increase and enhance our understanding of phenomena, we must build upon our present knowledge. One cannot, however, 'build upon' if one does not know what already exists. Volumes have been written on phenomena of interest to nurses, such as compliance, patient satisfaction, quality of life, social support, patient teaching, stress, bereavement, physical development, and so on. Some of these have more than one theory dedicated to them. By making use of the relevant ones in their studies, researchers can help to test them in practice.

You may have come across, while reading research articles, a sentence stating that 'a conceptual framework is used to underpin this study'. The *Oxford Dictionary* defines 'framework' as 'frame, structure, upon or into which casing or contents be put in' and 'underpin' as 'support from below with masonry . . . strengthen'. This reference to building and construction can equally apply to research. One can say that the function of a conceptual framework is to provide a structure that can strengthen the study. The nursing process is an example of a conceptual framework; it has four components (concepts): assessment, planning, implementation and evaluation. These components represent the structure to which nurses attach the contents (such as the information gathered in the process of assessing a patient). Thus, the nursing process can be used as a conceptual framework in a study of nursing care.

A conceptual framework for a research study can be derived from conceptual definitions, models or theories. For example, in a study on 'student nurses' views of health', the researcher can use the WHO (1946) definition of health as physical, mental and social well-being on which to underpin her study. These three components provide a guide to the researcher as to the areas of health on which to base her questions. She could have chosen Smith's (1981) 'progressive model of health which has four levels: clinical, role performance, adaptive and eudomonistic', on which Kenney based her study of 'the consumer's view of health' (Kenney, 1992). Our researcher could then base her questionnaire or interviews on each of these components. Alternatively, she could combine both definitions and provide her own conceptual framework.

The nursing research literature reveals a number of ways in which researchers make the link between previous knowledge and their own studies. These range from studies making no mention of a conceptual framework to those with a sound theoretical base. Below are some examples.

Russell (1996) carried out a small study on 'knowledge and practice of pressure area care' among a group of 30 qualified nurses. No mention is made of a conceptual framework. However, it is implicit rather than explicit that the author makes use of previous knowledge. For example, one of the 20 questions she asks the nurses in her study is, 'what are the stages of pressure sore development?' She assesses their answer against Torrance's classification of pressure sores (Torrance, 1983). In doing so, she is making a link with previous knowledge, although, in this case, Russell is not trying to test or build upon Torrance's classification, but only wants to find out whether or not nurses are aware of it. Similar other questions, such as those on 'capillary pressure' and 'factors which increase the risk of pressure sores', are based on existing knowledge. However, it is not clear how Russell derives her questions for her questionnaire.

This study does not test any propositions and does not have an identified conceptual framework. As the author states, the aim is, among other things, 'to identify nurses' needs for education in pressure sore prevention in relation to assessing, planning, implementing and evaluating care'. While the findings provide a valuable insight into the knowledge and practice of these nurses, they remain relevant mainly to them, although, as the author states, others 'may wish to implement' her recommendations.

Another study that has no identified conceptual framework but which draws on existing literature, especially research findings, is that of Woodward (1995) on 'psychosocial factors influencing teenage sexual activity, use of contraception and unplanned pregnancy'. According to the author, findings from the literature search into factors that influence teenage sexual behaviour and the use of contraceptives formed the basis of her study. The link with previous knowledge is made clear. For example, in her literature review, Woodward discusses previous work by Bury (1986), who stated:

> contraception may be more effectively and consistently used in established teenage relationships. This may be due to the increased communication about sex and contraception that exists in stable relationships as well as the anticipation of when sexual intercourse will occur.

Woodward (1995) included a question based on Bury's proposal in her questionnaire in order to find out whether it also applied to her sample. Her findings did not support this claim.

Although she does not mention a conceptual framework, Woodward bases her questions on research findings. She is in fact testing some of the ideas or proposals put forward by others. The findings of her study on 61 teenagers were used to support, reject or make suggestions on what was previously known about the subject. She has thus placed her study in the context of a wider discussion on psychosocial factors influencing teenage sexual activity. Woodward's conclusion makes this implicit:

> The findings of this study demonstrate that there is no simple model of teenage sexual or contraceptive behaviour which would assist in developing strategies to stem the continuing rise of unplanned pregnancy in the teenage years. Further studies to investigate the effects of family discord, unemployment and perception of future life prospects on use of contraception and unplanned pregnancy in their teenage years emerged as important areas for future research.

As the questionnaire is based on the existing literature, Woodward's study enters the general debate on the phenomenon she investigates. In contrast, the questionnaire of Russell (1996) is specific to her group of nurses and therefore focuses the discussion on her sample.

An example of a study based on a conceptual framework is that of Lutenbacher (2002) on relationships between 'psychosocial factors and abusive parenting attitudes in low-income single mothers'. The Transactional Model of Abuse (Cicchetti, 1989; 1994) served as the guiding framework for her study. As she explains:

> The multiple transactions among environmental factors, parent characteristics, and family characteristics are conceptualized as dynamic, reciprocal contributors to child maltreatment. This study examined material characteristics that contribute to potentially abusive parenting within the environmental context of low income female-headed households.

The factors on which data were collected and the tools selected for this study were based on the conceptual framework.

Conceptual frameworks in qualitative research

As explained earlier, qualitative research adopts the inductive approach. Therefore, conceptual frameworks have functions different from those in quantitative research. Researchers aim to develop their own concepts and theories from the data.

For example, Carter et al. (2004), in a study of the priorities of people living with a terminal illness, carried out qualitative interviews with ten participants. From the data, they identified 30 categories which were put in five interrelated themes, as shown in Figure 8.1. Other researchers can thereafter use them as a conceptual framework for their studies. Practitioners, too may find this framework useful for their practice.

It is also possible to derive questions or hypotheses from a conceptual framework using a quantitative approach and then collect data using qualitative methods such as unstructured interviews. This type of study would combine quantitative and qualitative approaches.

Another way in which a conceptual framework can be useful in qualitative research is when the researcher collects data qualitatively and tries to discover whether they support or reject existing theories. For example, Samarel (1992)

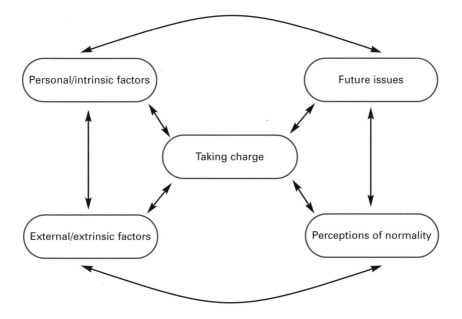

Figure 8.1 **Living with dying**

used a phenomenological approach to 'describe patients' experience of receiving therapeutic touch', and her 'findings were examined in the context of Martha Rogers' conceptual system' of unitary beings. The author states that 'no specific model or theory was used to guide the entire study'. Samarel (1992) concluded that 'the findings were not entirely consistent with Rogers' conceptual system'. Thus, the findings of qualitative studies can be discussed in the context of existing theories.

The function of the inductive process in qualitative research is summed up by Morse (1992), who states:

> the inductive process of qualitative methods provides a powerful means for us to develop and to modify theory, to examine the conceptual basis of our discipline as well as our own beliefs, and to (cautiously) move the discipline forward. Because in qualitative research theory is developed from data (rather than from the library) and is verified, it is usually quite solid. Sometimes, it is even surprising as new directions are identified and old concepts challenged.

Evaluating the use of conceptual frameworks in research

You can start this exercise by identifying the links that the researcher makes with previous knowledge. This may not be made explicit, as explained earlier. If previous knowledge is used, you can find out whether or not reference is made to conceptual definitions, theories, models, research findings or other material. In some cases, the researcher may refer to some or all of these in the same study. More important, however, is how researchers use previous knowledge to guide their study. It often happens that one or more theories or research findings are mentioned without any indication of how (if at all) they are integrated into the study. For example, there may be no indication of how the research questions were derived. In some cases, a theory is mentioned to embellish the study and raise its 'academic status' without any intention of integrating it into the study.

When research findings, conceptual definitions or theories are used to underpin a study, the researcher must justify her choice. There is sometimes more than one theory to explain the same phenomenon. For example, researchers have a choice between the health belief model and the theory of reasoned action to explain patient compliance with health advice. Similarly, if there is more than one conceptual definition of 'stress', why does the researcher choose one as opposed to another? The choice must be objective and appropriate.

To justify the claim that a conceptual framework underpins a particular study, the framework must, as explained earlier, guide every stage of the research process from the literature review to the analysis of data. You must therefore find out how the framework is reflected in the research questions or hypotheses and in the data collection and analysis methods.

The study must also 'feed back' to the conceptual framework on which it is based if it is to contribute to knowledge in general. You should look for discussions on how the current findings relate to the conceptual framework or other theories (even when these were not discussed earlier in the literature review). Unfortunately, this is not a frequent practice among researchers. As Downs (1994) notes, from her experience as the editor of the journal *Nursing Research*:

> Once a theoretical statement has been made, it is never referred to again. The discussion of the findings may go on at some length, but not even a tip of the hat is made to what presumably formed the basis for the work.

An example of a study in which the research findings are discussed in relation to the theoretical framework is by Kenney (1992) on 'the consumer's views of health'. The theoretical framework was based on the work of Smith (1981), Laffrey (1986) and Woods et al. (1988). In her discussion, Kenney shows how the findings supported some claims and questioned others. She concludes that the findings from her study 'provide some support for each of Smith's levels independently, but do not support the premise of an exclusive hierarchy model of health'.

To contribute fully to existing knowledge, nurse researchers must, on the basis of their findings, make clinical, methodological and theoretical recommendations.

SUMMARY

Summary and conclusion

In this chapter, we have explored the meaning, types, levels and functions of theories. The relationship between knowledge, theory, practice and research has been further examined. We have also looked at some examples of how researchers make use of previous knowledge, especially research findings and theories, to underpin their quantitative studies. Those adopting a qualitative approach often choose not to be influenced by existing knowledge but instead aim to generate their own concepts and theories. Nevertheless, they can still discuss their findings in the context of existing theories and research findings.

Not all research studies have an identified conceptual framework, and not all researchers believe they need one. To contribute to the pool of knowledge researchers must not only make use of what is already known, but also test it in practice. This deductive process, however, must not be at the expense of the efforts of others who seek to increase our understanding of phenomena by searching for new and fresh perspectives.

References

Ajzen I (2001) Perceived behavioural control, self-efficacy, locus of control and the Theory of Planned Behavior. *Journal of Applied Social Psychology*, **321**:665–83.

Billings J R (1995) Bonding theory – tying mothers in knots? A critical review of the application of a theory to nursing. *Journal of Clinical Nursing*, **4**:207–11.

Blue C L, Wilbur J and Marston-Scott M (2001) Exercise among blue collar workers: application of the theory of planned behaviour. *Research in Nursing and Health*, 24, 6:481–93.

Braden C J (1990) A test of the self-help model: learned response to chronic illness. *Nursing Research*, **39**:42–7.

Bury J (1986) Teenage and contraception. *British Journal of Family Planning*, **12**:11–14.

Carter H, MacLeod R, Brander P and McPherson K (2004) Living with a terminal illness: patients' priorities. *Journal of Advanced Nursing*, **45**, 6:611–20.

Cicchetti D (1989) How research on child maltreatment has informed the study of child development: perspectives from development psychopathology. In: D Cicchetti and V Carlson (eds), *Child Maltreatment: Theory and Research on the Causes and Consequences of Child Abuse and Neglect*, pp. 377–431 (New York: Cambridge University Press).

Cicchetti D (1994) Advances and challenges in the study of the sequelae of child maltreatment. *Development Psychopathology*, **6**:1–3.

Dodgson J E, Henly S J, Duckett L and Tarrant M (2003) Theory of planned behaviour-based models for breastfeeding duration among Hong Kong mothers. *Nursing Research*, **52**, 3:148–58.

Downs F S (1994) Hitching the research wagon to theory. *Nursing Research*, **43**, 4:195.

Fawcett J (1999) *The Relationship of Theory and Research*, 3rd edn (Philadelphia, PA: F A Davis).

Fawcett J and Gigliotti E (2001) Using conceptual models of nursing to guide nursing research: the case of the Neuman Systems Model. *Nursing Science Quarterly*, **14**, 4:339–45.

George J B (1985) *Nursing Theories – The Base for Professional Nursing Practice* (Englewood Cliffs, NJ: Prentice Hall).

Glaser B and Strauss A (1967) *The Discovery of Grounded Theory* (Chicago, IL: Aldine).

Homans G C (1967) *The Nature of Social Science* (New York: Harcourt and Brace).

Kenney J W (1992) The consumer's views of health. *Journal of Advanced Nursing*, **17**:829–34.

Kerlinger F N (1986) *Foundations of Behavioral Research*, 3rd edn (New York: Holt, Rinehart & Winston).

Klaus M H and Kennell J H (1976) *Maternal Infant Bonding* (St Louis, MO: C V Mosby).

Laffrey S C (1986) Development of a health conception scale. *Research in Nursing and Health*, 9, 2:107–11.

Layder D (1993) *New Strategies in Social Research* (Cambridge: Polity Press).

Le Fort S M (2000) A test of Braden's self-help model in adults with chronic pain. *Journal of Nursing Scholarship*, 32, 2:153:60.

Levin P F (1999) Test of the Fishbern and Ajzen models as predictors of health care workers' glove use. *Research in Nursing and Health*, 22, 4:295–307.

Lutenbacher M (2002) Relationships between psychosocial factors and abusive parenting attitudes in low-income single mothers. *Nursing Research*, 51, 3:158–67.

Merton R (1967) *On Theoretical Sociology* (New York: Free Press).

Moody L E (1990) *Advancing Nursing Science through Research* (Newbury Park, CA: Sage).

Morse J (1992) Editorial: The power of induction. *Qualitative Health Research*, **2**, 1:3–6.

Rosenstock I M (1974) The Health Belief Model and preventive health behavior. *Health Education Monographs*, **2**:354–86.

Russell L (1996) Knowledge and practice in pressure area care. *Professional Nurse*, **11**, 5:301–6.

Samarel N (1992) The experience of receiving therapeutic touch. *Journal of Advanced Nursing*, 17:651–7.

Skinner B F (1938) *The Behavior of Organisms* (New York: Appleton-Century-Crofts).

Smith J A (1981) The idea of health: a philosophical enquiry. *Advances in Nursing Science*, **3**, 3:43–50.

Torrance C (1983) *Pressure Sores: Aetiology, Treatment and Prevention* (Beckenham: Croom Helm).

Walker L O and Avant K C (1988) *Strategies for Theory Construction in Nursing* (East Norwalk, CT: Appleton & Lange).

Waltz C F, Strickland O L and Lenz E R (1991) *Measurement in Nursing Research*, 2nd edn (Philadelphia, PA: F A Davis).

Whitney J D, Stotts N A and Goodson W H III (1995) Effects of dynamic exercise on subcutaneous oxygen tension and temperature. *Research in Nursing and Health*, **18**:97–104.

WHO (World Health Organization) (1946) *Constitution* (Geneva: WHO).

Woods N F, Laffrey S, Duffy M, Lentz M J, Mitchell E S, Taylor D and Cowan K A (1988) Being healthy: women's images. *Advances in Nursing Science*, **11**, 1:36–46.

Woodward V M (1995) Psychosocial factors influencing teenage sexual activity, use of contraception and unplanned pregnancy. *Midwifery*, **11**:210–16.

9

Research Questions and Operational Definitions

OPENING THOUGHT

Questions are at the heart of all research and the nature and quality of the evidence depends largely on how the question is asked. Information may be the starting point but understanding must be the goal.

S. Lydeard

Introduction

The formulation of research questions is fundamental to the research process. It helps the researcher to clarify in her mind those questions which need to be answered. These can be formulated in a variety of formats, which often reflect the type of research carried out and the personal preference of individual researchers. Additionally, the terms and concepts used by the researcher must be defined in ways that can be understood by others who read the article or report. This chapter will help you to understand this important stage of the research process.

Formulating research questions

Research starts with a problem, which is often broad and multi-faceted. For example, if there is an increase in the incidence of pressure sores on a particular ward, the nurse researcher faced with this problem may ask several questions, such as:

- Is there a relationship between nursing care and the incidence of pressure sores?

- Is there a policy on the prevention and treatment of pressure sores?

- Is this policy effective?

- How does the current prevention practice compare with a new form of practice on another ward with a similar group of patients?

- Do nurses have the necessary knowledge and skills to prevent and treat pressure sores?

It is not possible, especially in a small project, to address all these issues. The researcher may have to settle for one or two of these questions and focus on them. The literature review can play an important part in narrowing the problem down to manageable proportions. By reviewing what has been written on the topic and how others have approached similar studies, the researcher is better informed about what needs to be done. The final choice of which aspect of the problem to focus upon depends on a number of factors, including the researcher's skills and interest, the lack of research on the topic and available resources.

The next step in quantitative research is for the researcher to state clearly what the purpose of the study is.

Aim or purpose of the study

The aim or purpose of the study is formulated so that researchers and readers are clear about what is being researched. Although the aim of most research is ultimately to improve practice, the aim of a study, in research terms, relates to the particular question(s) for which data can be collected. For example, the aim of the above study could be 'to find out if there is a relationship between nursing care and the incidence of pressure sores' on a particular ward. The long-term goal of a study may be to improve a particular practice, but the latter depends on more than research findings. Only in action research (see Chapter 10) do researchers aim to answer research questions and make changes (such as improving practice) at the same time. More often than not, the purpose of a study is stated earlier on in the article, but when this does not happen readers sometimes have to look for it. The 'aim' is itself broad and needs further explanation of how it is to be achieved. It should be further subdivided into specific questions, objectives or hypotheses.

Research questions

Research is about finding answers, and in order to do so questions must be posed. The purpose or aim of a study is usually formulated as a statement that begs many questions. For example, in the study, 'Nurses' autonomy: influence of nurse managers' actions' (Mrayyan, 2004), the aim was to 'examine the roles of nurse managers in enhancing hospital staff nurses' autonomy'. The aim was further broken down into the following research questions:

1. What aspects of autonomy do nurses perceive that they have in patient care and operational decisions about their units?

2. What are the actions of nurse managers that enhance staff nurses' autonomy?

3. What is the relationship between the perceived actions of nurse managers and nurse autonomy?

4. What are the three most important factors that hospital staff nurses perceive to encourage their work autonomy?

5. What are the three most important factors that hospital staff nurses perceive to hinder their autonomy?

As you can see, the aim only broadly hints at the topic to be studied. The research questions elaborate on the exact questions she wishes to answer.

By asking specific questions, the researcher has given more details about what the purpose of the study is. However, the above questions are not exactly or necessarily the questions that nurses in the study will be asked. These questions only provide a basis or framework from which further and final questions can be formulated in order to construct the tool of data collection, for example, a questionnaire. The broad research questions that emerge out of the purpose of the study must not be confused with detailed questions that the respondents are asked to answer.

Formulating the purpose or aim of a study in the form of questions is useful in helping to clarify exactly what the study is about and sets the parameters of the research project. It focuses the researcher's and the reader's mind on the task in hand.

Research objectives

Another way of detailing the purpose or aim of a study is in the form of objectives. Like research questions, objectives are set by the researcher in order to explain in some detail what the study is expected to achieve. In a study by Chan and Yu (2004) the overall aim 'was to investigate the quality of life (QoL) of clients with schizophrenia who resided in the community'. The following objectives were set:

● to provide a profile of QoL in clients with schizophrenia;

● to examine relationships between QoL and sociodemographic factors, such as gender, age, marital status, employment status and level of education; and

● to examine relationships between QoL and clinical factors such as mental status, number of hospitalisations and duration of illness.

They still had to ask specific questions in order to meet these objectives.

Hypotheses

Instead of asking questions or setting objectives, some researchers may go further in proposing what the answer to their main research question might be and then set out to look for evidence to support or reject their 'hunch'. In everyday life, people make educated guesses as to why certain things or events happen. For example, the increase in crimes by children is often blamed on violent behaviour in television programmes. Nurses hypothesise about the phenomena they deal with. For example, they may attribute the high incidence of pressure sores in obese patients to their weight, or blame constipation in older people on their lack of exercise. Some of these guesses may be influenced by their beliefs and experiences, and what they have read or heard.

Researchers, too, make educated guesses about the phenomena they investigate. However, unlike other people, they have to collect data in order to support or reject them. By proposing that there may be a relationship between pressure sores and obesity, the researcher is putting forward a hypothesis. By its very nature, a hypothesis is a tentative statement since the researcher is merely making an assumption before data are collected. A hypothesis can be defined as a tentative statement, in one sentence, about the relationship, if any, between two or more variables. A variable is anything that varies or can be varied. An example of a hypothesis is 'lack of exercise causes constipation in older people'. To be complete and comprehensive, a hypothesis must include three components: the variables, the population and the relationship between variables.

Variables

In the above example, 'exercise' and 'constipation' are the two variables for which a relationship is stated. In this case, it is a causal relationship because one (exercise) is assumed to cause the other (constipation). The variable 'exercise' can be varied (changed): older people can take more or less exercise. The other variable, 'constipation', may vary according to the presence or absence of exercise. The variable causing the change is referred to as the independent variable, and the one which is changed is known as the dependent variable. One way to remember which is which is to view the dependent variable as the one that depends on the other to be changed. These and other types of variables are further discussed in Chapter 11.

The population

For a hypothesis to be complete, the population to which the phenomenon is related must be stated. For example, in the above hypothesis, the population is older people. Later on more information or a definition of older people (i.e. the age group, the clinical area in which they are cared for or their gender) will be required to enable readers to identify the population to whom the hypothesis applies.

Relationship between variables

A hypothesis is a statement that normally specifies the relationship between variables. This relationship can be positive, inverse or of difference. Here are some examples:

- *Positive* – the more food people consume the more obese they become.

- *Inverse* or *negative* – the more information given to patients pre-operatively, the less anxiety they experience post-operatively.

- *Difference* – patients who exercise during the day sleep longer at night than those who do not.

Hypotheses are not only about cause and effect. Sometimes they point out that there is a relationship between two or more variables without any explanation of the exact nature of this relationship. This type of hypothesis is known as 'associative'. An example of an associative hypothesis is, 'there is a relationship between the amount of daily protein consumed and success in examinations'.

Evidence to support or reject hypotheses can be obtained through the collection of data and by statistical analysis. Hypotheses for research purposes are stipulated in two main formats: the null hypothesis (H_0) and the alternative hypothesis (H_1). An example of a null hypothesis is that there is no relationship between portion of meals and obesity. When a null hypothesis is not supported by research evidence, it gives rise to an alternative hypothesis. In this case, if the null hypothesis is rejected, then the alternative hypothesis is, 'there is a relationship between food portion and obesity'. Normally the null hypothesis is the one used because it is a simpler one than one which specifies that there is a relationship.

When a null hypothesis is tested, the results are expressed in terms of whether it is supported or rejected. However, it does not follow that because the null hypothesis is rejected, the alternative hypothesis is accepted. It merely shows that there is not enough evidence to support the null hypothesis. The new, alternative hypothesis has itself to be put to the test in further studies.

Hypotheses can also stipulate the relationships between more than two variables. These complex hypotheses are stated because, in real life, a number of factors or variables work together in order to produce an effect. Although it is common knowledge that high-fibre diets can prevent constipation, other factors such as mobility and fluid intake can also be implicated. By controlling mobility and fluid intake in an experiment focusing solely on fibre, the researcher creates an artificial situation. To make the experiment more like real life, the researcher may decide to study a number of variables at the same time. A hypothesis for this study may read as follows: 'Lack of dietary fibre and low fluid intake cause constipation among older people'. The independent variables are dietary fibre and fluid intake, and the dependent variable is constipation. See Research Example 13 for a study testing a hypothesis.

An oral care protocol intervention to prevent chemotherapy-induced oral mucositis in paediatric cancer patients: a pilot study   *Cheng et al. (2002)*

The purpose of the study was:

> to evaluate the use of a preventive oral care protocol during chemotherapy, in attempting to reduce the incidence and severity of chemotherapy-induced oral mucositis specifically in children with malignant disease.

The hypothesis was:

> a preventative care protocol systematically applied to paediatric cancer patients during chemotherapy would reduce the occurrence of oral ulcerative lesions, and alleviate the severity of oral mucositis and oral mucositis-related pain.

Comments:

1   A hypothesis should have three components: variables, a population and the relationship between the variables. The independent variable is: a preventative oral care protocol. The dependent variables are: occurrence of oral ulcerative lesions, the severity of oral mucositis and oral mucositis-related pain.

   The relationship between variables: the protocol (intervention) will affect the dependent variables. The population: children with cancer undergoing chemotherapy.

Finally, a hypothesis is either supported or rejected but not 'proven', because there may be many reasons or factors other than the independent variable that account for the results (see Chapter 11). Research findings must always be treated with caution.

In formulating questions, objectives or hypotheses, a number of terms or concepts are used. The next step in the research process is for these concepts to be defined so that readers (fellow researchers, practitioners and others) may be aware of the precise meaning of these terms and so that they can assess the validity and reliability of these definitions.

Ambiguities arise in the use of concepts used in everyday language. Such familiar terms as 'happiness', 'love', 'coping' or 'human rights' give rise to a multitude of definitions. A common and agreed understanding of these and other terms that we use can greatly enhance communication.

Operational definitions

If someone is asked if she is happy, the answer quite often is: 'It depends what you mean by happiness.' Such terms as 'happy' and 'happiness' are used daily in our lives and we are supposed to have a common understanding of what they mean. Yet when it comes to conveying their meanings to others, it is quite difficult. In nursing practice, too, we use a vast number of terms and concepts (e.g. 'pressure sore', 'fatigue', 'coping' and 'pain'). Professionals have to develop a common understanding of these terms to facilitate communication between themselves and with their clients. The definition of terms and concepts which nurses and other health professionals use is central to their practice. Without a consensus of what they mean, and in particular how they can be observed, nursing practice would be 'chaotic'. For example, a term like 'depression' may mean different things to different people. However, if nurses, as a professional group, are involved in assessing and treating this condition, they need to have a consensus of what it means and how it can be assessed. Thus whole books are dedicated to exploring, assessing, measuring and treating depression. Nonetheless our knowledge of some of the concepts used in everyday nursing practice still lacks clarification, let alone definition. Referring to the concept of 'fatigue', Trendall (2000) remarks that while it is a universally experienced concept, no universal definition was evident in the literature although 'we assume that we have shared understanding of something so common'. Tutton and Seers (2003) explain that there are many (historical) interpretations of the concept of 'comfort' and that there is a lack of clarity around the use of the term.

Researchers, too, have to be clear about the terms they use and the context in which they use them. In a study of the effects of therapeutic touch by nurses on depression, the researcher will need to define such terms or concepts as 'therapeutic touch', 'nurses', 'depression' and 'effects' (e.g. the outcomes to be measured).

If you think of research as an 'operation' or 'procedure', then an operational definition in a research study is the way the terms and concepts are defined for the purpose of the study. Although there is universal understanding of what the term 'nurse' is, the way in which 'nurse' is defined in a particular study depends on the context of the study. Researchers may define 'nurse' (for the purpose of the study) as only those qualified in the last five years or those working in hospitals or in particular clinical areas. Without this definition it is not possible for readers to know whom the researcher is referring to. This information is crucial for deciding if the study is rigorous enough and to whom the findings are generalisable. The more precise and adequate the description and definition of the nurses in the sample the easier it is for readers to know the exact population from whom data are collected. Researchers, therefore, set inclusion and exclusion criteria in order to define their samples. For example, in a study by Manias et al. (2004) on patients' perspectives of self-administration of medication in hospital, the eligible participants were defined as:

over 18 years of age; able to read, write and understand English; managing their own medications when not hospitalised and taking multiple medications on a regular and ongoing basis. In addition, they had been admitted to hospital at least twice for a medical illness in the past 2 years. People deemed by nursing staff to be too ill to participate, or not competent to provide informed consent, or not likely to be discharged to their preadmission were excluded.

Samples are relatively easy to define compared to other phenomena such as 'pressure sores' or 'drowsiness'. Researchers carrying out a study of the prevalence of pressure sores in a number of hospitals must ensure that the definition of the term 'pressure sore' is clear to everyone taking part in the study (i.e. those carrying out the observations) and those appraising the study. In a survey of pressure sore prevalence in hospitals in Iceland, Thoroddsen (1999) used the National Pressure Ulcer Advisory Panel's [NPUAP] (1989) definition of pressure sore as representing 'a continuum from an erythematous soft tissue lesion to an open wound extending into the deep tissues'. One can only imagine the difficulties which nurses might experience in trying to interpret this definition for the purpose of observing and measuring pressure sores in their hospitals. Therefore Thoroddsen (1999) adopted the following classification of pressure sores offered by Langemo et al. (1990) and Shea (1975) in order to facilitate observation:

Grade	Classification
I	Reddened area lasting more than 30 min after a change in position (no break in skin integrity).
II	Blister, break in skin.
III	Skin break with tissue exposing subcutaneous tissue. May be a deep crater with or without undermining.
IV	Skin break with tissue exposing muscle and bone with profuse drainage and necrosis. More extensively undermined.

Thoroddsen (1999) explained that the above operational definition is more simply worded than the NPUAP definition and would be more comprehensible and useful to nurses 'who may not be used to reading theoretical terms in a text'. However, there are still terms, such as 'reddened area', which could lead to different interpretations. Training and practice can enhance the reliability of pressure sore observations.

Other phenomena which nurses deal with, such as 'coping', 'comfort' or 'fatigue' are even more difficult to define operationally in research studies, mainly because they are not directly observable. Often dictionary definitions are of little use. One needs, as much as possible, to fully understand a phenomenon before it can be measured. For example, if a researcher wants to measure chronic fatigue, she needs to understand the concept in all its different manifestations, what gives rise to it, its main attributes or characteristics, how it differs from similar concepts (such as depression) or if it is a process, an outcome or both. This type of exploration is known as conceptual analysis, the outcome of which is a conceptual definition. Conceptual analyses are carried out mainly for the purpose of clarifying concepts which practitioners use in their practice. They are useful for researchers who can use them for defining concepts and as conceptual frameworks in their studies.

To fully explore, analyse and describe a concept a number of sources and methods are used. Those doing concept analysis draw mainly upon the literature, the experience of practitioners, case studies and research. The conceptual definitions which emerge as a result of this type of analysis contribute towards a fuller understanding of concepts. Such definitions can never fully capture the meaning of concepts. Trendall (2000), who carried out a concept analysis of 'chronic fatigue', concluded that while the exercise assisted with the understanding of the concept and future research, the complexity of chronic fatigue was still evident.

Although conceptual definitions shed more light on the use and meaning of concepts, they are not operational definitions as they do not specify what must be done in order to measure or assess them. Wang (2004), after completing a conceptual analysis of functional status, defined it as:

> activities performed by an individual to realize needs of daily living in many aspects of life including physical, psychological, social, spiritual, intellectual, and roles. Level of performance is expected to correspond to normal expectation in the individual's nature, structure and conditions.

If a researcher wants to measure functional status using this conceptual definition she has to operationalise it for use with specific populations and with specific conditions. Fortunately for researchers, tools have been developed to measure these concepts. For example, functional ability of children and young people with myalgic encephalopathy can be measured by the Moss Scale (Moss, 2005).

To summarise, operational definitions are important in order to convey to readers the meaning researchers give to the terms or concepts used in a study.

Evaluating operational definitions

There are a number of criteria that can be used to evaluate the efficacy of operational definitions. The main ones (adapted from a list from Waltz et al., 1991) include clarity, precision, validity, reliability and agreement/consensus.

Clarity

If the operational definition is not clear, it cannot be put into practice. The process of operational definition is precisely to reduce a complex or abstract concept into simple instructions that can be understood in the same way by everyone. Hall and Lanig (1993) gave the following definitions of spiritual care, spiritual activities, integration and comfort in their study of 'spiritual caring behaviours as reported by Christian nurses'. As they explained:

> The investigators defined spiritual care as those activities the nurse might use to meet perceived spiritual needs. The behaviors of talking about spiritual concerns, praying, and reading Scripture were selected as the most common spiritual activities that a nurse might use with a person to demonstrate care. Integration was defined as the harmonizing and inclusion of personal spiritual values into regular nursing activities. Comfort was defined as the degree of ease, readiness, and/or spontaneity the nurse experienced during these times.

While most of this is fairly clear, new concepts such as 'harmonising', 'spiritual values' and 'degree of spontaneity' are themselves abstract.

Precision

Operational definitions must be as precise as possible, so that a degree of consistency is achieved when put into practice. For example, H S Wilson (1989), in a study of 'family caregiving for a relative with Alzheimer's dementia: coping with negative choices', defined a 'family caregiver' as:

> a member of the patient's informal support system (family/friend) who: (a) carried primary responsibility for providing a range of care to the patient at home, (b) was identified by a referral source as having ongoing responsibility for the patient's care, (c) was not financially reimbursed for caregiving activities, and (d) had been a caregiver for a minimum of 6 weeks not more than 3 months prior to the interview.

This can be compared with the definition of 'chief carer' in a study by Brocklehurst et al. (1981) on 'social effects of stroke', which reads as follows:

> the person most totally involved in looking after the patient (if the patient was at home) or who seemed to be the person most likely to be involved in home care should the patient leave hospital in future.

The second definition may still serve the purpose of the study. However, by being precise and as detailed as possible, operational definitions offer readers a chance to compare whether the population in the study is similar to their own client groups, thereby increasing the applicability of the findings to their own settings.

Validity

To be valid, the operational definition must represent what it is supposed to represent. There is the danger in translating a broad conceptual definition into a number of constituent parts that it may not represent the concept being defined. One can ask whether, in fact, when a researcher sets out to measure a particular concept, she actually measures that concept or something else. As J Wilson (1989) explains:

> there is a logical gap between the concept with which the researcher begins and the subsequent research. To take an absurd (but, believe it or not, real life) example, researchers interested in what makes happy marriages decided to assess a marriage as happy if the partners called each other 'darling' more than a certain number of times a day. As many married couples know, one can say 'darling!' *con amore*, or through clenched teeth: as a candidate for a reasonable way of verifying, or explicating the concept 'happily married', this is a non-starter.

One of the common ways of operationalising such conditions as schizophrenia or depression is to rely on medical diagnosis. Although it saves the researcher the effort of providing her own definitions, using medical diagnoses as operational definitions is not without problems. If, in a study measuring the 'level of social support available to Chronic Fatigue Syndrome (CFS) sufferers, the latter are defined as persons diagnosed by their general practitioners as having CFS', it is possible that some general practitioners may overdiagnose, underdiagnose or misdiagnose CFS. Some people with CFS may not even have consulted a general practitioner, anyway. Therefore, in some instances, the validity of using medical diagnoses as operational definitions is questionable.

Another aspect of the validity of an operational definition is its appropriateness for the specific population for whom it is formulated. Concepts may have different meanings for different groups due to class, cultural, geographical, gender, age and social differences. Such a concept as 'touch' or 'bereavement' can be manifested and interpreted differently in different cultures or even according to gender. Grant and Kinney (1991) explain that:

> although it may be appropriate to assess tiredness in adults who have a sleep pattern disturbance by asking whether they feel tired, weary, or fatigued, it would not be appropriate to use this method with infants or very small children. However, tiredness potentially could be measured in a population of 2–4-year-olds by focusing on behaviours such as rubbing or closing eyes frequently, irritability, crying, or holding a favourite object such as a blanket or teddy bear.

Reliability

The question to ask about the reliability of an operational definition is whether it will be consistently interpreted (in the same way) by all those who have to use it. Sometimes two or more researchers carry out observations in the same study; they must be able to interpret operational definitions in the same way. In the above example of a study on pressure sores, Dealey (1991) defined a grade 1 pressure sore as 'redness which does not fade and blanches under light pressure'. There are a number of concepts, such as 'redness', 'fading', 'blanching' and 'light pressure', which can be interpreted differently by different nurses. Training and monitoring those who have to carry out observations can increase inter-rater reliability (i.e. agreement between all those who make the observations and recordings). However, this is not always done. Dealey (1991) comments that a weakness in the methodology of her surveys was that 'there was no system for checking the accuracy of the information collected' and that 'previous studies had shown that there could be difficulty in recognizing grade 1 sores'. Misinterpretation of definitions could lead to the under- or overreporting of grade 1 sores, thereby giving inaccurate results on which subsequent decisions on nursing practice might depend.

It is not possible to offer absolutely perfect operational definitions, nor is it possible to offer further definitions of each of the terms that operational definitions generate. The problem with definitions is explained below by Bertrand Russell (1918):

> It is rather a curious fact in philosophy that the data which are undeniable to start with are always rather vague and ambiguous. You can, for instance, say: 'There are a number of people in this room at this moment'. This is obviously in some sense undeniable. But when you come to try and define what this room is, and what it is for a person to be in a room, and how you are going to distinguish one person from another, and so forth, you find that what you have said is most fearfully vague and that you really do not know what you meant.

Agreement/consensus

For some terms such as 'students' or 'patients', researchers can offer their own definitions to suit their studies. No consensus or agreement is necessary for the term, provided that the researcher makes it very clear how the population is defined and that the definition is not absurd. On the other hand, there are concepts such as 'anxiety' or 'stress' for which there must be a consensus for their definitions, otherwise the validity of the findings will be seriously in question. To achieve consensus, operational definitions must reflect the concept in all its complexities and must be informed by the current state of knowledge on the concept. To gain consensus, researchers may provide a rationale for their definitions.

In some cases, researchers use operational definitions from previous studies. This allows for comparisons of the findings to be made and may lead to further refinement of the definition. The drawback of this is that sometimes no fresh contribution towards defining concepts is offered.

Operationalising concepts that figure in research questions, objectives or hypotheses is an important but often difficult part of the research process in quantitative research.

Research questions in qualitative research

Different approaches within qualitative research mean that one cannot generalise about them. Purists, however, would see qualitative research as inductive rather than deductive. As the deductive approach involves the testing of hypotheses and theories, these have to be formulated and the variables they contain must be operationally defined. With the inductive approach, hypotheses and theories are expected to emerge out of the data. In phenomenological research, the researcher collects data from the respondent's perspective, and formulating questions or hypotheses at the start of the study is therefore not appropriate. However, in order to focus the study, some broad aims and even objectives are sometimes formulated. For example, in a qualitative study exploring 'the communication that takes place between nurses and patients whilst cancer chemotherapy is administered' (Dennison, 1995), the following objectives were set:

- to describe the content of the communication that took place between the nurses and the patients using meaningful categories;

- to describe the process of communication;

- to identify the environmental factors that may have influenced the conversations; and

- to identify those characteristics of the participants which may have influenced the conversations.

In a study of mature women's experiences of preregistration nurse education (Kevern and Webb, 2004) the following research questions were set:

- What are the experiences of mature women in preregistration nurse education?

- Could their needs be more appropriately addressed?

Although aims and objectives can be set, qualitative researchers tend to use these as broad areas on which to focus.

In some qualitative studies, however, broad questions are not set in advance, although researchers choose a starting point to focus on certain aspects of a phenomenon. During fieldwork (when researchers are out there collecting data), they may be more attracted to some aspects than others. In a study by Millman (1976) of the 'backrooms of American medicine', the broad area of study was 'features of the everyday world of the hospital that adversely affect the quality of patient care'. As she explains:

> At first, my research interests were quite general. I soon found, however, that my attentions were drawn toward two intriguing issues. One was the variety of ways that doctors define, perceive and respond to medical mistakes – both their own mistakes and those made by hospital colleagues . . . The second major issue I came to focus on is the competing interests and conflicts among various groups of doctors within the hospital.

Millman (1976) carried out this ethnographic study of 'doctors and staff at work in a private, university-affiliated hospital'.

The ethnographic approach, which uses participant observation as its main data collection method (see Chapter 15), provides the opportunity for starting with a broad topic and thereafter focusing on particular aspect(s). In phenomenological studies, which use the unstructured interview method (see Chapter 14), it is also possible for researchers to select broad topic areas that they want to cover, but they may find their attention drawn to certain specific issues. Although the purpose of the study or broad questions are reported at the start of qualitative research articles, one cannot be certain that they were in fact the original aspects on which the researchers set out to focus.

In quantitative research, the measurement of concepts, whether in surveys or experiments, is central to the research process, and therefore these concepts require precise operational definitions. In qualitative research, the respondents' conceptualisation of the phenomenon is often the outcome of the study. Therefore, according to purists, operational definitions have no place in qualitative research. In fact, the researcher's conceptualisation of the problem is 'bracketed' to prevent it from influencing respondents. However, it is possible to find qualitative studies in which concepts are operationally defined. In a study on 'the process and consequences of institutionalising an elder', Dellasega and Mastrian (1995) offer these operational definitions of the following concepts: 'specific stressors', 'family members' and 'decision making/placement'. As they explain:

> In this study, specific stressors were defined as emotionally difficult events and feelings that were described by subjects in connection with the decision-making process, the placement process, or both. Family members were a spouse, a sibling, or a child of an elderly nursing home resident who was intimately involved in the decision-making or placement process and who

consented to be interviewed. Decision making/placement was defined as considering alternatives and making choices that led to admission of an elder to a skilled nursing facility.

These definitions are broad and serve to explain the areas on which the researchers focused. They are not operational definitions in the 'quantitative' sense as they do not specify how these concepts are to be precisely measured; they merely delineate the areas of study. They are sometimes called 'inclusion' or 'exclusion' criteria. They specify who/what to include or exclude from the study.

In quantitative research, all questions must be decided in advance. This assumes that researchers know what questions to ask or the attributes of the phenomenon to be observed. However, it is possible that by just talking to or observing respondents, we come across new ways of thinking on certain topics. The view often taken by qualitative researchers is that not only do we not know the answers, but also we do not know what questions to ask.

Qualitative researchers work with the assumption that operational definitions fail to capture the essence of what is studied. For example, such a concept as 'intelligence' is reduced to being measured by a set of responses to a questionnaire called an intelligent quotient test. By defining the attributes or symptoms, we can miss the essence of the phenomena we seek to study.

The dilemma of operational definitions is aptly expressed by Bertrand Russell (1918):

> Everything is vague to a degree you do not realise till you have tried to make it precise, and everything precise is so remote from everything that we normally think, that you cannot for a moment suppose that is what we really mean when we say what we think.

Critiquing research questions and operational definitions

It is important to identify the purpose of the study, the research questions, objectives or hypotheses. Sometimes these are not reported under their respective headings; more often, readers have to tease out what they are. In one experimental study published in a reputable journal, the hypotheses were stated in the 'findings' sections. Readers cannot fully evaluate the methodology (and the literature review) that comes earlier in the article if they do not know what hypotheses or objectives are set.

Also, do not be surprised if the objectives are presented as aims (the distinction between these terms was made earlier in this chapter) or the conceptual definitions as operational definitions, as frequently happens. Terminologies do not always convey exactly what researchers did; they have to provide the relevant information clearly and precisely. It is essential for you to be clear about what questions are posed, how the variables are defined for the purpose of the study, what the researchers did to find answers to the questions and what the findings to these questions are. One useful exercise is to divide a page into three columns, and list the research questions in column 1, the method of data collection in column 2 and the findings in column 3. In this way, you can find out whether the purpose of the study, as expressed through research questions, objectives or hypotheses, has been achieved. It is not unusual to find that not all the research questions set at the beginning of an article are dealt with in the results and discussion sections. Sometimes new findings unrelated to the original research questions creep into the results and can surprise you.

To assess the value of operational definitions in quantitative research, you can use the five criteria discussed in this chapter: clarity, precision, validity, reliability and agreement/consensus. Although specific questions and operational definitions are not normally stated in qualitative research, the article or report must give a clear account of the broad area of study, the concepts investigated, the methods used and the findings.

SUMMARY

Summary and conclusion

In quantitative research, the formulation of the purpose of the study, research questions and operational definitions is a crucial part of the research process. These facilitate the readers' understanding of the nature and magnitude of the task undertaken by the research. They inform readers of what the study is about, and what is being measured, assessed or explored and how. Research is a private enterprise that is made public for it to contribute to existing knowledge. Reporting research questions and operational definitions facilitates the communication between researchers and those who subsequently read and use the report.

Most qualitative researchers only formulate broad questions or identify a broad area of study. During the study, questions emerge as the researcher learns more about the area and decides what to focus on. Concepts constructed from the data can thereafter be operationalised.

References

Brocklehurst J C, Morris P, Andrews K, Richards B and Laycock P (1981) Social effects of stroke. *Social Science and Medicine*, **15A**:35–9.

Chan S and Yu I W (2004) Quality of life of clients with schizophrenia. *Journal of Advanced Nursing*, **45**, 1:72–83.

Cheng K K F, Molassiotis A and Chang A M (2002) An oral care protocol intervention to prevent chemotherapy-induced oral mucositis in paediatric cancer patients: a pilot study. *European Journal of Oncology Nursing*, 6, 2:66–74.

Dealey C (1991) The size of the pressure-sore problem in a teaching hospital. *Journal of Advanced Nursing*, 16:663–70.

Dellasega C and Mastrian K (1995) The process and consequences of institutionalizing an elder. *Western Journal of Nursing Research*, 17, 2:123–40.

Dennison S (1995) An exploration of the communication that takes place between nurses and patients whilst cancer chemotherapy is administered. *Journal of Clinical Nursing*, 4:227–33.

Grant J S and Kinney M R (1991) The need for operational definitions for defining characteristics. *Nursing Diagnosis*, 2, 4:181–5.

Hall C and Lanig H (1993) Spiritual caring behaviors as reported by Christian nurses. *Western Journal of Nursing Research*, 15, 6:730–41.

Kevern J and Webb C (2004) Mature women's experiences of preregistration nurse education. *Journal of Advanced Nursing*, 45, 3:297–306.

Langemo D K, Olson B, Hanson D, Burd C, Cathcart-Silbergerg T and Hunter S (1990) Prevalence of pressure ulcers in five patient care settings. *Journal of Enterostomal Therapy*, 17, 5:187–92.

Manias E, Beanland C, Riley R and Baker L (2004) Self-administration of medication in hospital: patients' perspectives. *Journal of Advanced Nursing*, 46, 2:194–203.

Millman M (1976) *The Unkindest Cut* (New York: Morrow Quill).

Moss J (2005) Development of a functional ability scale for children and young people with myalgic encephalopathy (ME)/chronic fatigue syndrom (CFS). *Journal of Child Care*, 9, 1:20–30.

Mrayyan M T (2004) Nurses' autonomy: influence of nurse managers' actions. *Journal of Advanced Nursing*, 45, 3:326–36.

National Pressure Ulcer Advisory Panel (NPUAP) (1989) Pressure ulcers, prevalence, cost and risk assessment: Consensus Development Conference statement. *Decubitus*, 2, 2:24–28.

Russell B (1918) The philosophy of logical atomism. In: R C Marsh (ed.) (1971) *Bertrand Russell: Logic and Knowledge* (London: George Allen & Unwin).

Shea J D (1975) Pressure sores: classification and management. *Clinical Orthopedics and Related Research*, 112:89–100.

Thoroddsen A (1999) Pressure sore prevalence: a national survey. *Journal of Clinical Nursing*, 8:170–9.

Trendall J (2000) Concept analysis: chronic fatigue. *Journal of Advanced Nursing*, 32, 5:1126–31.

Tutton E and Seers K (2003) An exploration of the concept of comfort. *Journal of Clinical Nursing*, 12:689–96.

Waltz C F, Strickland O L and Lenz E R (1991) *Measurement in Nursing Research*, 2nd edn (Philadelphia, PA: F A Davis).

Wang T J (2004) Concept analysis of functional status. *International Journal of Nursing Studies*, 41, 4:457–62.

Wilson H S (1989) Family caregiving for a relative with alzheimer's dementia: coping with negative choices. *Nursing Research*, 38, 2:947–58.

Wilson J (1989) Conceptual and empirical truth: some notes for researchers. *Educational Research*, 31, 3:176–80.

Research Designs

Introduction

The next step in the research process after the literature review and the formulation of the research questions is the planning or designing of strategies for the collection and analysis of data. In practice, while the aims and objectives or hypotheses are being formulated, the researcher must also give prior thought to the possible design to be used to avoid setting unachievable objectives. The literature review should help the researcher to identify research designs and related issues in similar studies. Researchers have coined a number of terms to describe research designs in quantitative and qualitative research, with which you should become familiar if you are to fully understand the research process. Such terms as 'prospective', 'longitudinal', 'cross-sectional' or 'ex post facto' may mean little at present; this chapter will explain these and other terminologies commonly used in order to enhance your interest in, and understanding of, research articles and reports.

Research design

The term 'research design' means a plan that describes how, when and where data are to be collected and analysed. The design of a study comprises the following aspects:

- the approach (qualitative, quantitative or both, with or without a conceptual framework);
- the method(s) of data collection and ethical considerations;
- the time, place and source of the data;
- the method of data analysis.

However a design does not only specify the steps and actions to be taken but represents the thinking, beliefs and strategies of the researcher/s and the logic of the enquiry.

Sometimes the terms 'design', 'methods' and 'methodology' are used interchangeably. Methods of data collection are the tools (e.g. questionnaires or scales) and techniques (e.g. interviews or observations). Methodology is the study of methods.

Selecting a design

In order to meet the aims and objectives of a study, researchers must select the most appropriate design. In practice, the selection of the design depends largely on the beliefs and values of the researcher (she may, for example, place particular value on the quantitative approach), the resources available (cost, time, expertise of the researcher), how accessible the respondents are and whether the research is ethically sound. Resources often influence the choice of questionnaires over interviews. While such practices may be acceptable, readers must bear in mind that there is no short cut to knowledge. Making compromises and selecting strategies other than the most appropriate has implications for the validity and reliability of the data.

The purpose and types of quantitative research

You will recall from Chapter 2 that the steps of the inductive process comprise the following: description, classification, correlation, causation, prediction and control. Using this framework, one can group quantitative studies into three overlapping categories: descriptive, correlational and causal. In quantitative descriptive studies researchers aim to describe phenomena about which little is known. Descriptive studies tend to answer questions such as: What is the attrition rate on a particular course? What is the pattern of alcohol consumption among third-year student nurses? What is the bed occupancy rate in an intensive case unit? What is the attitude of health visitors towards teenage mothers? In quantitative descriptive studies, researchers use measurements to answer these questions (see Chapter 3). From the data, patterns or trends may emerge and possible links between variables can be observed, but the emphasis is on the description of phenomena. For an example of a quantitative descriptive study see Research Example 14.

Correlational studies (see Research Example 15) seek deliberately to examine or explore links between variables. The purpose is often to develop hypotheses that can be tested later in experiments. Sometimes the term 'exploratory' is used to denote descriptive or correlational studies. To some extent, all research explores phenomena.

Causal or experimental research is concerned with cause and effect. It sets out to confirm or reject the effect of one variable on another.

Research designs depend on the research questions. For example, a descriptive study of postoperative stress may reveal how people experience stress, what factors they perceive as causing or relieving their stress and how they cope with it. Such a study may also give an indication that patients who are given information prior to surgery are less stressed afterwards. A correlational study can be carried out

Tobacco use and baccalaureate nursing students: a study of their attitudes, beliefs and personal behaviours
Chalmers et al. (2002)

A quantitative descriptive study

This survey of the total population of baccalaureate nursing students in one Canadian province aimed to provide quantitative descriptive data on their attitudes, beliefs and personal behaviour in relation to tobacco issues.

Comments:

1 Chalmers et al. (2002) used a number of quantitative methods to collect data. These include:

   ● A 22-item questionnaire on demographic factors, smoking history of family and friends, perceived influences on smoking behaviours, resources used in attempts to quit smoking, and satisfaction with resources.
   ● A scale 'to assess the level of nicotine addiction' in those participants who reported that they were smokers.
   ● A 14-item beliefs and attitudes questionnaire.
   ● A 52-item scale to assess the health promotion attitudes and behaviours of the participants.

2 Data were analysed using descriptive and analytic procedures.

3 Descriptive studies tend to collect a wide range of data on the phenomenon being surveyed, as shown above. In contrast, correlational studies focus on two or three variables, as do experiments.

4 This is a quantitative study because of the measuring tools employed to collect data. These are analysed and reported quantitatively to provide a descriptive profile of nursing students in relation to tobacco.

5 Descriptive studies can generate ideas that can be further explored or tested in other studies.

to collect data specifically to examine the connection between the two variables (information and stress). A questionnaire may be administered to a large number of patients to find out whether there is a difference in the self-reported levels of postoperative stress between those who received information and those who did not.

RESEARCH EXAMPLE 15

Relationships between partners' support during labour and maternal outcomes
Ip (2000)

A correlational study

This study sets out to measure the relationship between women's ratings of partners' participation during labour and maternal outcomes.
    Two null hypotheses were formulated to test these correlations.

1   There is no statistically significant relationship between ratings of fathers' support during labour and maternal outcomes as measured by anxiety level, pain perception, dosage of pain-relieving drugs used and length of labour.

2   There is no statistically significant relationship between women's rating of fathers' support and duration of fathers' presence during labour.

Comments:

1   The author's main objective was not to describe the level of anxiety or pain perception but to find out if perception of fathers' support correlated with the quality of the women's birth experience.

2   Although two hypotheses were formulated, this is not an experimental study since the researcher did not introduce any intervention (independent variable) and measured the outcome (dependent variable). There was also no experimental or control group.

3   The findings show no significant correlation or association between level of emotional support and maternal outcome measures. However, perceived practical support of the partners was positively related to a number of variables including dosage of pain-relieving drug and length of labour.

Although correlational studies may seek to establish links between variables, no firm conclusions can normally be drawn as, for example, in the above study the researcher had no control over the information given and had to rely retrospectively on respondents' reports. To be able to make more definite statements about the relationship between preoperative information and postoperative stress, an experimental design may be used, in which the researcher controls or manipulates the information given and measures the level of stress while trying to control for other factors that may influence postoperative stress. The next chapter gives examples of various types of experiments.

Descriptive and correlational studies, perhaps the most common forms of research in nursing, are no less important or difficult than experimental ones. All research studies require rigour, and all have a contribution to make which can be assessed by the 'added understanding' they bring to the phenomenon being investigated. Although research is described here as having three neat, distinct categories, studies may in practice combine elements from each of them. It is not unusual, therefore, to find descriptive studies that are also correlational.

Types of research designs

There is no consensus among researchers on the classification of designs (Castles, 1987); what seems to emerge is that, broadly speaking, there are three types of design:

- experimental (including quasi-experimental)

- survey

- case study

Experiments examine and establish causal links between variables. In its basic form, an experiment consists of a researcher introducing and manipulating a variable (for example, information giving prior to surgery) and measuring its effects, if any, on another variable (for example postoperative stress), while making sure that there is no interference from other variables (for example, drug intake or information from other sources). In quasi-experiments, the researcher has less control over certain variables than in a true experiment.

A survey is designed to obtain information from populations regarding the prevalence, distribution and interrelationship of variables within those populations (Polit and Hungler, 1995). As such, the survey is appropriate for descriptive and correlational studies. Surveys are generally associated with the collection of a wide range of data from large, representative samples. Sometimes the entire population is surveyed (as in the case of a census) or a representative sample may be drawn. According to Polit and Hungler (1995), the central focus of a survey is very often 'on what people do: how or what they eat, how they care for their health needs, their compliance in taking medications, what types of family-planning behaviours they engage in, and so forth'. The main methods of data collection in surveys are questionnaires and structured and semi-structured interviews, although observations can also be used, as in the case of a survey on dressing practices or pressure sores. Survey methods are discussed in Chapter 13.

The survey is also a choice design for correlational studies. As explained earlier, links between variables suggested by data from descriptive studies can be followed up in correlational studies. Correlational studies using the survey design aim to establish links without introducing an intervention. A survey can be carried out to find whether or not there is a link between lung cancer and people who smoke. The survey may comprise a large number of smokers and non-smokers. Data may show that indeed those who smoke have a higher prevalence of lung cancer. In this case, the researcher did not introduce 'smoking' to a group of people, but simply investigated the link after the smoking had taken place. Such a design is also known as ex post facto or 'after the fact' (Kerlinger, 1973). In correlational studies, researchers commonly collect demographic details such as age, occupation, gender and educational background and seek to establish links between these and other characteristics of respondents, such as their beliefs and behaviours. It is easy to see how surveys are suitable for descriptive as well as for correlational studies.

Case studies focus on specific situations. Using this design, the researcher studies individuals, groups or specific phenomena. Creswell (1994) explains that, in case studies, the researcher 'explores a single entity or phenomenon ("the case") bounded by time and activity (a program, event, process, institution, or social group) and collects detailed information by using a variety of data collection procedures during a sustained period of time'.

The type of data produced is mainly descriptive, although attempts are made to find correlations between variables. As a design, it lends itself well to both quantitative and qualitative approaches. For example, a researcher may evaluate a particular health promotion programme or find reasons why some women do not comply with advice from midwives at an antenatal class using the quantitative approach. Another researcher may carry out an ethnographic study of patient–nurse interactions on a particular ward.

The cases on which researchers focus need not necessarily be unusual; they can, and often are, typical of others. Using the case study approach, data can be collected in the past, present or future. For example, a researcher may investigate the events that led to the closure of hospital X in 1980 by interviewing some of those who were involved in the closure and by studying newspaper and television reports of what happened. A researcher can also 'follow' a group of mothers from the time they give birth to 18 months afterwards, to find out about infant feeding practices. While surveys involve large populations and use samples for the purpose of generalising their findings, case studies tend to be more specific, in-depth and holistic. The emphasis is on understanding a particular case or group of people, although the data gathered may be useful to other similar cases.

Experiments, surveys and case studies broadly describe the main research designs in social, health and nursing research. There are also different types of experiment, survey and case study, as will be shown later in this and the next chapter. Not all research fits neatly into this classification, as, for example, the Delphi technique. The purpose of classification, however crude, is to simplify things and thus facilitate understanding. It has few implications for the reliability and validity of the data if a survey is wrongly described as a case study. What is crucial is for researchers to explain the research process in detail for readers to understand what was done. However, confusion can be created if appropriate terminologies are not used.

Variations on research design

Not all experiments, surveys and case studies are the same. Some surveys collect data on one occasion only, others do so at intervals. Case studies can investigate current as well as past phenomena; some experiments may have only two groups, while others may have three or more. Research designs can be further classified according to their data sources (longitudinal and cross-sectional, retrospective and prospective) and their functions (evaluative or comparative). Other variations include the Delphi technique and action research.

Longitudinal and cross-sectional studies

Some nursing phenomena evolve over time, and it seems appropriate that data should be collected at intervals in order to capture any change that may take place. For example, people coming to terms with the loss of a spouse may go through different phases. Collection of data at three- or six-month intervals from the time of bereavement up to two years afterwards would probably provide a better picture of the bereavement process, than would collection of data on only one occasion. People's attitudes, beliefs and behaviours may change over a period of time. A researcher may be interested in studying the impact of patient education on the subsequent behaviour of postmyocardial patients. It is possible that a month after the infarction patients may be following nurses' advice, but there is no guarantee that this behaviour will be sustained.

Researchers who want to know whether the effects of patient education are durable will have to collect data at intervals over a period of time. Such a design is called longitudinal (see Research Example 16). It is appropriate for phenomena that change over time. The intervals at which data are collected must be justified and this should be on the basis that they are the most appropriate times to capture the phenomena under investigation. The term 'cohort' is used to describe the same group of respondents who are 'followed' over a period of time. Thus, if your class of students takes part in a longitudinal study to find out how their careers progress over the next ten years, your class constitutes a cohort. This type of design is also called 'cohort study'. Two or more groups can also be 'followed' for comparative purposes. One of the problems with cohort studies is the likelihood of a 'cohort effect'. This is described as the effects on a particular cohort as a result of sharing common life experiences. The particular time and context in which a cohort live and interact influence attitudes, beliefs and behaviour.

RESEARCH EXAMPLE 16

A longitudinal study of perceived level of stress, coping and self-esteem of undergraduate nursing students: an Australian case study
Lo (2002)

A longitudinal study

Lo (2002) investigated the perception and sources of stress, coping mechanisms, and self-esteem in a cohort of nursing students during three years of their undergraduate nursing programme. She used a number of measuring instruments (General Health Questionnaire, Self-esteem Scale and the modified Ways of Coping Scales) to find out how they performed on the selected variables.

The results showed that first-year students experienced 'significantly less transient stress compared with year 2 students'. In year 3 they had more positive self-esteem than in year 2. There were no significant differences with regard to chronic stress, avoidance and proactive coping, and negative self-esteem.

Comments:

1   The reason for choosing this design is because of the 'lack of longitudinal studies of the perceived stress, coping and self-esteem of nursing students going through their nursing programme'. Data were collected at three time points (one in each of the three years). This seems to be natural intervals to monitor their progress.

2   The attrition rate can be high in longitudinal studies. It was particularly low in this study (120 in year 1, 112 in year 2 and 101 in year 3). The lower numbers in year 2 and year 3 were attributed to drop-outs and absence of students on days when questionnaires were distributed. The low attrition rate is mainly due to the sample in this study being a 'captive' population (i.e. on a particular programme, for the duration of the study).

One of the main problems with longitudinal studies is that those supplying the data may drop out of the project. This is referred to as 'mortality' or 'attrition'. Respondents may actually die, but more often they withdraw or cannot be traced. This affects the original composition of the sample and may have implications for the generalisability of the findings. If the project lasts for several years, it is not unusual for the original researchers to cease to be involved in the project, often as a result of a career move.

Most research has the potential to influence the subsequent behaviour of respondents, although the extent to which this happens depends on the methods the researcher uses and the nature of the research. The effect of the observer on the observed is well documented (see Chapter 15). Surveys also can raise issues and trigger reactions among respondents. Longitudinal studies, because of their prolonged nature, are more likely not only to raise respondents' awareness, but also to give them time to change their attitudes and behaviours, thereby preventing researchers from studying behaviours as they would have been if there was no research interference. While studying 'the changing situations of a panel of family caregivers of elderly relatives in the home' using a longitudinal design, Collins et al. (1989) became 'increasingly aware of the unintended effects that study participation has had on the family caregiver'. They concluded from their study that:

> through the research process researchers actively influenced the experiences of many of the family caregivers in the study. Caregivers seem to have been stimulated to evaluate and change their appraisals of their care-giving situations and, at times, their use of external resources and patient management strategies.

Another problem with longitudinal studies is that they take time and are costly since they may span a number of years. To get round these problems to some extent, it is sometimes possible to survey a cross-section of respondents, who can provide data to describe the changing nature of the phenomenon. For example, instead of interviewing a group of people experiencing bereavement at six-monthly intervals, the researcher can choose to collect data from people who are at different stages of bereavement. She will interview a group at one month after the loss, a group who are bereaving at six months and another group who are at the one-year stage. All these data will be gathered only once from each group and together will provide an insight into the process of bereavement.

A cross-sectional design is one in which data are collected from different groups of people who are at different stages in their experience of the phenomenon. Its limitation lies mainly in the fact that the same group is not studied over time and that the various groups may not have similar characteristics. For example, various designs have been used to find out whether intelligence and problem-solving ability decline with age. Much of the research that supports the cognitive decline in aging hypothesis is cross-sectional, whereas longitudinal studies often report no decline or much more subtle effects (Robbins, 1991). In these studies, the performance of older people in intelligence tests and other problem-solving exercises were compared with that of younger people.

Comparing generations who had different upbringing, opportunities (especially educational) and stimulation (from toys, audiovisual media, and so on) is unlikely to yield valid results. A more appropriate design would be a longitudinal one in which the same person's level of intelligence is measured every 10 or 20 years. Such a study, by its nature, has practical, financial and other implications, including attrition (the loss of participants to the study). This is why cross-sectional designs are preferred when researchers need answers now rather than in 10 or 20, let alone 60 or 70, years' time.

Retrospective and prospective studies

Phenomena that have already occurred have their explanations in the past. Researchers have to 'work backwards' and search for variables or factors to account for them. A wealth of valuable information resides in people and documents, which can help to shed some light on many current concerns. Records are kept for the purpose of describing, and accounting for, what people do. For example, community nurses' diaries contain information that can help towards the understanding of what they do. Patients' notes give information on the treatment and progress of their illnesses and a considerable number of demographic and other personal details. These were not collected for the purpose of research but can be used retrospectively to explain and inform current phenomena.

A retrospective design is one in which researchers study a current phenomenon by seeking information from the past. For example, Cheater (1993) carried out a retrospective document survey 'to investigate the extent to which urinary incontinence had been identified as a problem, and to examine the nature of its assessment and management'. As part of the survey, she examined '229 nursing and medical records of patients identified as incontinent of urine by the nurses-in-charge, in 14 acute medical wards and 26 health care of the elderly wards'. This study was mainly descriptive. However, a study can also be correlational, as when the researcher investigates a condition or illness that has already occurred and searches for variables in records or personal accounts that may be associated with it. For example, researchers have looked at upbringing, lifestyles and life events (information from the past) in an attempt to find causes that may be related to patients currently suffering from schizophrenia (i.e. which have already occurred). For an example of a retrospective study see Research Example 17.

Retrospective studies must be differentiated from historical studies. If one takes the view that everything that has gone before us is history, all retrospective studies can be termed historical. The crucial difference, in research terms, between the two is that retrospective studies aim to describe or explain a current phenomenon by examining factors that are associated with it or gave rise to it. A historical study, however, does not need to have a 'foot in the present'. It seeks to understand phenomena as embedded in that particular period in history. For example, a nurse historian may carry out a study of leadership styles of matrons in the nineteenth century or describe moral treatments that psychiatric patients received in asylums. Although some comparisons can be made with current leadership styles or psychiatric treatments, the aim of these studies is to focus on these events only as they happened at the time, with or without relevance or reference to what happens now. Here are some examples of historical research:

The nursing record as a research tool to identify nursing interventions
Hale et al. (1997)

A retrospective study

Hale et al. (1997) carried out this study 'to identify the nursing interventions given to two groups of patients: those who had suffered a myocardial infarction and those who had sustained a fractured neck or femur'.

Comments:

1   Three methods of data collection were used: retrospective case note data abstraction, interviews with 'a nurse who had looked after the same patient' and interviews with a senior ward manager about actual policy practices.

  The first two methods are retrospective because entries in the case notes were made before the study started. Interviews aimed to find out what 'nursing staff said they did'.

●   A historical study of men in nursing (Mackintosh, 1997)

●   The historical context of addiction in the nursing profession: 1850–1982 (Heise, 2003)

●   Careful nursing: a model for contemporary nursing practice (Meehan, 2003)

●   Profiling Black South African nurse pioneers: promoting the Black biography . . . Thembani Grace Mashaba (Mhlongo, 2004).

One of the main drawbacks of retrospective designs is that the researcher relies on existing data that were, most probably, not collected for research purposes and therefore lack the rigour with which research is carried out. Description of past behaviour may be highly subjective. Records may be incomplete, or difficult to make sense of or even to decipher. Relying on respondents' memory also has its limitations. Apart from forgetting important details, respondents can be selective in how they view the past. Despite these shortcomings, retrospective studies have been useful in, for example, making links between lung cancer and smoking, and heart disease and fat intake.

A prospective design is one in which researchers study a current phenomenon by seeking information from the future (see Research Example 18). Nurses

RESEARCH EXAMPLE 18

Waiting for coronary artery bypass surgery: a qualitative analysis
Fitzsimons et al. (2000)

A prospective study

As the authors explain, this prospective study 'aimed to investigate the experience of waiting for Coronary Artery Bypass from a qualitative perspective'. Interviews were conducted with 70 randomly selected patients at three intervals over the first year on the waiting list: at referral for surgery ($n = 70$), after waiting six months ($n = 49$) and after waiting one year ($n = 28$).

Fitzsimons et al. point out that this was the first known qualitative study which specifically examined patients' perception of the waiting period prior to bypass surgery.

Comments:

1 'Waiting' is a process which takes place over a period of time. Therefore a prospective design is most appropriate for capturing patients' experience over the one-year period.

2 Attrition (loss of participants due to mortality, severe morbidity or withdrawal from the project) is one of the drawbacks of the prospective design. Researchers must estimate how many participants they are likely to 'lose', and therefore recruit more at the start of the project.

may want to know the effects of their practices on patients' behaviour over time, or how the diagnosis of a condition such as breast cancer subsequently affects the lifestyle of its sufferers. Researchers using a prospective design can have some control over whom they want to include in their study and how data are collected. To ensure that the lifestyle of the newly diagnosed cancer patients would not have changed anyway, another group of people without breast cancer can be studied at the same time. With this design, data are collected at one or more points in the future, as is the case in longitudinal studies. In fact, the two designs have a lot in common. The main difference between them is that longitudinal studies can be both prospective and retrospective. Williams et al. (1994) used a prospective design to study 'early outcomes after hip fracture among women'. Outcomes were compared in three groups of formerly community-living women: 'those discharged home from the hospital, those discharged to a nursing home and staying there for more than 1 month, and those staying for less than 1 month'.

Evaluative studies

In the era of evidence-based practice and client-centred care, evaluative studies assume great importance. Practitioners can evaluate their practice by reflecting on what they do. The difference between this and an evaluative study is that the latter is a systematic appraisal using research methods. Evaluative studies tend to focus on a particular practice, policy or event. They are normally carried out when the researcher wants to find out if, how and to what extent the objectives of particular activities have been or are being met. These activities could be the provision of service, a teaching programme or a series of therapeutic sessions. By focusing on these specific, well-defined activities, evaluative studies tend to take the form of case studies.

In Young's (1994) evaluative study of a community health service development, 'surveys of patients and staff in the health authority were conducted about a range of issues, defined by the original aims of the scheme'. The researcher may also decide to select aspects she wants to evaluate no matter what the original objectives were. However, if the purpose of the evaluation is to improve that particular activity or to be 'wiser next time', it makes sense that the aims and objectives should provide the benchmark against which the success of the programme or activity can be measured.

In evaluative studies, researchers can use quantitative and/or qualitative methods. In Davis et al.'s (1994) study of 'nursing process documentation' in one hospital, the quantitative methods comprised 'a documentation Questionnaire, constructed and used by the researcher, and a self-administered Ward Manager Questionnaire, also constructed by the researcher'. On the other hand, Jennings (1994) used semi-structured interviews in her study of 'hospital at home'. The main limitation of evaluation studies lies in the fact that they are aimed at understanding specific practices and policies. Their contribution to knowledge in general, and research methodology in particular, remains a secondary objective.

There are many similarities and differences between audit and research (Closs and Cheater, 1996). Evaluative studies seem to resemble audit mainly because both tend to address issues in specific settings. Audit and evaluation research must use rigorous methods to collect and analyse data. Finally, the contribution of audit and evaluative studies to the development of theory is rather limited.

The main difference between them is that the research evaluation of a project can sometimes be an afterthought, although the original aims and objectives can be used as benchmarks. Audit, on the other hand, is a cycle that 'involves setting standards for practice, monitoring that practice, comparing actual practice with the standards set, if necessary making changes to practice and then remonitoring practice to see if the agreed standard is attained' (Closs and Cheater, 1996). This important practice element is not usually present in evaluative studies. Research Example 19 gives an account of an evaluative study.

RESEARCH EXAMPLE 19

An evaluation of a local clinical supervision scheme for practice nurses
Cheater and Hale (2001)

An evaluation study

Cheater and Hale (2001) carried out an evaluation of a local clinical supervision scheme for practice nurses. The aims of the study were to:

- assess the level of uptake of clinical supervision by practice nurses;

- identify factors which hindered/facilitated uptake;

- evaluate how far clinical supervision had influenced (i) quality of clinical care; (ii) organisation of care; (iii) professional development.

Comments:

1   Evaluation studies are undertaken in order to find out the extent to which a scheme, service or policy has achieved its intended objectives. The authors explained that this study aimed to 'find out how far the objectives of the local scheme had been met during the first year of implementation'.
    It is likely that 'up-take levels' and 'outcomes' of the scheme were set at the implementation stage. Evaluation studies also provide opportunities to explore why people use a particular service or not.

2   To measure the performance of a service it is important that baseline data are collected. In this study Cheater and Hale sent a questionnaire to all practice nurses and general practitioners involved, at the start of the scheme. Twelve months after, a second questionnaire was administered to the same sample to 'find out about their experience of the scheme and to assess how supported they felt to undertake their role'. The second questionnaire contained additional items to explore 'the level of uptake; perceived GP support; the benefits and difficulties experienced in participating in the scheme; and intentions for future involvement'.

3   The evaluation of a service is a complex exercise often requiring a combination of methods and the collection of data from numerous sources. In this study, two questionnaires were administered and two focus groups were carried out. Data were collected from practice nurses as well as from general practitioners.

4   The evaluation of service guidelines, policies and interventions is central to clinical governance. This study was carried out by the authors on behalf of the Clinical Governance Research and Development Unit of a Health Authority.

Comparative studies

Many research designs involve some forms of comparison. Experimental studies compare results of experimental and control groups. Surveys collect data that allow comparisons according to demographic factors such as age, gender or class. The difference between these and comparative studies is that the purpose of the latter, at the outset, is to compare – whether it is people's characteristics, policies, practices or events.

As the main purpose of comparative studies is to compare, the rationale for this must be provided. The reasons given by Tiwari et al. (2003) in their study of 'critical thinking disposition of Hong Kong Chinese and Australian nursing students' include a lack of understanding of how critical thinking may vary across cultures.

Comparative studies can be quantitative, qualitative or both. Research Example 20 describes a comparative study in which a quantitative approach is used. While and Wilcox (1994), on the other hand, used qualitative methods to explore 'the experience of children admitted to a day-case unit with that of children admitted to a general paediatric ward'. Their study 'aimed to provide an in-depth description of the experience' of the children. The methods used included non-participant observation, interviews and a diary. Comparative

RESEARCH EXAMPLE 20

A comparison of hospital- and community-based mental health nurses: perceptions of their work environment and psychological health

Fielding and Weaver (1994)

A comparative study

This study compares hospital- (*n* = 67) and community-based (*n* = 55) mental health nurses in relation to their perceptions of the work environment and also their psychological health. Measures include: the General Health Questionnaire, the Maslach Burnout Inventory and the Work Environment Scale. The data, obtained from self-returned questionnaires, show that community nurses rated their work environments higher for the dimensions of Involvement, Supervisor Support, Autonomy, Innovation and Work Pressure. Hospital nurses saw their environments as being higher in (managerial) Control. There were no differences between the groups for the dimensions of Peer Cohesion, Task Orientation, Clarity or (physical) Comfort. Furthermore, there were no overall differences between the two groups in relation to psychological health, although the pattern of factors associated with emotional well-being differed. Finally, analysis

➤

→

of the community data revealed that those nurses with 'flexitime' arrangements evaluated their work environments less positively and showed higher levels of psychological strain than did those working 'fixed-time' schedules. The findings suggest that the hospital and community environments make different demands on nursing staff, and that this should be considered when organising nursing services if stress is to be avoided.

Comments:

1   The above abstract shows that the purpose of the research was to compare the two groups. They did not collect data from psychiatric nurses in a variety of settings, which incidentally showed differences between hospital- and community-based nurses.

2   Care must be taken to compare 'like with like'. In this study: in order to ensure that the two groups being compared were equivalent with respect to other major work variables, all participants met the following criteria: (a) they held professional nursing qualifications (SRN or RMN), (b) they were employed at grade 'H' (the top clinical grade) or below, and (c) they worked the equivalent of 37.5 hours per week.

   The differences in the data between groups can sometimes be due to the differences in their characteristics. You must pay particular attention to this aspect of the study when you set out to evaluate it. Sometimes the different conditions or settings in which the tools are administered or observations are carried out can also produce different data. In this study, the response rate for community-based nurses was 72 per cent and for the hospital-based ones, 45 per cent. Fielding and Weaver suggest that it was likely that 'the lack of personal contact at the point of distributing the questionnaires for the hospital-based nurses is responsible for the difference in return rates for the two groups'.

3   Fielding and Weaver gave many reasons why this comparison was necessary. They relate to the NHS changes affecting the role and practices of both hospital- and community-based mental health nurses. As they explained:

   although both groups of nurses are likely to feel the impact of change and its resulting stress, the particular stressors (and means for their amelioration) may be quite different for each group.

A quantitative approach was used in this comparative study. The tools of data collection included: the Maslach Burnout inventory, the general health questionnaire, the work environment scale and a questionnaire for personal and work-related details.

studies are a useful way of learning about people and practices. In health care, it is well known that there are different treatments and approaches to the same condition. While evaluation studies provide data on the effectiveness of particular treatments, comparative studies make it possible to compare different treatments. Since comparative studies adopt a variety of designs, such as experiments, surveys or case studies, they have the same strengths and limitations as these.

The Delphi technique

Another form of research, which is a variation of the survey design, is the Delphi technique. It consists of gathering the views of experts on a particular issue with the added agenda of seeking an agreement or consensus on the issue. This necessarily entails 'going back' to the experts until consensus is reached. There are many issues in nursing that some researchers believe can be enlightened by experts.

The Delphi technique consists mainly of seeking the views of a panel of experts on a particular issue, usually by means of a questionnaire. After analysis of the data, the same experts are given feedback from the findings and asked to reconsider their views with a view to reaching consensus. This exercise is repeated until the researcher is satisfied that the study has achieved its aims. This type of design is particularly useful when setting priorities, clarifying roles, defining concepts and identifying competencies (see Research Example 21 for an example of the Delphi technique).

For example, Lopez (2003) sought consensus among critical care nurses in Hong Kong on their research priorities. The main reason given by the author for using this type of approach is because of the lack of knowledge of 'the most significant problems or questions affecting the welfare of critically ill patients in Hong Kong'. In this study, critical care nurses were defined as 'experts' because they were expected to be most aware of research questions or issues in that area.

There are different versions of the Delphi technique although the core principles should include a panel of experts, more than one round of questionnaires, an attempt to reach consensus of opinion through feedback and the assurance of anonymity (between experts) throughout the process (Beretta, 1996).

The Delphi technique has the advantage of collating the views of experts using questionnaires without incurring the cost of getting the experts together. The fact that these people do not meet and are not aware of who the others are means that they do not have the opportunity of influencing one another, therefore allowing diverse opinions to be expressed. According to Reid (1988), 'the method removes the influence of the dominant personalities in achieving consensus'. The disadvantages include the subjective bias in the researcher's choice of 'experts' and the pressure on respondents to agree, thereby introducing the possibility of hasty decisions being taken. There is also the problem of low response rates, especially in the later rounds of the questionnaire, which

The ideal attributes of Chief Nurses in Europe: a Delphi study
Hennessy and Hicks (2003)

A Delphi study

The purpose of this Delphi study was 'to identify the characteristics considered to be most relevant in a Chief Nurse, in order to inform and systematize recruitment'. According to the authors, the Delphi technique has the capability to establish core attributes of various occupational roles in health care and 'it has international applicability'.

Hennessy and Hicks (2003) sent a questionnaire to a panel of 330 key experts in 22 countries (15 in each country) and sent a revised questionnaire (based on feedback from the first questionnaire) to the same 15 key experts ($n = 180$) in each of the 12 countries which responded in the first round.

Comments:

1 One of the difficulties with the Delphi technique is about the definition and recruitment of 'experts'. In this study 'expert' 'was agreed with senior personnel at WHO/Europe to mean appropriate stakeholders in government-level health departments, including a range of senior health professionals and executive officers of national organisations, and other people acknowledged as having an important perspective on this subject'. Deciding on the panel size depends on who is available and on the subjective judgement of researchers. The non-response rate can be high in studies in which participants have to answer more than one questionnaire. In the first round of this study the individual response rate was 23 per cent; in the second round it was 84 per cent.

2 The number of 'rounds' of questionnaires vary according to studies. Here only two rounds were thought sufficient to identify the attributes of these nurses.

3 The first questionnaire generated 4273 attributes (of Chief Nurses), and after analysis these were reduced to 16 themes (e.g. leadership, political astuteness etc.) which were used in the second round. Participants were asked to rate each of these attributes on a visual analogue scale. It was therefore possible to quantify the degree of importance which these experts from different countries attached to each of these attributes.

4 The authors recognised the 'relatively low response rate' and suggested that there may have been some bias both in geographical location (because only experts from 12 of the 22 countries responded) and 'in the nature of expert opinion provided'. However, the findings can still be useful in informing policies for recruiting these nurses and 'for developing critical pathways for the development of postholders'.

casts doubt on the 'consensus' reached. Could it be that those who drop out do so because they do not want to change their initial views?

According to Powell (2003), the findings of a Delphi study 'represent expert opinion rather than indisputable fact' and that 'further inquiry to validate the findings may be important'. For further discussion of the technique see Beretta (1996), Hasson et al. (2000) and Powell (2003).

Action research

Action research, as the term suggests, has two main components – action and research. The purpose of conventional research is mainly to contribute to the body of knowledge. Some of this knowledge could eventually, but not necessarily, be used in practice. With action research, the emphasis is on 'action', and research methods are used to inform this action. Defining action research is problematic since there are a number of models (see for example Hart and Bond, 1995). In essence, it involves a collaboration between researcher and practitioner in:

- identifying a practice problem;
- using research methods to assess this problem;
- planning and implementing the change;
- evaluating the outcome.

And so the cycle continues. The number of steps depends on whose model one uses.

In its conventional form, research is normally carried out by outside researchers on practitioners and their practice to advance the researchers' cause. They use the practice setting to collect data, and rely on the goodwill of practitioners but give little back. In action research, there is more 'give and take' in the relationship between these two protagonists. With conventional research, findings are often couched in research terminologies that can remain incomprehensible to practitioners. Often the researcher's interpretation of practice phenomena does not coincide with the practitioner's perception of the same. Action research has the advantage that researcher and practitioner can enter into a dialogue, discuss their different interpretations and produce more valid findings by drawing from each other's special knowledge and experience. Research findings in conventional research can take up to two years before they are published. In action research, the emphasis is on the 'here and now'. Solutions to problems are immediately implemented and evaluated.

Action research is not possible without the collaboration of all those involved in, or affected by, the introduction and implementation of change. This has led to the narrow belief that all action research involves participation, hence the term Participatory Action Research (Fals-Borda and Rahman, 1991). There are different views surrounding collaboration and participation (see e.g. Fraser, 2000). Potentially action research can be empowering and emancipatory if participants (e.g. practitioners or carers) have control over what they want to change and how this should happen. In reality the degree of real participation in action research varies according to individual projects. Participation ranges from token, minimal, moderate to full. Increasingly there is the recognition that change is more difficult when it comes 'from above'. By listening, and understanding people's needs, motives and circumstances, it is possible to develop interventions or programmes which suit them best. This is why action research is also associated more with qualitative than quantitative approaches, although both can be useful.

Action research has a number of limitations including the difficulties in getting all those involved motivated enough to see the project to its successful completion. It is time-consuming as, unlike conventional research, it involves an (or several) implementation stage. When action research is carried out in a particular clinical setting, there may be little choice for some to 'opt out', as the project may have to involve all of them. 'Reluctant' participants may feel pressurised to conform. In conventional research, the decision to participate or not is up to the individual. Action research is about change and change has political dimensions and implications. The potential for conflict of interest between researchers (often seen as outsiders) and practitioners, and between practitioners themselves is real (see e.g. Williamson and Prosser [2002] for a discussion of the political and ethical aspects of action research).

Despite these limitations, action research is gaining popularity in health and nursing at a time when there is increasing concern about the research–practice gap (Meyer, 2000; Williamson and Prosser, 2002).

Examples of action research studies include an evaluation of the clinical practice facilitator role for junior nurses in an acute hospital setting (Kelly et al., 2002), nursing staffs' perceptions of persons suffering from mania in acute psychiatric care (Hummelvoll and Severinsson, 2002) and the development and evaluation of an information booklet (Hendry and Cabrelli, 2004). In Research Example 22 Walker and Poland (2000) show how they used action research to develop nursing practice in a rehabilitation setting.

Qualitative research approaches

Qualitative researchers do not carry out experiments as they aim mostly to describe phenomena. They do not normally use the term 'survey' to describe their research, although they study people's beliefs, attitudes, intentions, and so on, mainly perhaps because of the survey's association with structured methods, such as questionnaires. Some may describe their designs as case studies. In general, they do not subscribe to these terms but instead describe their approach as ethnographic, phenomenological or grounded theory, and they go on to explain what they do.

Using action research to develop reflective nursing practice in a rehabilitation setting

Walker and Poland (2000)

An action research project

This project was aimed at changing nurses' 'perceptions of nursing and their role, from a "doing for" to an "enabling, rehabilitative" style of nursing'.

Comments:

1   Action research involves collaboration between researchers and practitioners. In this project the Director of a hospital made the initial request to a researcher from a local university. Some of the researcher/s can also be from the practice setting (i.e. internal).

2   A participative action research approach was adopted. As Walker and Poland (2000) explained:

> As changes were clearly intended, this influenced the selection of participative action research for the project. This approach was chosen particularly because it helped promote the ownership by nurses of the intended developments, and because of its potential to maintain changes beyond the involvement of the researcher.

The Director felt that enforced changes could be counterproductive.

3   The project had a number of phases. There were three rounds of questionnaires and a group interview. Each phase was guided by the previous one and was evolutionary. Staff had opportunities to discuss the findings, to question their own perceptions and to check out the researcher's interpretations. Thus the research methods provided data on which nurses could explore, reflect and examine their (and the organisation's) roles and values.

   As the authors explain, this action research project 'provided a means for participants to explore their own practice through examining data generated by themselves'.

4   Sometimes the involvement of an outsider researcher can be an advantage. Walker and Poland (2000) explain that 'given the situation at the time, there would have been suspicion of ulterior management motives if an inside researcher had attempted to carry out this study'.

Ethnographic studies

As explained in Chapter 4, ethnography is concerned with understanding human behaviour in the cultural and social context in which it takes place. This means that the ethnographer has to spend some time in the company of those being studied. This is what is often referred to as 'fieldwork'. As Hammersley and Atkinson (1983) explain:

> The ethnographer participates, overtly or covertly, in people's lives for an extended period of time, watching what happens, listening to what is said, asking questions; in fact collecting whatever data are available to throw light on the issues with which he or she is concerned.

The purpose of participating is to obtain a holistic view of respondents' behaviour. The ethnographer can not only ask questions, but also observe and, to some extent, share some of the respondents' experiences. The researcher's aim is to understand the way in which people live from their point of view (Spradley, 1980). Observations and interviews are the two main data collection tools. Hughes (1992) points out that question asking, however, does not stand alone as a primary data-gathering tool, and direct questions are often ancillary to participant observation. According to him, 'the researcher uses the senses – vision, hearing, touch, smell, taste – as much as cognition as primary data-gathering tools to characterize important physical and social features of a given field of human behaviour'.

Data from other sources, such as overheard conversations, case notes and information on notice boards, are all part of data collection. For example, in a study of the effects of 12-hour shifts on nurses, the researcher can carry out participant observation (see Chapter 15) on a number of 12-hour shifts and is thus able to ask questions, observe nurses' behaviour in the ward, canteen and social club, and, to some extent, perhaps experience the fatigue and loss of concentration that nurses may also experience.

In ethnographic studies, researchers are supposed not to impose their own interpretations in their attempt to understand and explain respondents' behaviour. In practice, researchers, as anyone else, need a framework in order to make sense of phenomena; they can only use their experience to do this. What differentiates ethnography and the hypothetico-deductive approach of quantitative studies is that in the former, the researcher is prepared to look at phenomena through the lenses of respondents, whereas in the latter, the researcher sets out mainly to test out her ideas.

It is not possible to generalise from data analysis processes in qualitative research, largely because the researcher analyses data during data collection as well as thereafter. While fieldwork notes and transcriptions can be systematically analysed and described, what happens during the interaction between researcher and respondent is a unique process that is usually difficult to convey to readers.

The best that researchers can do is to offer their thoughts and reflections on aspects they perceive as influencing data collection.

Ethnographic data analysis, therefore, involves the researcher's analysis and synthesis of data during interviews and observations. Categories, concepts, themes, patterns, hypotheses or theories that may emerge during the early part of data collection are constantly compared, reviewed and explored further. Field notes provide additional opportunities to continue this process of making sense of respondents' behaviour. A number of computer programmes, such as TAP (Text Analysis Package), QUALPRO and the Ethnograph (see Tesch, 1990) have been developed to facilitate qualitative data analysis. The analysis of data from qualitative interviews and unstructured observations is further discussed in Chapter 16.

Some of the limitations of ethnographic studies include the possibility that the researcher may immerse herself in the particular culture she studies to the extent that she is unable to have an objective view of the situation even after the fieldwork has been completed. Another problem is that it is not possible for the ethnographer to be in all places at the same time. She needs to be very enterprising to observe and experience as much as possible. The large amount of data that ethnographic studies may generate can make data analysis a laborious, time-consuming and challenging task. There are also ethical implications in collecting data on or from people without their awareness and consent. These are discussed in Chapter 15. An account of an ethnographic study is given in Research Example 23.

Phenomenological studies

While ethnography has its roots in cultural anthropology, phenomenology, as explained in Chapter 4, is based on the philosophy of Husserl (1962). The researcher is interested in how respondents give meaning to their experience and, in particular, in how they perceive their world. As Koch (1995) explains, 'one of Husserl's directives to phenomenology was that it should be a descriptive psychology, which would "return things to themselves" and to the essences that constitute the consciousness and perception of the human world'. Phenomenology, as a research method, is especially suited to the study of peoples' experience of illness and the care they receive. The client-centred approach requires nurses to take the perception of each client into account. According to Beck (1994), 'phenomenology affords nursing a new way to interpret the nature of consciousness and of an individual's involvement in the world'.

Not all researchers use the work of Husserl to guide their studies. For example, in a study of 'critical nurses' use of technology in intensive care unit', Alasad (2002) was guided by the work of Heidegger. The philosophy of Ricoeur influenced another phenomenological study of the meaning of lived experiences of giving touch in care of older patients (Edvardsson et al., 2003).

RESEARCH EXAMPLE 23

Meaningful social interactions between older people in institutional care settings
Hubbard et al. (2003)

An ethnographic study

In this study Hubbard et al. (2003) use an ethnographic approach to explore 'the reasons for and types of social interaction in institutional settings, and the ways in which the context of peoples' lives shapes social interaction'. Four different settings in Scotland were studied: 'a dementia unit of a nursing home, a floor of the same nursing home designated for older people with physical impairments, another nursing home and a residential home'.

Comments:

1   Interactions in natural settings are well suited to the ethnographic approach. As the authors explained:

> Naturalistic observations were carried out so that the researchers were immersed in the ways in which residents socially interacted and made sense of their own and each other's actions.

2   In this study, the researchers spent prolonged lengths of time in the company of the participants. Observations were carried out in each setting, over 24 hours for approximately four weeks. Two-hour observation periods were conducted during the daytime, between 8 am and 9 pm, and one session on the night shift which was usually from 9 pm until 8 am.

3   As is common in ethnographic studies, data can be collected in every practicable and ethically permissible situation. In this study the observations were conducted in public places, including dining rooms, corridors and lounges. Some observations were, however, carried out in a bedroom if agreed to by a resident.

   Ethnographic studies provide numerous occasions for data collection. For example, in this study, the residents 'drew the researchers into their social worlds', thus providing opportunities, through casual conversations, to explore the participants' interpretations.

4   To minimise interference with the residents' social interactions and activities, the researchers took the role of 'observer as participant'. They also reminded residents that they (researchers) were there to observe. Note pads were made visible and note taking was overtly carried out to emphasise the observers' role as researchers.

5   Data were analysed with the use of 'the data software package, Nud*ist'.

The primary tool of data collection in a phenomenological study is the interview, during which the researcher seeks to gain insight into how respondents make sense of their experiences. The emphasis is on facilitating respondents to talk freely about the topic; questions are asked in an attempt to seek clarification, illustration or further exploration. As explained in Chapter 4, the phenomenological researcher tries to bracket her own presuppositions about the phenomenon under study. For a discussion of 'bracketing' see Beech (1999).

Phenomenological data can be analysed by searching for themes, patterns or trends. These themes are then put together to describe the 'essence' of the phenomenon. Findings are often presented in the form of verbatim quotes (in the exact words of participants) from respondents. A number of authors (Vankaam, 1966; Colaizzi, 1978; Giorgi, 1985) have developed their own methods to describe phenomenological data. Beck (1994) points out that there are differences in their approaches and disagreements over how data should be processed. According to her:

> Colaizzi is the only one who calls for a final validation to be achieved by returning to each participant. Only Vankaam requires intersubjective agreement be reached with other expert judges. In contrast to both of these phenomenological methods, Giorgi's analysis relies solely on the researcher.

Beck (1994) was referring to ways in which these phenomenologists validated the data they had collected. These disagreements suggest that there are different phenomenological methods.

Colaizzi, Giorgi and Vankaam operate within the discipline of psychology, which explains why the focus is on individual's perceptions, while ethnography is the domain of anthropologists, who place emphasis on culture. It is the standpoint from which they operate that distinguishes phenomenology from ethnography.

Many of the limitations of phenomenological studies are the same as those of qualitative approaches in general. Bracketing is not easy to achieve as it is not possible for people to suspend totally their presuppositions nor to account for all of them, especially if they are not aware that they are using them. The conduct of interviews and the analysis of data requires skill and sensitivity. See Research Example 24 for an example of a phenomenological study.

Grounded theory

Grounded theory (see Research Example 25) is an approach which seeks to develop hypotheses and theories out of data from interviews and observations of people in their own environments. The main characteristics of grounded theory are: the interplay between induction and deduction, the use of theoretical sampling and constant comparisons. The aim of grounded theory is to develop substantive theories by studying the social psychological processes

RESEARCH EXAMPLE 24

Successful adherence after multiple HIV treatment failures
Enriquez et al. (2004)

A phenomenological study

'The aim of this phenomenological study was to describe and understand the experience and decision-making processes of people who became adherent to their HIV medication regimens after previously failing treatment because of non-adherence' (Enriquez et al., 2004).

Comments:

1 To gain an insight into participants' experiences, 'Husserlian phenomenology was selected' as it enables researchers 'to capture the essence of what a non-adherent person experiences in order to incorporate the behaviour of adherence'.

2 A purposeful sample of 11 men and 2 women was selected for this study.

3 The researchers in this study sought responses from participants in the form of narratives. As they explain: participants were asked to 'tell their story'. There was 'little or no prompting'.

   Phenomenological researchers typically use a broad or overarching question to enable participants to talk about their experience. In this study the overarching question was, 'What made you successful and keeps you successful with adherence to your HIV treatment now, when you weren't before?'

4 The researchers tried to use bracketing in an attempt 'to prevent bias in this study'.

5 The Giorgi method was used to analyse the data.

6 Three themes emerged out of the data. These were: 'cycle of non-adherence', 'the trigger' and 'readiness for adherence' (which had five sub-themes). As common in phenomenological studies, these themes were then put together to form the essence of 'the phenomenon of readiness for HIV treatment adherence'.

which people experience in order to make sense of their world. Glaser and Strauss (1967) describe substantive theories as those

> developed for a substantive, or empirical area of sociological inquiry, such as patient care, race relations, professional education, delinquency, or research organisations.

The experience of fatigue for people living with hepatitis C
Glacken et al. (2003)

A grounded theory study

The aim of this study was to explore the nature of the fatigue that individuals with hepatitis C experience using a grounded theory approach. The rationale for this choice of design is based on the underdevelopment (at the time of the study) of the concept of fatigue for people with hepatitis C and because grounded theory is suitable 'for eliciting processes and changes over time, allowing appreciation of the possible evolving nature of the concept under examination' (Glacken et al., 2003).

Comments:

1   The authors followed the methodological principles of grounded theory of Strauss and Corbin (1990).

2   Theoretical sampling was used in this study. Glacken et al. (2003) pointed out that:

> In contrast to other forms of sampling, the principal concern of sampling was with the representativeness of the emerging concepts in their varying forms. The researcher was looking for events and incidents that were indicative of the phenomena being studied, and was not counting individuals.

3   Data collection consisted of in-depth interviews, and 'data generation was not distinct from data analysis'. The researcher also used constant comparisons and induction and deduction techniques throughout the study. As they explained:

> Two analytical procedures served as the mutual bedrock for all coding processes, namely making constant comparisons and asking questions of the data. The questions generated were subsequently posed as hypotheses, with verification being sought in the data. It is believed that these procedures enabled the researcher to give the emerging concepts depth and specificity. Throughout the study, the first author kept written memos and used diagrams to help formulate her thoughts and make visual links between emerging categories.

Grounded theorists begin by developing themes and hypotheses, from the data (i.e. by induction). Thereafter these hypotheses can be verified against further observations (i.e. by deduction). However, the emphasis in grounded theory should always be on induction. Theoretical sampling means interviewing or observing participants according to the emerging themes or ideas from the data. For example, in a study of 'information needs and information seeking behaviour of newly diagnosed cancer patients', McCaughan (2002) found that patients accessed lay sources (e.g. the local hairdresser, members of the clergy or herbalists). She decided to interview these people to find out more about this topic. Constant comparisons, in grounded theory, means comparing similar and different instances in the data to gain a multi-dimensional view of phenomena.

The principles and procedures of grounded theory were explained originally by Glaser and Strauss (1967). Later Strauss and Corbin (1990, 1998) described, step by step, the procedures for developing their brand of grounded theory, and in particular the analysis of grounded theory data.

Discourse analysis

The design of a study using discourse analysis is similar to that of a phenomenological study. The difference between them is that phenomenology focuses on the experience or perceptions of participants as narrated by them whereas in discourse analysis the focus of study is discourse through words, phrases or sentences and the manner and context in which they are expressed. As explained in Chapter 4, language is not just a medium of conveying what we mean; it is a way of constructing social reality. By learning language we learn values, beliefs and social norms from the particular culture or sub-culture in which it is embedded. Through language we also transmit our view of the world and seek to shape it according to our beliefs.

Sources of data in discourse analysis are texts in the forms of transcribed interviews, recorded conversations, diary entries, letters, books, songs and other similar media. The frameworks which discourse analysts use to analyse data vary according to the preference of researchers. Conversation analysis is often based on the work of Potter and Wetherell (1987). Foucault (1972) is popular with critical analysts, in particular those who want to explore power relationships between participants.

Discourse analysis, as an approach, has been used to study a number of topics in health and nursing including nursing documentation (Traynor, 1996), the policy of special observation of psychiatric patients (Horsfall and Cleary, 2000) and the redistribution of medical work in primary care (Charles-Jones et al., 2003). White (2004), Stevenson (2004) and Campbell and Arnold (2004) also offer useful insights into the use of discourse analysis in nursing research. Research Example 26 is a description of a study based on discourse analysis.

Community nurses' perceptions of patient 'compliance' in wound care: a discourse analysis

Hallett et al. (2000)

A discourse analysis study

The purpose of this study was to explore 'community nurses' perceptions of quality in their work'. Sixty nurses were interviewed, and although 'compliance' was not the focus of study, these nurses gave numerous examples of 'non-compliance' which they perceived as a serious obstacle to wound care. As the authors explained, 'it became clear that these examples were so numerous that they were of interest and importance in their own right'.

Comments:

1   As explained earlier, usually discourse analysis is based on one or more theoretical framework. This study draws on the work of a number of theorists and philosophers. The view taken is that of the researcher looking for 'hidden meanings in the text' and that 'language is used to make sense of experience'.

2   The texts which Hallett et al. refer to are the interview transcripts. As they explain:

> Interview transcripts are viewed as texts for interpretation, and the interpretations drawn from them are guided by the attempt not only to understand the meanings which certain events hold for participants but also appreciate how these meanings are socially constructed in terms of professional–client relationships.

3   The authors found that non-compliance could be explained by nurses in a number of ways ranging from 'passive resistance', through 'overt refusal' to 'deliberate interference' in order to prolong treatment.

Summary and conclusion

In this chapter, some of the common terminologies used to describe research designs have been explained. Different levels and types of designs in quantitative research have been identified, as have the four most popular designs in qualitative research. To facilitate

➜

➔

understanding, it was felt necessary to present each one as distinct and separate from the others. In practice, there is considerable overlap between, for example, descriptive and correlational studies. Experiments can be prospective, and a comparative study can be both descriptive and retrospective. What is important, however, is not what terminology is used but that the most appropriate design is selected and described in enough detail to make sense of what was done and to assess the reasons for, and implications of, such actions.

References

Alasad J (2002) Managing technology in the intensive care unit: the nurses' experience. *International Journal of Nursing Studies*, **39**, 4:407–13.

Beck C T (1994) Phenomenology: its use in nursing research. *International Journal of Nursing Studies*, **31**, 6:499–510.

Beech I (1999) Bracketing in phenomenological research. *Nurse Researcher*, **6**, 3:35–51.

Beretta R (1996) A critical review of the Delphi technique. *Nurse Researcher*, **3**:79–89.

Campbell J and Arnold S (2004) Application of discourse analysis to nursing inquiry. *Nurse Researcher*, **12**, 2:30–41.

Castles M R (1987) *Primer of Nursing Research* (Philadelphia: W B Saunders).

Chalmers K, Seguire M and Brown J (2002) Tobacco use and baccalaureate nursing students: a study of their attitudes, beliefs and personal behaviours. *Journal of Advanced Nursing*, **40**, 1:17–24.

Charles-Jones J, Latimer J and May C (2003) Transforming general practice: the redistribution of medical work in primary care. *Sociology of Health and Illness*, **25**, 1:71–92.

Cheater F M (1993) Retrospective document survey: identification, assessment and management of urinary incontinence in medical and care of the elderly wards. *Journal of Advanced Nursing*, **18**:1734–6.

Cheater F M and Hale C (2001) An evaluation of a local clinical supervision scheme for practice nurses. *Journal of Clinical Nursing*, **10**:119–31.

Closs S J and Cheater F M (1996) Audit or research – what is the difference? *Journal of Clinical Nursing*, **5**:249–56.

Colaizzi P (1978) Psychological research as the phenomenologist views it. In: R Valle and M Kings (eds), *Existential Phenomenological Alternative for Psychology* (New York: Oxford University Press).

Collins C, Given B and Berry D (1989) Longitudinal studies as intervention. *Nursing Research*, **38**, 4:251–3.

Creswell J W (1994) *Research Design: Qualitative and Quantitative Approaches* (Newbury Park, CA: Sage).

Davis B D, Billings J R and Ryland R K (1994) Evaluation of nursing process documentation. *Journal of Advanced Nursing*, **19**:960–8.

Edéll-Gustaffson U, Arèn C, Hamrin E and Hetta J (1994) Nurses' notes on sleep patterns in patients undergoing coronary artery bypass surgery: a retrospective evaluation of patient records. *Journal of Advanced Nursing*, **20**:331–6.

Edvardsson J D, Sandman P and Rsamussen R H (2003) Meanings of giving touch in the care of older patients: becoming a valuable person and professional. *Journal of Clinical Nursing*, **12**, 4:601–9.

Enriquez M, Lackey N R, O'Connor M C and McKinsey D S (2004) Successful adherence after multiple HIV treatment failures. *Journal of Advanced Nursing*, **45**, 4:438–46.

Fals-Borda O and Rahman M A (1991) *Action and Knowledge: Breaking the Monopoly with Participatory Action Research* (London: Intermediate Technology Publications).

Fielding J and Weaver S M (1994) A comparison of hospital- and community-based mental health nurses: perceptions of their work environment and psychological health. *Journal of Advanced Nursing*, **19**:1196–1204.

Fitzsimons D, Parahoo K and Stringer M (2000) Waiting for coronary artery bypass surgery: a qualitative analysis. *Journal of Advanced Nursing*, **32**, 5:1243–52.

Foucault M (1972) *The Archaeology of Knowledge* (London: Routledge).

Fraser D M (2000) Action research to improve the pre-registration midwifery curriculum – Part I: an appropriate methodology. *Midwifery*, **16**:213–23.

Giorgi A (1985) *Phenomenology and Psychological Research* (Pittsburg, PA: Duquesne University Press).

Glacken M, Coates V, Kernohan G and Hegarty J (2003) The experience of fatigue for people living with hepatitis C. *Journal of Clinical Nursing*, **12**:244–52.

Glaser B and Strauss A (1967) *The Discovery of Grounded Theory: Strategies for Qualitative Research* (Chicago, IL: Aldine).

Hale C A, Thomas L H, Bond S and Todd C (1997) The nursing record as a research tool to identify nursing interventions. *Journal of Clinical Nursing*, **6**, 3:207–4.

Hallett C E, Austin L, Caress A and Luker K A (2000) Community nurses' perceptions of patient 'compliance' in wound care: a discourse analysis. *Journal of Advanced Nursing*, **32**, 1:115–23.

Hammersley M and Atkinson P (1983) *Ethnography: Principles and Practice* (London: Tavistock).

Hart E and Bond M (1995) *Action Research: A Guide to Practice* (Buckingham: Open University Press).

Hasson F, Keeney S and McKenna H (2000) Research guidelines for the Delphi survey technique. *Journal of Advanced Nursing*, **32**, 4:1008–15.

Heise B (2003) The historical context of addiction in the nursing profession: 1850–1982. *Journal of Advanced Nursing*, **14**, 3:117–24.

Hendry P and Cabrelli L (2004) Meeting patient and relatives' information needs upon transfer from an intensive care unit: the development and evaluation of an information booklet. *Journal of Clinical Nursing*, **13**, 3:396–405.

Hennessy D and Hicks C (2003) The ideal attributes of Chief Nurses in Europe: a Delphi study. *Journal of Advanced Nursing*, **43**, 5:441–8.

Horsfall J and Cleary M (2000) Discourse analysis of an 'observation levels' nursing policy. *Journal of Advanced Nursing*, **32**, 5:1291–7.

Hubbard G, Tester S and Downs M G (2003) Meaningful social interactions between older people in institutional care settings. *Ageing and Society*, **23**:99–107.

Hughes C C (1992) 'Ethnography': what's in a word-process? Product? Promise? *Qualitative Health Research*, **2**, 4:439–50.

Hummelvoll J K and Severinsson E (2002) Nursing staffs' perceptions of persons suffering from mania in acute psychiatric care. *Journal of Advanced Nursing*, **38**, 4:16–424.

Husserl E (1962) *Ideas: General Introduction to Pure Phenomenology* (New York: Collier).

Ip W Y (2000) Relationships between partners' support during labour and maternal outcomes. *Journal of Clinical Nursing*, **9**:265–72.

Jennings P (1994) Learning through experience: an evaluation of 'Hospital at Home'. *Journal of Advanced Nursing*, **19**:905–11.

Kelly D, Simpson S and Brown P (2002) An action research project to evaluate the clinical practice facilitator role for junior nurses in an acute hospital setting. *Journal of Clinical Nursing*, **11**, 1:90–8.

Kerlinger F N (1973) *Foundations of Behavioural Research*, 2nd edn (New York: Holt, Rinehart & Winston).

Koch T (1995) Interpretive approaches in nursing research: the influence of Husserl and Heidegger. *Journal of Advanced Nursing*, 21:827–36.

Lo R (2002) A longitudinal study of perceived level of stress, coping and self-esteem of undergraduate nursing students: an Australian case study. *Journal of Advanced Nursing*, **39**, 2:119–26.

Lopez V (2003) Critical care nursing research priorities in Hong Kong. *Journal of Advanced Nursing*, **43**, 6:578–87.

Mackintosh C (1997) A historical society of men in nursing. *Journal of Advanced Nursing*, **26**:232–6.

McCaughan E (2002) Information needs and information seeking behaviour of newly diagnosed cancer patients. Unpublished doctoral thesis. University of Ulster, Northern Ireland.

Meehan T C (2003) Careful nursing: a model for contemporary nursing practice. *Journal of Advanced Nursing*, **44**, 1:99–107.

Meyer J (2000) Using qualitative methods in health related action research. *British Medical Journal*, **320**:178–81.

Mhlongo T (2004) Profiling Black South African nurse pioneers: promoting the Black biography . . . Thembani Grace Mashaba. *Nursing Times Research*, **9**, 1:65–72.

Polit D F and Hungler B P (1995) *Nursing Research: Principles and Methods*, 5th edn (Philadelphia, PA: J B Lippincott).

Potter J and Wetherell M (1987) *Discourse and Social Psychology* (London: Sage).

Powell C (2003) The Delphi technique: myths and realities. *Journal of Advanced Nursing*, **41**, 4:376–82.

Reid N (1988) The Delphi technique: its contribution to the evaluation of professional practice. In: R Ellis (ed.), *Professional Competence and Quality Assurance in the Caring Professions*, 2nd edn (London: Chapman & Hall).

Robbins S E (1991) The psychology of human ageing. In: S J Redfern (ed.), *Nursing Elderly People* (Edinburgh: Churchill Livingstone).

Spradley J (1980) *Participant Observation* (New York: Holt, Rinehart & Winston).

Stevenson C (2004) Theoretical and methodological approaches in discourse analysis. *Nurse Researcher*, **12**, 2:17–29.

Strauss A and Corbin J (1990) *Basics of Qualitative Research: Techniques and Procedures for Developing Grounded Theory* (London: Sage Publications).

Strauss A and Corbin J (1998) *Basics of Qualitative Research: Techniques and Procedures for Developing Grounded Theory*, 2nd edn (London: Sage).

Struthers J (1999) An investigation into community psychiatric nurses' use of humour during client interactions. *Journal of Advanced Nursing*, **29**, 5:1197–1204.

Tesch R (1990) *Qualitative Research: Analysis Types and Software Tools* (New York: Falmer Press).

Tiwari A, Avery A and Lai P (2003) Critical thinking of disposition of Hong Kong Chinese and Australian nursing students. *Journal of Advanced Nursing*, **44**, 3:298–307.

Traynor M (1996) Nursing documentation and nursing practice: a discourse analysis. *Journal of Advanced Nursing*, **24**:98–103.

Vankaam A (1966) *Existential Foundations of Psychology* (Pittsburg, PA: Duquesne University Press).

Walker G and Poland F (2000) Using action research to develop reflective nursing practice in a rehabilitation setting. *Quality in Ageing – Policy, Practice and Research*, **1**, 2:31–43.

While A E and Wilcox V K (1994) Paediatric day surgery: day-case unit admission compared with general paediatric ward admission. *Journal of Advanced Nursing*, **19**:52–7.

White B (2004) Discourse analysis and social constructionism. *Nurse Researcher*, **12**, 2:7–16.

Williams M A, Obserst M T and Bjorklund B C (1994) Early outcomes after hip fracture among women discharged home and to nursing homes. *Research in Nursing and Health*, 17:175–83.

Williamson G R and Prosser S (2002) Action research: politics, ethics and participation. *Journal of Advanced Nursing*, **40**, 5:587–93.

Young K R (1994) An evaluative study of a community health service development. *Journal of Advanced Nursing*, **19**:58–65.

11 Experiments

> **OPENING THOUGHT** ▶ Man is a cause-seeking creature; in the order of spirits he might be called the 'cause-seeker'. Other spirits conceive of things in relations different from us and incomprehensible to us.
>
> G C Lichtenberg

Introduction

In the previous chapter, we identified three levels of research in quantitative studies: descriptive, correlational and causal. The experiment as a research design corresponds to the third level. Its aim is to establish causal links between variables. It is the principal method in the natural sciences for testing hypotheses and theories, and it uses the deductive approach to data collection (hence the label 'hypothetico-deductive').

In this chapter, we will explore the meaning and purpose of experiments, the difficulties and limitations of using the experimental design in social and health research, the strategies that researchers use to enhance the validity and generalisability of their findings, the ethical implications of experiments involving humans as 'subjects', and the use and value of experiments in the study of nursing phenomena.

The current emphasis on systematic reviews of randomised controlled trials (RCTs) in itself warrants a closer examination of the experiment as a viable design in nursing research; this is why it is given a lengthy treatment here.

The meaning and purpose of experiments

The term 'experiment' conjures up images of scientists mixing chemicals in a laboratory or observing the behaviour of rats in conditions induced by a researcher. Television adverts often show a man or woman in a white coat making such statements as 'test after test proves that' a particular brand of detergent or cat food is better than others. In everyday life, too, we also 'experiment'. A spice may be added to our usual recipe to find out whether it makes it taste better.

Painkillers are taken to relieve headaches or sleeping tablets to induce sleep. The aim in each case is to attempt to produce a change (improve taste, relieve pain or induce sleep) by doing something (adding a spice, or taking painkillers or sleeping tablets). Whether or not we know it, we unwittingly carry out experiments, more often on ourselves, with the aim of making our lives more comfortable. Most people are particular about the type of painkiller they take for a headache. They have probably arrived at this choice by 'trying out' several brands. Some people with back pain will 'try' different forms of treatment, such as medication prescribed by a general practitioner, herbal medicine or the services of an osteopath. They know how they felt before and after each of these treatments and are thus able to make up their minds about its effectiveness. In 'trying out' these drugs or treatments, people have in fact engaged in a 'trial' or experiment.

Professionals, too, experiment during the course of their work. To enhance learning, teachers may 'experiment' with seminars, group discussions or lectures. Nurses may try a different type of dressing or introduce a different approach to the organisation of patient care, such as primary nursing or team nursing. If these do not produce the desired effect, they may try other approaches. By basing their practice on 'trial and error', some nurses unwittingly 'experiment' on their clients, and the negative implications of this can be serious.

In Chapter 2 it was explained that people need to know why things happen. A headache is explained by pressure at work, a hot summer may be attributed to global warming and an increase in child violence is often blamed on the type of television programme children watch. Even when we cannot explain a phenomenon such as winning a lottery, we put it down to 'lady luck'. In fact, we are constantly preoccupied with 'cause and effect'. The relationship between cause and effect is the essence of an experiment.

Clinical trials

The difference between the types of experiment that lay people and practitioners unwittingly carry out and 'research experiments' is that, in the latter, the researcher, systematically and rigorously, studies cause-and-effect relationships between variables, by taking steps to ensure that the results obtained (the effect) can only be attributed to the intervention (the cause).

In health care, experiments are normally referred to as clinical trials. They are carried out mainly to study the effects of interventions (including drugs, psychosocial therapies, educational programmes, services and diagnostic tests). Trials of health care interventions are often described as either explanatory or pragmatic (Roland and Torgerson, 1998). Explanatory trials study the efficacy of interventions. They seek to understand why and how an intervention works so that we can gain a scientific (biological, physiological or psychosocial) understanding of the intervention. These types of trials are normally carried out under ideal circumstances. Participants are carefully selected according to narrow sets of criteria. While the results may show how and why an intervention works, they may not have wide generalisability.

In normal everyday practice, some patients with a certain condition such as rheumatism may differ in characteristics, attributes and background from others. Frequently they have multiple concurrent illness conditions. Clinicians are interested to know if their interventions can work with the type of patients they encounter in their daily work. Pragmatic trials investigate the effectiveness of interventions in real-life situations. This means that few patients are excluded (only those for whom the intervention may be inappropriate). In pragmatic trials the intervention is made to suit the patient condition, while in explanatory trials the patient is selected to suit the intervention.

The results of pragmatic trials may be questionable because researchers have little control over the conditions in which the intervention is administered and evaluated, but the results have wider applicability.

Effectiveness, in pragmatic trials, is often patient-centred and includes, for example, evaluation of safety, comfort, side-effects as well as symptom reduction, healing and cure. Research Example 27 (see p. 223) is an example of a pragmatic trial. For a comparison of explanatory and pragmatic trials see Roland and Torgerson (1998).

The logic of experiments

Suppose a nurse observes that constipation is rife among patients on her ward. Having read in the literature that lack of fibre may be responsible for constipation, she decides to put this to the 'test'. After finding out that the amount of fibre in her patients' current diet is in fact low, she increases it and observes whether there is a reduction in the incidence of constipation. However, a colleague may be sceptical and say that these results would have been obtained with or without an increase in fibre and that other factors, such as medication, mobility, age or nursing care, may be implicated. To rule out the possibility that the reduction in constipation would have happened anyway, the nurse can decide to have two groups of patients: one receiving the current diet, and the other the new diet. Additionally, she may account for or 'control' the other factors by making sure that patients in both groups are, in general, similar in the amount and type of medication they take, in their degree of mobility, and in age, and that they are nursed by the same team of nurses. To avoid the possibility of bias in the selection of patients, the researcher can randomly assign them to either group. In so doing, she has carried out a research experiment. She has:

- put a hypothesis to the test (that a high-fibre diet reduces constipation);
- introduced an intervention (a new high-fibre diet) and measured the outcome (a reduction in constipation);

- compared the pre-test scores (the level of constipation before the experiment) with the post-test scores (the level of constipation after the experiment);

- compared the scores of the group of patients on whom she experimented (experimental group) with those of the group receiving the usual diet (control group);

- controlled other factors that may work for or against a reduction in constipation (by making sure that one group does not receive more laxatives than the other);

- randomly allocated patients to the two groups (to ensure that both groups are similar (equivalent) in relevant factors except in the amount of fibre in their diets).

Our nurse has in effect met the three requirements of a true experiment: intervention, control and randomisation.

Intervention

Without intervention, there is no experiment. A researcher has to do something to produce an effect or outcome. In the above example, the intervention is the introduction of a new diet, and the outcome is a reduction in constipation. In a correlational study, the researcher would not actively have intervened by introducing the new diet but instead could have, for example, carried out a survey of the fibre content of patients' diets and their bowel habits to find out whether or not there was a link between these two variables. Portsmouth et al. (1994) give us an example of a correlational study on the relationship between 'dietary calcium intake and energy intake of 113 eighteen-year-old university students in Western Australia'. They did not introduce any intervention but instead asked the students to record what they consumed over a period of four days. The analysis of these records showed that there was a strong positive association between these two variables (dietary calcium and dietary energy intake). In experimental studies the researcher attempts to make things happen, while in correlational ones she studies phenomena as they are. In health research, the term 'treatment' is often used instead of 'intervention'.

The experiment is the design of choice to test hypotheses and theories. In Chapter 9, a hypothesis was defined as 'a statement in one sentence, about the expected relationship between two or more variables'. In its simplest form, the hypothesis has two variables: independent and dependent. Moore (2001) carried out an experiment to test the following null hypothesis: topical Amethocaine will have no effect in reducing behavioural and physiological responses in neonates. The independent variable was treatment with Amethocaine gel and the dependent variables were the behavioural and physiological responses to intravenous cannulation (Moore, 2001).

The purpose of an experiment is to collect data to support or reject the null hypothesis. Although experiments should have a formal hypothesis you will find when reading research articles that many of them express the purpose of their studies in the form of questions.

For example, Pearson and Hutton (2002), in their study comparing the ability of foam swabs and toothbrushes to remove dental plaque, used an experimental design to answer the following questions:

● Is there a difference between the ability of foam swabs and a toothbrush to remove dental plaque from approximal and crevice surfaces?

And, if there is a difference,

● What is the magnitude of the difference between the ability of foam swabs and a toothbrush to remove dental plaque from approximal and crevice surfaces?

On the other hand, Robbins et al. (2003) in their study evaluating the effectiveness of a home visit and booklet in providing education to parents about infant illnesses, formulated their research questions in the form of objectives. As they explain, the objectives of the study were to evaluate the effects of the intervention on:

● use of health services;

● parental feelings of confidence and knowledge of common childhood illnesses;

● parents' intention of carrying out home care activities for their child's symptoms;

● parents' intention of seeking professional advice.

One can see that the above questions and objectives have the potential of being translated into hypotheses such as 'foam swabs are more effective in removing dental plaque than toothbrushes'. 'A visit and a booklet will increase the use of health services by parents'.

See how many hypotheses you can develop from the above questions and objectives.

Many authors do not state their hypotheses, questions or objectives. This does not facilitate the task of the reader, who has to piece together information from different sections of the article, including the results section, to find out what the author should have stated clearly in the first place.

Control

Experimental and control groups

To make sure that the intervention which she has introduced is the only variable responsible for the outcome, the researcher can devise strategies to control extraneous variables. These are variables other than the experimental intervention that may also affect the outcome. Suppose that a researcher uses an experimental design to test the effectiveness of counselling in the treatment of a group of depressed patients. She may find that after a series of counselling sessions, their conditions have improved. She cannot be certain, however, that 'with the passing of time' they would not have got better anyway or that other factors such as the drug treatment they were also receiving or their nursing care did not contribute to their improvement. To find out whether the counselling sessions were indeed the only contributing factor, she could have compared her group of patients with another group receiving no treatment. However, in health care settings it is likely that patients are receiving some form of treatment. She can, therefore, compare the group of patients receiving the counselling sessions with another group receiving the usual treatment. The group that is receiving the new intervention is called the *experimental group*, and the group with which the comparison is made is called the *control group*.

Because there is a possibility that some of the patients in one group may be more acutely ill or one group may have more women than men, for example, the researcher has to make sure that the two groups are similar in the main relevant characteristics, such as age, gender, social class, type and duration of depression, that may affect the recovery from depression. In this way, she will have more confidence that her results are unaffected by these variables. She has, therefore, exerted control over these extraneous variables.

Between-subject or parallel groups design

By allocating subjects to either the experimental or control group, the researcher is making a comparison between the two parallel groups of subjects. This type of control is known as between-subject or parallel groups design. It is the most common design in randomised controlled trials.

In Robbins et al.'s (2003) study of 'minor illness education for parents of young children', the parents in the experimental group received a visit and booklet by the research nurse. The parents in the control group received only the service offered routinely by the health visitor.

Between-subject designs can have more than two groups. The number of groups depends on the purpose of the experiment. For example, in a study of the effects of relaxation, music and the combination of music and relaxation on postoperative pain, Good et al. (2001) allocated participants to one of the following four groups: group 1: relaxation only; group 2: music only; group 3:

music and relaxation only; group 4: casual conversation (preoperatively) and ambulated with the data collector and lay quietly for 15 minutes during rest (postoperatively).

The most important consideration in parallel groups trials is ensuring that the two groups are similar in key characteristics. If there are differences in, for example, age, gender, or illness conditions in the profile of the two groups then it would be difficult to attribute the results to the intervention only. One way to achieve equalisation of groups is to randomly allocate participants. Randomisation is the objective process of allocating participants to groups. This is explained further in the next section. For an example of parallel design see Research Example 27.

Within-subject or crossover design

Despite the efforts of researchers to select subjects with similar characteristics for the experimental and control groups, the fact remains that they are different groups of individuals and we can never be sure whether or not some of their differences, however negligible, account for differences, if any, in the outcome. To overcome this problem, the same group of people can sometimes serve as both the control and experimental groups. For example, if a researcher wants to find out whether aromatherapy can induce sleep in patients with sleeping problems, she can select a group of 20 patients, administer aromatherapy to 10 patients and give the other 10 their usual sedatives for a period of three weeks. She then changes this over, giving the first group their usual sedatives and the other group the aromatherapy. By comparing the results for each patient, the researcher can assess the effects of the new intervention. This type of allocation is called a crossover or within-subject design as it involves the same subjects 'crossing over' to the new intervention after receiving their usual treatment and vice versa.

Pearson and Hutton (2002) used a crossover design in their study on the effectiveness of foam swabs to remove dental plaque. They explain that participants were allocated to one of two groups (foam swabs or toothbrushes) for one week. In the second week treatments were reversed. This was done to 'ensure that any learning effect resulting from the order of treatment (tooth brushing or using foam swabs) could be assessed'. This design minimised the possibility of differences between groups as 'each person acted as their own control' (Pearson and Hutton, 2002).

The advantage of this type of design is that 'subjects are paired with themselves and the influence of patient characteristics can be eliminated' (Beck, 1989). Also each participant counts as two because they receive both the intervention and the usual treatment. One of the main problems with the crossover design is related to the carry-over effect which happens when the effect of the first treatment continues into the second treatment period. In the above example of aromatherapy and sleeping problems, it could happen that the aromatherapy

Prescribed exercise in people with fibromyalgia: parallel group randomised controlled trial

Richards and Scott (2002)

A between-subject or parallel groups design

This parallel groups randomised controlled trial evaluated the effectiveness of cardiovascular fitness exercise, in people with fibromyalgia, in reducing 'tender point counts', pain, and in increasing their well-being.

Comments:

1   This trial comprised two groups: control and experimental. The control group received 'relaxation and flexibility'. The experimental group received 'prescribed graded aerobic exercise'.

2   One hundred and thirty-six participants were randomised to either the control or experimental group. As the authors explain:

> Participants were randomly assigned in equal proportion to either graded aerobic exercise or relaxation. An independent researcher not involved in the assessment used a random number table for allocation.

The purpose of random allocation is to prevent bias in selecting participants. The profile of participants in each (after random allocation) was shown to be similar, in terms of such factors as age, gender, marital status, analgesics, antidepressants and mental and physical well-being. This means that any differences in outcomes would not be attributed to these factors.

In parallel groups trials, it is essential that the two groups are similar in key characteristics.

3   This study is an example of a pragmatic trial. This choice of design was based on the rationale that previous trials of exercise therapy in fibromyalgia had characteristics of 'explanatory' trials as they 'excluded many cases, and lacked generalisability because the interventions took place in hospitals and were supervised by highly experienced healthcare professionals'.

On the other hand, this trial was 'pragmatic' as 'it evaluated the prescription of a community based exercise programme in patients with fibromyalgia who were seen in a hospital outpatient rheumatology clinic'. Richards and Scott explain that because their trial was inclusive of all cases, their findings were 'widely generalisable'.

that the first group of patients received was so effective in relaxing them that its effects continued for a while even after the therapy was discontinued. If this group were to have their usual sleeping tablets immediately after the aromatherapy was stopped, it would be difficult to assess whether their sleep was helped by their usual drug therapy or by the carry-over effects of aromatherapy. Researchers must pay particular attention to this problem and often leave a time gap between the two interventions. Another limitation is that crossover design can only be used for chronic conditions. Passmore et al. (1993) show in Research Example 28 how this can be done.

While in the crossover design the same patient receives the two interventions consecutively, it is possible in some cases for the same patient to receive two interventions at the same time. In McMahon's study of submammary lesions, two interventions were carried out on the same subject at the same time (McMahon, 1994). For example, a subject was treated with Drapolene cream on one breast and soap and water on the other. This avoids the need for a control and an experimental group and ensures that extraneous variables are reduced to a minimum since it involves the same patient and almost the same type of lesion. However, there are very few cases where this type of experiment would be possible.

Single-subject design

One of the problems of experiments involving people in health care settings is finding large samples. Even when this is possible, it is difficult to allocate them into groups that are identical in relation to the relevant variables. The problem is further exacerbated when subjects, for various reasons, drop out of the experiments. A single-subject or single-case design, on the other hand, minimises these logistical problems since it involves only one participant at a time (although obviously if the one participant drops out, the experiment has to be scrapped). In its simplest form, it involves a pre-test followed by an intervention and a post-test. For example, a single-subject design could be used in an experiment to find out the effect of relaxation therapy on stress in one particular patient. Baseline measurements can be taken to find out how stressed the patient is before receiving relaxation therapy. A post-test measurement will then determine whether or not the therapy has been effective. Such a design is known as the AB design, where A is the pre-test, B the post-test and the intervention the middle.

It will, however, take more than just one intervention for a firm conclusion on the effect of relaxation therapy to be drawn. This will have to be repeated many times, especially on different days and if possible in different circumstances, to avoid other influences. Bithell (1994) points out that some researchers require data to be collected on at least ten occasions 'if statistical analysis is to be performed'.

Single-case designs give researchers the opportunity to focus on an individual

Chronic constipation in long-stay elderly patients: a comparison of lactulose and a senna–fibre combination
Passmore et al. (1993)

A crossover design

This multi-centre study, conducted in long-stay elderly patients in hospitals or nursing-home care (five hospitals and two nursing homes), compared the efficacy and cost-effectiveness of a senna–fibre combination and lactulose in treating constipation. As the author explains:

> According to a randomised, double-blind, cross over design, patients (77) received active senna–fibre combination 10 ml daily with lactulose placebo 15 ml twice daily, or active lactulose 15 ml twice daily with senna–fibre placebo 10 ml daily for two 14-day periods according to a computer generated randomisation code.

Passmore et al. (1993) made sure that 'before entry into the first phase, and between treatments, subjects had a three- to five-day period free of laxatives'.

Comments:

1   Each patient received two consecutive treatments: (a) active senna–fibre with lactulose placebo, and (b) active lactulose with senna–fibre placebo. The order in which they took them was determined by a computer.

2   Before crossing over to the second treatment, the researchers allowed a period of 3–5 days 'laxative free' to avoid any carry-over effect the first treatment might have had.

3   To avoid the possibility of the participants and researchers knowing which treatment was the senna–fibre combination and which was the lactulose, a placebo was used for each situation. Thus, the 'senna–fibre combination with lactulose placebo' would have been similar to the 'active lactulose and senna–fibre placebo', especially as the two were administered in the same doses. The term 'double blind' is explained later on.

and therefore pay more attention to details. It is particularly suited to the principle of patient-centred care, since the interaction between the individual and the treatment is unique, although lessons learnt can be applied to other cases as well. Riddoch and Lennon (1994) remind us that the single-case experimental method has been well established in psychology and educational research since the late 1800s and early 1900s. This type of design is useful when little is known about the effectiveness of interventions coupled with difficulties in undertaking a large-scale conventional experiment. Selkowitz et al. (2002), who used a single-case design to study the efficacy of pulsed low-intensity ultrasound in wound healing, explained that there was limited clinical research available and no consensus on the efficacy of this treatment for pressure ulcers.

Much of child psychology developed from the work of Piaget, who based many of his theories on observations of his own children. In the field of learning, Skinner, Pavlov and Thorndike emphasised the importance of the intensive study of an individual in deriving an understanding of conditioning.

One of the major limitations of single-case designs is that their findings cannot be generalised to similar populations, since they are individual cases. Bithell (1994) questions the scientific credibility of single-subject experiments. According to her, if we wish to demonstrate the general effectiveness of a treatment for patients with a particular problem, then a group study must be carried out with a representative sample drawn from that patient group. A series of case studies will not do. Riddoch and Lennon (1994) disagree with Bithell's arguments and claim that 'a series of case studies may provide strong evidence for the efficacy of a particular treatment manipulation provided every attempt has been made to control for threats to internal validity'. Internal validity and external validity are explained below. In Research Example 29 Cross and Tyson (2003) use a single-case design to study the effect of a slider shoe on hemiplegic gait.

Solomon four design

Sometimes the purpose of more groups is not to have more interventions but rather to have more control over extraneous variables. Earlier, it was explained that a pre-test and a post-test are normally carried out to find whether the independent variable (or intervention) has caused a change in the dependent one (outcome). It may happen, however, that the act of pre-testing may itself influence the outcome. For example, it could be that by assessing how depressed subjects are at the beginning of an experiment (pre-testing), some may become more aware of their condition and thereafter motivate themselves to get better. To avoid such influences, a Solomon four design can be used. This consists of four groups, of which two are control and two are experimental. Pre-tests and post-tests are carried out with one control and one experimental group only, and post-tests only for the other control and experimental group:

Experimental group 1	Pre-test	Intervention	Post-test
Control group 1	Pre-test	Usual treatment	Post-test or no intervention
Experimental group 2	No pre-test	Intervention	Post-test
Control group 2	No pre-test	Usual treatment	Post-test or no intervention

RESEARCH EXAMPLE 29

The effect of a slider shoe on hemiplegic gait

Cross and Tyson (2003)

Single-subject design

A single-case design was used to test the effects of the slider shoe in improving the efficiency and speed of walking in people undergoing gait rehabilitation post-stroke.

Comments:

1   Four clients were selected to take part in this study. Single-case study design can be carried out with one or more participants. The results of the study are normally reported according to each individual rather than as a group.

2   In this study the ABA design was used, as explained below:

A: Participants walked without the slider shoe
B: Participants walked with the slider shoe on their weak foot
A: Participants walked without the slider shoe again

The experiment lasted six days (two days per phase). Each individual's gait was measured six times per day.

3   The authors recognised that such a study is 'a preliminary exploration' and that 'any attempt to generalise must be treated with caution'. They indicated that a larger group study was planned.

This type of design eliminates the effects that a pre-test may have on the outcome. By comparing the results of these groups, it is possible to discover whether such influences have indeed crept in.

Quasi-experiments

For a number of reasons, ethical and practical, it may sometimes not be possible to carry out true experiments in nursing and midwifery. For example, if a researcher introduces a new model of nursing in a ward, it is not feasible to randomly allocate patients to two groups in the same ward or even to allocate them to different wards because of clinical, organisational and ethical considerations. The best she can do is to compare the ward introducing the new model with a similar ward in the same hospital. Although the researcher has a new intervention, she does not have a 'proper' control group but a comparison group as she cannot randomise subjects to each group. She has only partly met the criteria of a true experiment. In effect, she has carried out a quasi-experiment, a design that must have a new intervention but not necessarily a control group and has no randomisation (see Research Example 30 for a study using a quasi-experimental approach).

This type of experiment is appropriate in cases where the researcher seeks to introduce minimum disruption in a natural setting. Because in quasi-experiments researchers do not have the high degree of control over extraneous variables that is seen in true experiments, it is not possible to state with confidence that any new intervention is actually responsible for the effects measured. In other words, quasi-experiments cannot establish cause-and-effect relationships with certainty but they can establish strong links.

There are a variety of quasi-experimental designs. At the very least, the researcher can introduce a new intervention into a group and measure the outcome. For example, relaxation therapy may be introduced to a group of patients, and the researcher may want to find out whether they report a decrease in their level of anxiety. This is the weakest form of experiment since there are

RESEARCH EXAMPLE 30

The utility of cognitive behavioural therapy on chronic haemodialysis patients' fluid intake: a preliminary examination
Sagawa et al. (2003)

A quasi-experiment

The hypothesis for this study was: Cognitive behavioural therapy (CBT) will assist chronic haemodialysis participants to achieve their personal fluid intake objectives.

One group of 10 patients were given the intervention (CBT). Baseline measurements (weight recorded daily for four weeks) were followed by a programme of CBT for six weeks. Post-intervention, the weights of the patients were recorded daily for four weeks.

Comments:

1   In this study there was an experimental but no control group. This means that it would be difficult to credit the outcome (weight gain after CBT) to the intervention only.

2   This was a preliminary study and the author suggested that a larger study would be required to identify all of the potential benefits of CBT for this condition. More importantly, a randomised controlled trial would add credibility to the findings by controlling other factors which may account for the outcomes.

3   This type of design was described by the author as 'one group before and after quasi-experiment'.

no baseline scores (pre-test) and no other groups with which to compare the final scores.

The next step up is when a researcher measures the anxiety level prior to and after the introduction of relaxation therapy. This time, there is more confidence that a change has happened (if it has), although it is still difficult to establish with certainty that relaxation therapy is the cause, because a number of other factors may be implicated. To be more certain, the researcher may decide to have two groups: one experimental and one comparison. She measures the anxiety level on the experimental ward before and after the intervention. She also carries out the same measurements at the same time with patients on a similar ward (comparison group) who did not receive relaxation therapy. She can begin to have more confidence in her results. This last design is called a non-equivalent groups design. It may be that the subjects in both groups are similar in many respects but that the researcher did not have enough control over their selection and allocation to ensure that they were in fact equivalent. These three designs are depicted in Figure 11.1.

One group:	no pre-test	intervention	post-test
One group:	pre-test	intervention	post-test
Two groups:			
Experimental (non-randomised)	pre-test	intervention	post-test
Comparison group	pre-test	intervention	post-test

Figure 11.1   Quasi-experimental designs

Another quasi-experimental design is the interrupted time series (ITS) (Cook and Campbell, 1979). This involves only one group (experimental) and a series of measurements before and after the intervention. This can be illustrated as shown in Figure 11.2 (Polit and Hungler, 1983). O_1 to O_4 represent the four baseline measurements at time intervals selected by the researcher, X represents the time at which the new intervention takes place and O_5 to O_8 represent the four post-intervention measurements at time intervals selected by the researcher.

Suppose that a nurse wants to carry out an experiment by introducing primary nursing onto a ward to find out whether or not it increases patient satisfaction with nursing care. She can measure patient satisfaction on four occasions, monthly for four months, prior to the introduction of primary nursing, and can carry out four measurements at the same intervals afterwards. Her reason for the multiple measurements could be that one measurement may not be reliable since any event happening on that day or immediately prior to it might influence the results. By having four measurements at reasonable intervals, it is hoped that the

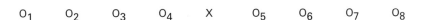

$$O_1 \quad O_2 \quad O_3 \quad O_4 \quad X \quad O_5 \quad O_6 \quad O_7 \quad O_8$$

Figure 11.2   One-group interrupted time series

same events may not be present each time. A better picture of patient satisfaction (which can fluctuate over time) can be obtained by more than one measurement. Multiple post-intervention measurements have similar functions. It can detect, among others, the 'novelty effect' of new interventions. Most of the phenomena with which nurses deal are dynamic and evolving and can be better studied over time.

There are a number of variations on the ITS (Cook and Campbell, 1979), including the two-groups design, depicted in Figure 11.3. One of the strengths of the ITS is that multiple measurements over a period of time give a more accurate representation of phenomena that fluctuate. Its main weakness is that the extended period of time required for multiple measurements increases the opportunity for extraneous variables to creep in.

Experimental group: O_1 O_2 O_3 O_4 X O_5 O_6 O_7 O_8

Comparison group: O_1 O_2 O_3 O_4 X O_5 O_6 O_7 O_8

Figure 11.3 Two-groups interrupted time series

Factorial designs

Experiments typically investigate the effect of one variable (independent) on another (dependent). To prevent bias other variables are 'controlled'. For example, in investigating the effect of exercise on constipation, other factors such as fluid and fibre intake will have to be the same in both control and experimental groups. While it is important to know if exercise has an effect on constipation, it is likely that in real life, many factors interrelate to produce an outcome. In this case it could be hypothesised that exercise, fluid and fibre intake may, in combination, produce an effect on constipation. This hypothesis can be investigated by means of a factorial design.

A factorial design is one in which the effect of two or more independent variables on one or more dependent variables can be tested in the same study. The term 'factor' in factorial designs refers to 'variables'. Factorial designs are particularly suited to the study of interactions between variables and of the 'added' value of using a combination of interventions. This type of design also allows for treatments (e.g. drugs or psychosocial interventions) to be varied. The strength of the approach is that it can all be done in one study. For an example of a factorial design see Research Example 31.

Randomisation

Controlling extraneous variables with the use of a control group whose subjects are similar in the relevant characteristics to those in the experimental group does

Randomised factorial trial of falls prevention among older people living in their own homes

Day et al. (2002)

A factorial design

In this study, Day et al. (2002) tested the effectiveness of, and explored the interactions between, three interventions to prevent falls among older people.

Comments:

1   The rationale for choosing a factorial design given by the authors was that only one trial had examined the interactive effects of multiple interventions in the same study.

2   The three interventions tested in this study were: group-based exercise, home hazard management and vision improvement. There were seven experimental groups and one control group. The allocation of interventions was as follows:

Group 1:	Exercise
Group 2:	Home Hazard Management (HHM)
Group 3:	Vision
Group 4:	Exercise and HHM
Group 5:	Exercise and Vision
Group 6:	Vision and HHM
Group 7:	All three interventions
Group 8 (Control group):	No intervention

3   While a factorial design is appropriate for studying the effects of single and combined interventions, the complexity and logistical problems of managing the study can be enormous. One potential difficulty (not experienced in this study) is obtaining adequate samples for each group.

4   In this study, group-based exercise was 'the most single potent intervention', but the 'strongest effect was observed for all three interventions combined'.

not necessarily ensure that biases are absent in the allocation of subjects to the two groups, and those more likely to respond positively to the new intervention may be assigned to the experimental group. The researcher may have 'hand-picked' subjects for the two groups. A random allocation can go some way towards removing any subjective bias that a researcher may show in selecting subjects. In experimental terms, randomisation means that subjects have equal chances of being allocated to a particular group.

There are different ways in which randomisation can be carried out. If all eligible subjects are known in advance, it is possible, if the numbers are small, to pick names out of a box and allocate them alternately to groups. With large numbers, a computer package may be of assistance. More often, subjects are entered into an experiment at the time of admission to treatment. Each subject is given an opaque envelope containing either the letter 'A' or the letter 'B'. Neither the researcher nor the participant knows which 'letter' the envelope contains until it is opened. This is called concealed allocation.

Other methods of allocation are: matched pairs and cluster randomisation.

Matched pairs

One strategy that has been useful in ensuring that the subjects in the two groups are similar in the relevant characteristics is 'matching'. If a researcher requires an equal distribution of the following characteristics – women aged between 48 and 50, middle class and newly diagnosed with breast cancer – in her experimental and control groups, she will look for two subjects who meet these criteria and allocate one to each group until the required sample size is reached. This matched-pairs allocation technique is usually appropriate when the researcher knows in advance which variables to control. Also, as Dane (1990) points out, 'there is no end to the number of potential variables that may require matching, and therefore you can never be sure you have matched participants on all relevant characteristics'. Another limitation of this approach is that it can take a long time to find enough matched pairs for an adequate sample size. To partly overcome this problem, the researcher may try to match groups instead of pairs.

Cluster randomisation

Instead of randomising and allocating individuals to groups, researchers increasingly randomise clusters (e.g. hospitals or schools) instead of individuals. For example, in Meyer et al.'s (2003) study of the effect on hip fractures of increased use of hip protectors in nursing homes, a cluster was defined 'as a nursing home in itself or an independently working ward of a large nursing home'. Forty-nine clusters agreed to take part and, by randomisation, 25 clusters (with 459 residents) were allocated to the intervention group, and 24 clusters (with 483 residents) constituted the control group (Meyer et al., 2003). The Medical Research Council (2002) gives several reasons to explain when cluster randomisation is appropriate. These include:

● The intervention to be studied is itself delivered to and affects groups of people rather than individuals. Examples include changes in general practice organisation and use of local radio for health promotion.

- The intervention is targeted at health professionals with the aim of studying its impact on patient outcomes. An example would be education about guidelines for a particular medical condition; it would be difficult for professionals receiving such education not to let this affect the management of all of their patients.

- The intervention is given to individuals but might affect others within that cluster – i.e. contamination. For example, recipients of a behavioural intervention to promote weight loss or reduce smoking might share their information with others attending the same clinic.

- If the intervention involves supplying equipment or staff to an administrative unit, then by randomising these units rather than individuals only a subset of the units would receive the equipment or staff. This may be cheaper or administratively more convenient.

The unit of analysis can be the clusters or individuals. If analysis is at the level of individuals, the sample size has to be increased in order to compensate for the differences between clusters. Informed consent could be a problem but the need for individual informed consent should not be ignored in cluster randomisation.

There has been a large increase in the numbers of trials using cluster randomisation. For bibliometric surveys on cluster randomisation trials, see Bland (2004).

The random block design

Conventional randomisation may produce groups which have similar profiles. For example, after randomisation, the average age of participants in the control group and experimental group may be similar. However, age distribution may not be similar. Therefore, although it looks as if the groups are similar in 'average' age, in fact one group may comprise mainly middle-aged people and the other, half younger and half older people (Ross, 1999).

The randomised block design may offset this weakness in conventional randomisation by grouping participants who share the same characteristics (e.g. age, gender, condition, behaviour) so that 'like' can be compared with 'like'. Participants are matched and put into groups. The groups are then randomly selected to be either control or experimental. The number of groups depends on the purpose of the study. One of the limitations of this design is the difficulties involved in managing a large number of groups and in getting adequate sample sizes for each.

The Zelen design

In the conventional RCT, participants who meet the inclusion criteria are randomised after they consent to take part. This may lead to some withdrawing from the trial because they are not allocated to the group (control or experimental) they hoped for. Some may be so disappointed that they may not comply fully with the protocol, and this may affect how they respond to their allocated treatment. The Zelen design (Zelen, 1979, 1990; Homer, 2002) offers an alternative approach which consists of randomising everyone (who meet the inclusion criteria) before consent is sought. In the conventional RCT the details of the trials are made known to all prospective participants when consent is sought. The process of seeking informed consent in the Zelen design depends on whether the single- or double-consent approach is used (Homer, 2002).

In the single-consent version, participants in the control group are not asked for consent and they are not made aware of the trial. However, they are all included in the analysis of data. All those in the experimental group are asked for consent to participate. Those who refuse the new treatment are offered the usual treatment but are not included in the trial. Data analysis includes only patients who retain their original allocation (Torgerson and Roland, 1998).

In the double-consent version, all participants (control and experimental groups) are asked for their consent. If some in the control group refuse, they are offered the experimental treatment, if this is available outside the trial (Homer, 2002). If some in the experimental group refuse, they can be offered the usual treatment or available alternatives. Only those who retain their original allocation are kept in the trial.

There are ethical issues involved in the use of the Zelen design. For example, not informing the control group of the experimental treatment (in the single-consent design) is unethical. Those who have used this design point out that making control group participants aware of the new, potentially beneficial treatment, which they cannot receive (as is the case with conventional RCTs), can lead to disappointment and dissatisfaction (Dennis, 1997).

Placebos and blind techniques

Two other strategies to control extraneous variables are the use of placebos and blind techniques in experimental designs.

Placebos

The idea of receiving a new form of treatment can itself make some people feel better. If some subjects in an experiment have high expectations of a new drug or other form of treatment being tested, this can affect the results of the study. To overcome the possible suggestive effect of the new intervention, a placebo – a substance that has no pharmacological or therapeutic property – can be administered to one group for comparison purposes. It is made, as much as possible, to resemble the new drug or treatment. Kleijnen et al. (1994) point out that in any medical intervention there are placebo effects to some degree and these include perception of the therapist by the patient, the effect of the therapeutic setting, and the credibility of the medication itself (size, shape, colour, taste).

It often is not possible to devise a placebo to match a psychosocial intervention, such as counselling. For this reason, the use of placebo is uncommon. Most clinical trials test the best known (usual) treatment against the new treatment.

For an example of the use of placebos in an experiment see Moore's (2001) study comparing the effectiveness of Amethocaine gel with a placebo in the management of procedural pain in neonates.

Single-blind and double-blind techniques

Being aware of which interventions the control and experimental groups are receiving may introduce bias on the part of the subjects and researchers. Patients may have a preference for a particular drug with which they are familiar or may have high expectations of the new therapy being tested. These may influence their assessment of the interventions. Researchers, too, may be biased in favour of the intervention being tested, and this may affect their observations and recording of data. To avoid these types of influence, it is possible, especially when two 'drugs' look and taste similar, as when placebos are used, not to let the subjects know whether they are in the experimental or the control group. For ethical reasons, their informed consent for taking part in the experiment must be obtained. A single-blind trial is one in which either the participants or the researchers are unaware of the allocation to groups. A design in which both the subjects and the researchers are unaware of which drug each group is receiving is called a double-blind trial. Dumas (1987) describes a triple-blind design as one in which 'persons other than the experimenters evaluate the response variables without knowing the group assignments of the subject'.

Cook and Campbell (1979) explain how the need for the placebo control group and double-blind experiments arose:

> In the earlier medical experiments on drugs, the psychotherapeutic effect of the doctor's helpful concern was confounded with the chemical action of the pill. So, too, were the doctor's and the patient's belief that the pill should have helped. To circumvent these problems and to increase confidence that any observed effects could be attributed to the chemical action of the pill alone, the placebo control group and the double-blind experimental design were introduced.

Internal and external validity

A randomised controlled trial (RCT) is an experiment in which subjects are randomly allocated to one or more control groups and to one or more experimental groups, depending on the number of interventions. It is a popular type of experiment for testing the effectiveness of drugs and other forms of therapies, and is increasingly being used to assess the effectiveness and cost efficiency of other types of interventions, services and policies as well. The uses and limitations of RCTs are discussed later in this chapter.

The purpose of experiments in nursing and health care in general is ultimately to contribute to better treatment, care and other services. The usefulness of their findings, however, depends on their internal and external validity. Internal validity is the extent to which changes, if any, in the dependent variable can be said to have been caused by the independent variable alone. External validity is the extent to which the findings of an experiment can be applied or generalised to other similar populations and settings.

Internal validity

A number of unwanted factors internal to the study can, on their own or combined, interfere with the experiment and make it difficult to conclude with confidence that the findings reflect the true relationship between the two variables being investigated and nothing else. The purpose of control is precisely to eliminate or minimise these unwanted effects. Brennan and Croft (1994) ask two questions that can be used to assess the internal validity of an experiment:

1 To what extent might flaws in the study design have biased the study result?

2 If the result is thought to be free from bias, to what extent might other causes have confounded the observed association?

From these questions emerge two terms central to the understanding of internal validity: biases and confounders. Biases can be present at every stage of an experiment, from the admission of subjects to the experiment to the interpretation and reporting of findings. On the other hand, some factors in the study may work in the same or opposite direction to the independent variable and therefore affect the dependent variable. These factors or variables are known as confounders or confounding variables. The following hypothetical experiment gives an example of confounders.

A teacher carries out an experiment to investigate the effectiveness of a new study method: self-directed learning. She allocates 20 students to the experimental (self-directed learning) group and 20 students to the control group, who were exposed to their usual teaching method (lectures). The teacher then compares the students' knowledge at the end of the module and finds that those receiving lectures have a higher knowledge score than do the self-directed learning students. She had 'controlled' other variables such as age, gender and educational level to prevent these from influencing the results by making sure that, on average, both groups had students of the same age and educational level and had an equal number of males and females.

However, one variable of which she may have been aware but which she found difficult to control was the 'learning ability' of each student. It could be that the learning ability of those receiving lectures was higher than that of the other group. The researcher cannot state with confidence that the lecture is the better method of imparting knowledge, nor can she know whether the difference in the two groups' learning abilities is responsible for the difference in knowledge scores. In this experiment, 'learning ability' may be a confounding variable as it may be confounding, or confusing, the results. On the other hand, the researcher may also find that some members of the lecture group have also been exposed to a television programme on their module topic during the course of the experiment. She was powerless to do anything to prevent this as she learnt about it after the experiment was completed. Therefore 'exposure to the TV programme' is a confounding variable. Researchers may be aware of such variables and unable to control them, or be unaware of them. Their task is to speculate on the effects of all possible confounders as they are more familiar with their study than are those reading the report.

The random allocation of subjects should remove possible confounders by making the groups more or less similar in relevant characteristics, but it does not always do so. It may happen, for example, that by randomly allocating patients with the same type of illness to two groups, one group ends up with some patients who are more acutely ill than the other group. The severity or acuteness of the illness can therefore constitute a confounding variable. It has the potential to affect the results, especially if a drug or therapy is the subject of an experiment. It is sometimes possible to make allowance for such effects when data are analysed and interpreted. However, such undesirable interference from confounding variables can and must be avoided. According to Brennan and Croft (1994), samples in clinical trials can be made as large as necessary 'to ensure that imbalances in randomisation are extremely unlikely'.

Biases and confounders threaten the internal validity of experiments, hence the term 'threats to internal validity'. Cook and Campbell (1979) have identified a number of factors that can affect study findings. Some of these will be used here to assess the internal validity of experiments. These are history, maturation, testing, instrumentation, selection, mortality and statistical regression.

History effects

A history effect is produced whenever some uncontrolled event alters participants' responses (Dane, 1990). In the above experiment on teaching methods, the uncontrolled event is the television programme that was shown during the time the experiment took place. According to Dane (1990), the event is a commonplace event, not necessarily a 'truly historical' one. It may not come to the attention of the researcher and thus its effects may remain unknown, but it may not confound the results if both groups are exposed to it. An example of a historical effect comes from a study by Berg et al. (1994) on 'nurses' creativity, tedium and burnout', in which the authors speculate that the 'results may have been affected by factors of an individual or social type'. They explained that 'there was a large organizational change in the public sector during the intervention which meant that both wards were completely reorganized from the county council to the community and also Sweden, in general, was facing increasing unemployment'.

Maturation effects

Some changes in people's behaviour and attitudes can happen over time with or without a specific intervention. For example, an intervention designed to reduce anxiety of newly admitted patients to hospital may account for a reduction in anxiety when the pre-test scores and the post-test scores are compared. However, it could be that with the passing of time, patients were less anxious because they became more familiar with their surroundings and with staff. This type of effect is known as maturation. It is a threat to internal validity 'due to the respondent's growing older, wiser, stronger, more experienced, and the like between pretest and posttest' (Cook and Campbell, 1979). Maturation effect can sometimes be controlled by randomisation.

Testing effects

The process of repeated testing can itself affect performance. People can alter their answers in the post-test, if they obtained low scores in the pre-test. They may also have thought about their performance in between tests or become more familiar with the test format. Differences in scores may only partly be due to the intervention. Therefore testing is a threat to internal validity if it is not 'controlled' as part of the experiment.

Instrumentation effects

The measuring process itself can be biased. Operational definitions of independent and dependent variables can be subjective (see Chapter 9). The choice of data collection methods may also reflect the researcher's preference and may not be the most appropriate for the study. For example, Allen et al. (1992), in their study of 'the effectiveness of a preoperative teaching programme for cataract patients', admitted that the questionnaire they had developed had some limitations. They explained:

> the areas of knowledge tested may not be the most important ones despite a content review by ophthalmic nurses and ophthalmologists. A true–false format was perceived by the researchers to be the most appropriate for elderly subjects. Although subjects did not have difficulty in answering this kind of question, it may be that another format would be more appropriate.

The measuring process can also undergo changes that can bias the results. Smith (1991) points out:

> Observations, questionnaires, and interviews are commonly used in experimentation as measuring instruments. Observers and interviewers are particularly subject to changes in instrumentation – they learn, in the process of observing or interviewing, how to make different measurements, and their temporary motives (hunger, fatigue) may change the measurements. To the extent that they unwittingly make measurement changes during pretests and posttests, they contribute to instrumental invalidity.

A common problem with measuring tools is that they are sometimes not sensitive enough to measure the small differences between experimental and control group scores. A study by Martin et al. (1994), comparing patients receiving the 'home treatment team' nursing care and those receiving 'appropriate conventional community services', found that:

> The assessment scales chosen may have been insufficiently sensitive. If patients who benefited were those at the threshold of managing at home, a smaller change than we could detect with this study might nevertheless have resulted in a favourable outcome.

Selection effects

There are at least two points in the choice of participants at which bias can 'creep in'. Although the experimenter can set inclusion criteria (such as patients of a certain age group and not seriously ill), she still has to make a judgement about whom to include or exclude. Assessing the severity of illnesses is not as straightforward as it seems: it involves a degree of subjectivity. The allocation of subjects to groups can also give rise to bias. The more objective the allocation of subjects, the less likely it is to be biased. In quasi-experiments, researchers often have to 'work' with the people who are available. These may comprise, in the words of Smith (1991), 'volunteers, hypochondriacs, scientific do-gooders, those who have nothing else to do, and so forth'. Random allocation can avoid many of the selection effects.

Mortality effects

Researchers take care in allocating subjects so that groups are as far as possible similar in all the important characteristics. When subjects drop out, either because they die, cannot tolerate treatment or simply want to stop taking part, it can create an imbalance between the groups. The loss of participants to a study is known as mortality or attrition. Not only do groups become smaller in size, but they may also become dissimilar in the relevant characteristics. In fact, the benefits of randomisation can be undermined by mortality, especially in cases where drop-outs are not even between groups. The reasons why subjects fail to complete the experiment must be made clear and must be taken into account in the analysis of data.

Internal validity is the crucial test that every experiment should pass. As Cook and Campbell (1979) explain:

> Estimating the internal validity of a relationship is a deductive process in which the investigator has to systematically think through how each of the internal validity threats may have influenced the data. Then, the investigator has to examine the data to test which relevant threats can be ruled out. In all of this process, the researcher has to be his or her own best critic, trenchantly examining all of the threats he or she can imagine.

Your task as a reader is to assess the extent to which the researcher does this and to think of possible biases and confounders that may have been overlooked but which may have affected the findings.

Internal validity is not an all-or-nothing issue. It is more a question of the extent to which an experiment has internal validity, as it is not possible to be aware of, or eliminate the effects of, all biases and confounders. The validity of the findings is determined by checks on biases and extraneous variables. The list of all possible confounders must be exhausted before a causal relationship between the variables under study can be established.

Statistical regression

Statistical regression, also known as regression to the mean, has been used to explain differences between pre-test and post-test scores. It is a statistical phenomenon that can make natural variations in repeated data look like real change (Barnett et al., 2005). Statistical regression is the tendency of high or low scores (outliers) to come closer to the mean (regression) when measured for the second time. This is because it is believed that very high scores and very low scores occur by chance, and the chances of this happening is lower than for scores which reflect the mean or average. This can be illustrated by an example from the television card game show: *Play your cards right*. Participants are asked to guess whether the next card is higher or lower than the previous one. Inevitably when, for example, a ten of hearts is shown, the next card is predicted to be lower. Participants seem to estimate that the chances of a lower number coming up is greater than for a higher number (as there are fewer cards above than under ten).

Statistical regression has implications for clinical practice as well. If patients with very high blood pressure (BP) are treated with a particular medication, it can lead to reduction in BP. This could be because the medication is effective, or because the BP was so high, that the next reading was likely to be low anyway.

The size of the reduction in BP could also be a combination of the effect of the drug and statistical regression. According to Morton and Torgerson (2003), regression to the mean 'can result in wrongly concluding that an effect is due to treatment when it is due to chance'.

In research, statistical regression can be a threat to validity, in particular, in single-group trials. The absence of a control group makes it difficult to ascertain if the difference in pre-test and post-test scores is due to the intervention or to chance. As very high or very low scores have a tendency to regress to the mean, one should be careful in interpreting results of trials when pre-test scores are unusually much higher than the mean.

External validity

The internal validity of a study is a necessary but not sufficient condition for its findings to be generalisable to other similar populations and settings; it must also have external validity. An experiment takes place in a particular setting with a specific group of people at a particular time. Together, these factors contribute to make the experiment a unique happening. The question to ask is, 'Can its findings apply readily to similar populations in different settings?' For this to be possible, the population and setting of the experiment must closely approximate the population and setting where the findings are to be used. For example, if a study shows that giving relevant information prior to surgery relieves postoperative stress, does this mean that giving information to preoperative surgical patients in hospitals other than where the experiment was carried out would also relieve their postoperative stress? Does information giving have the same effect in a ward where the atmosphere is relaxed and nurses are attentive to patients' concerns as in another ward where the atmosphere is tense and the nurse–patient relationship leaves a lot to be desired?

The main threat to external validity comes from the selection and allocation of subjects. Randomisation in experiments means the random allocation of available subjects to groups. It does not mean that the samples are representative of the target populations (see Chapter 12). Subjects in experiments are typically recruited at the time of diagnosis or admission to hospital. They can be described as accidental samples and are convenient, since the potential subjects happen to present themselves at the time of recruitment. Seldom are sample frames available from which representative samples can be drawn. RCTs also recruit volunteers, who are then randomly allocated to groups. In Cupples and McKnight's (1994) study of health promotion in general practice for patients at high cardiovascular risk, 'letters were sent to 1431 patients'. Those who responded and were eligible were then randomly allocated to the control or experimental group using a computer programme. This example shows that the sample starts by being 'volunteer' and therefore not necessarily representative of people at 'high cardiovascular risk'. The target population of people at high cardiovascular risk consists of people of different gender, class, educational background, lifestyle and personality. Some may be more positive towards health promotion than others. It may be that by taking subjects who are available or who volunteer, most of those who come forward are from an educated, middle-class background and see the experiment as an opportunity to do something about their health. What randomisation does is simply to allocate randomly those who come forward, for the purpose of having equal groups. The generalisation of the findings to everyone at high cardiovascular risk is therefore limited.

Not all those who are available or who volunteer are recruited to an experimental study. The researcher normally selects a sample by specifying inclusion or exclusion criteria. In this way, the sample is 'sanitised'. For example, Koh et al. (1994) describe those who were excluded in their study of the effect of a mental stimulation programme on the mental status of elderly patients with dementia as: below 55 years of age, or were noisy, violent or irrational, on medication such as sedatives and tranquillisers, known to have marked impairment of vision or hearing, severely incontinent or insufficiently mobile, i.e. unable to walk 50 yards to the room where the sessions were held.

The sample is further 'sanitised' when those who cannot complete the experiment drop out or are withdrawn. The findings of studies such as Koh et al.'s (1994) may not be generalisable to all elderly patients with dementia. In real life, many of these patients are 'noisy', 'insufficiently mobile' and receiving medication. Studies of 'sanitised' samples can only have external validity for people who meet the criteria set by the researchers for inclusion in the experiment.

According to Britton et al. (1999), external validity can be affected if those participating are 'unrepresentative of the reference population for whom the intervention in question is intended'. They carried out a systematic review 'to assess the extent, nature and importance of excluding subjects or the unwillingness of particular centres, clinicians or patients to participate'. They found that many RCTs have blanket exclusions, such as the elderly, women and ethnic minorities, but reasons for these exclusions are seldom given (Britton et al., 1999).

Oldham (1994) puts the issue of internal and external validity of experiments in context:

> Maximising internal validity by exerting a high degree of control may, however, provide an artificial situation reducing the external validity of the results. In the clinical environment, it is often necessary to reach a compromise between the two or ensure that the studies are replicated in a new setting and with different subjects. Much greater confidence can be placed in the findings if the results can be replicated in differing environments.

When evaluating an experiment, you can use the different aspects of internal and external validity discussed here as a 'checklist'. You will find that not all authors provide enough information on their experiments for you to carry out an evaluation effectively. One of the common omissions is information related to the intervention received by the control group. While a detailed description of the new intervention may be provided, the control group's intervention is simply described as the 'current treatment'. Some researchers forget that while they may be familiar with the 'current treatment', many readers are not. For example, in one study on the effect of an educational programme on the knowledge and attitude of patients to a particular topic, the teaching methods, the content and the duration of the programme that the experimental group received were described in detail. No such information was available about the control group. When no significant difference in knowledge and attitude was found, the researcher was at pains to explain why this was so. Attempts were made to explain what the control group 'would have received' rather than what they 'actually' received. It was not clear how much attention the researcher gave to finding out what the control group was exposed to. It is difficult to assess the internal validity of an experiment that sets out to compare two interventions when information on one intervention is not adequate.

One study which paid attention to what the control group received was that of Moore et al. (2002). They use qualitative research methods to investigate both 'how the intervention was delivered in practice and what constituted normal care'.

Information about randomisation is also often lacking. According to Fetter et al. (1989), 'randomisation, a key element, is one of the least reported aspects of clinical trials'. Readers must be made aware of the precise method of random allocation and its implication for the internal or external validity of the findings.

Ethics of experiments

A number of ethical issues raised here apply equally to non-experimental research. Because experiments involve interventions by the researcher, they have more potential for causing physical and mental harm. There is an unequal distribution of power between the experimenter and the subject, more power resting with the former. Dane (1990) makes this point when he states that 'the power differential between researcher and participant is often greater in experimental research than in other research methods, if for no other reason than the experimenter can manipulate some aspect of the participant's environment'. The researcher also has power over whom to enter into the experiment and who should receive the current or the new treatment, except where randomisation is used. This unequal power relationship is evident in the fact that researchers possess information about the experiment and its implications, and control how much is given to participants. Sometimes participants actively seek to be included in clinical trials if they perceive they will receive better treatment.

There are, however, rules of ethical conduct which, if followed, can to some extent prevent abuse on the part of researchers. Ethical research committees exist for the purpose of ensuring, at least on paper, that participants' rights and well-being are protected. Many would like such committees to have a policing role as well. Clinicians and managers can and should also act as gatekeepers in order to protect the interest of patients.

Often when ethical issues of research are discussed in articles and reports, the main aspects dealt with are anonymity and confidentiality. While these are undoubtedly important, researchers must also be concerned with the physical and mental harm that can be done to participants in experiments. Causing them to worry is stressful enough. As regards clinical trials, Fetter et al. (1989) ask 'three central questions': 'is experimentation with human subjects justified?', 'do the possible benefits of conducting the study outweigh the potential risks?' and 'has informed consent been respected?' Let us now look at each of these questions.

Is experimentation with human subjects justified?

Clinicians 'do things' to people all the time without being fully aware of their effectiveness. As explained earlier in this chapter, this form of trial and error is itself a form of 'back door' and uncontrolled 'experimentation'. At least research experiments are more in the open, with the result that participants' rights can be more protected. The purpose of clinical trials is to assess the effectiveness of particular treatments and to learn more about them for the benefit of more people than those included in the experiment.

Experiments should only be carried out when necessary. Just because patients are a captive population does not mean that they should be used by anyone wishing to 'prove' anything. Newell (1992) raises doubts also about the ethical implications of using a small number of subjects in experiments. As the author explains:

> The ethical aspect of sample size is that if a trial is of insufficient size to detect (for the benefit of future patients) a better treatment, it can hardly be ethical to include a patient in the trial, particularly as this will often involve discomfort, disturbance or some small element of risk to the patient.

Do the possible benefits of conducting the study outweigh the potential risks?

If clinical trials are carried out to assess the effectiveness of particular drugs or other therapies, it stands to reason that in cases where this information is already available, there is no need for the experiment unless the evidence is inconclusive and the intention is to replicate the study. No experiment can be justified if patients are denied the best available treatment for the purpose of experimentation. When an experiment is carried out, researchers must ensure that control groups are given the best available treatment. On the whole patients included in trials do better than those who are not irrespective of whether they are in the control or the experimental group. For a debate on the ethical basis for entering patients in randomised controlled trials see Weijer et al. (2000).

Has informed consent been respected?

Patients entering trials are often in a vulnerable position as well as being a captive population. They may be in a confused state, especially if they have just learnt that they have an illness. One can also ask whether or not they are in a position to refuse to take part in an experiment, especially in cases where the clinicians treating them are also the researchers involved in the study. As Silverman (1994) observed:

> many patients (often the majority of those eligible) refuse to participate in a trial in which the treatment is to be decided by the play of chance. In some instances, it was noted, patients enrol only because an exciting new form of treatment is not available outside the trial. Consequently, these patients may be disappointed, less cooperative, and more likely to drop out before completing the assigned regimen if they are randomly allocated to receive the treatment alternative they do not prefer.

Sometimes randomization takes place before consent to participate is obtained. One study which used this approach was by García de Lucio et al. (2000). They found that several randomised people refused to take part.

In some cases participants may not understand what randomisation is. Featherstone and Donovan (1998), in their interviews with participants from an RCT, reported that many found 'the concept of randomization difficult'. They concluded that 'patients may need to discuss the purposes of randomization in order to understand them fully enough to give truly informed consent'.

While researchers may believe that randomisation is a fairer way to allocate subjects to control or experimental groups, some patients want to have a choice of groups. It also shows that patients are not as 'passive' as one might think. However, there is no doubt that some may feel obliged to take part for one reason or another.

People approached to take part in a study should be fully informed of its implications and of their rights to refuse or withdraw at any time during the experiment. Their informed consent should be sought prior to the study, and this consent must be offered free from pressure of any kind. Researchers have a vested interest in recruiting participants to their study. Giving information on the negative implications of the experiment may lead to refusal to participate. Where the number of potential participants is large, this may not be an issue, but when participants are hard to recruit, it must create a tension between the obligation to provide 'balanced' information and the need to recruit.

In the case of single- or double-blind experiments, the question of telling patients which treatment is the placebo negates the purpose of blindness in the study. However, giving a tablet of no pharmacological property or an injection of sterile water in an attempt to deceive patients into thinking that they are real treatments is an infringement of their rights. Researchers must, however, tell patients that a placebo is used and leave it to them to accept or refuse to take part.

Beside the possibility of withholding information from patients, researchers may be tempted to 'lean on' them. McMahon (1994) describes the dilemma that he and the other researchers in his study faced between recruiting fairly and using persuasion:

> Both my researcher associates and I had the experience of patients who refused to take part whom we felt that if we had 'pushed' would have consented. The issue of how persuasive one ought to be is not often discussed and this may be affected by whether one feels that the patient has a moral obligation to participate (Sim, 1991). Our experience demonstrated to us how easy it would have been with a largely elderly and vulnerable sample to, in our view, break the rules for the personal gain of having adequate numbers in the study.

Debriefing participants can help to bring them back to earth. However, one can still question the ethics of intensive monitoring of patients during the period of the experiment, only to leave them alone feeling abandoned once the data are collected. The security afforded during their interactions with researchers is suddenly removed at the end of the experiment. Sometimes drug manufacturers may make 'compassionate supplies' freely available to participants who leave a trial, if the treatment has been beneficial.

No experiment is more important than the right of individuals to privacy and safety. Researchers must examine their own conscience and motives when taking decisions that can affect the participants' well-being. The role of ethics committees, practitioners and managers as gatekeepers and advocates for patients and others who take part in experiments is of the utmost importance.

Problems in conducting experiments

Setting up, and conducting, an experiment requires rigorous standards that are not easy to attain. One of the problems frequently mentioned in the literature is the recruitment of subjects to trials. Silverman (1994) reports on comments made at a workshop held at the UK Cochrane Centre in Oxford by some participants who argued that randomisation 'is often responsible for poor recruitment'. According to them, 'many patients (often the majority of those eligible) refuse to participate in a trial in which the treatment is to be decided by the play of chance'.

The difficulty of recruitment is further exacerbated when subjects drop out or are withdrawn during trials. Although some of the problems caused by subject mortality can be taken into account in the analysis of data, they by and large pose a threat to the rigour of experimentation, not least because researchers can be tempted to treat drop-outs as incidental and may not discuss the implications for the findings.

Blindness in clinical trials poses methodological problems, apart from the ethical implications discussed earlier. The researcher can never be sure that those who should be 'blind' in trials are necessarily so. Dale and Cornwell (1994), in their study 'of the role of lavender oil in relieving perineal discomfort following childbirth', found that, of the three interventions used, 'the GRAS compound' was distinguishable from the other two. As they explained, 'in a "perfumery" sense the GRAS compound did not smell as "pleasant" as the lavender and synthetic lavender oils'. These and other clues negate the intended effects of blindness in experiments and pose a threat to internal validity.

Ethical objections, recruitment and mortality problems, difficulties in achieving blindness, the dilemma between seeking informed consent and putting pressure on people to participate, and the reactions of subjects when being studied are some of the challenges that researchers face in trying to achieve their objectives, maintain rigour and keep within ethical boundaries all at the same time.

Randomised controlled trials in nursing

Nursing, like all other health professions, needs to justify its practice on sound evidence. The RCT is considered the gold standard of research designs to evaluate effectiveness of interventions (Centre for Reviews and Dissemination, 2001). Variation in nursing practice for the same condition is well documented in the literature (see Chapter 19). The RCT has the potential to compare existing practices or to evaluate new ones. Yet a number of authors have pointed out that there are few RCTs in nursing (Shuldham and Hiley, 1997; Bonell, 1999). In a Medline and hand search, Cullum (1997) found 522 'reports of RCTs' which evaluated aspects of nursing care between 1966 and 1994 (28 years). This is relatively low compared to other designs such as the survey and qualitative approaches. In a recent content analysis of Australian nursing research published from 1995 to 2000, only one randomised controlled trial was found out of 495 studies. Webb (2003) found that out of 138 empirical papers (which explicitly stated their methodology) published in 2001 and 2002 in the *Journal of Clinical Nursing*, six were RCTs. In a similar analysis of all papers in the *Journal of Advanced Nursing* in 2002, only eight RCTs out of 256 empirical papers were identified (Webb, 2004). Although more extensive analysis is needed, these findings give a clear indication of the low proportion of RCTs in nursing research.

Shuldham and Hiley (1997) suggest that the 'apparent antipathy of nurses and midwives to the RCT is due to the lack of experience, education and understanding of this method of research'. Bonell (1999) believes that nursing has been hesitant in its adoption of quantitative and experimental research because of nurses' stereotyped views of these methods.

The relative lack of RCTs in nursing can partly be explained by the nature of some nursing interventions. For example, 'giving information to patients prior to discharge' cannot be as neatly packaged, as can tablets or injections. The number of confounding variables involved in the 'information giving' sessions and the problems in standardising the content of the intervention and context in which it takes place make it difficult to account for the outcomes.

Medical treatments such as drugs, surgical interventions or the use of diagnostic and screening equipment can to some extent be studied by means of RCTs. The less the number of confounding variables the easier it is to control or to account for them. The less involvement professionals and researchers have with an intervention in RCTs, the more likely it is that the results will be attributed to the intervention itself rather than to other factors. Cochrane himself was diffident about encouraging 'widespread RCTs in the care sector' because the objectives are more difficult to define and the technique (RCT) was less developed in that sector (Cochrane, 1972).

The more control researchers exert over variables, which may work with or against the experimental intervention, the less the experiment resembles the real situations in which health professionals work. Closs and Cheater (1999) explain that 'depending on the aim of the research, less tightly controlled research designs produce findings of a different nature which may be equally valuable'. Thus quasi-experiments and single-case designs also have the potential to produce evidence for nursing interventions.

The planning, implementation and successful completion of an RCT can be demanding in terms of time, skills and resources. There are also problems in relation to recruitment, consent attrition, implementation of intervention and contamination.

A number of papers have provided useful insights into the process of RCTs and some of the problems which arise. Brooker et al. (1999) report on some of the factors including poor recruitment, stress and poor morale of staff, inadequacy of staff training for the study which led to the abandonment of an RCT of problem drinkers in an accident and emergency department. Ellis et al. (2000) describe an attempt to set up an RCT to evaluate the extent to which pre- and post-registration educational programmes prepare practitioners to promote patient/client autonomy and independence in the delivery of care to older people. They encountered a number of difficulties such as 'lack of a standard intervention', 'difficulty in measuring practice outcomes', 'managers' perceptions of the effect of the random allocation of participants to each arm of the study' and problems with recruitment. As a result, Ellis et al. (2000) chose a quasi-experimental design instead. Plant et al. (2000), in their RCT of a nursing intervention for breathlessness, also encountered a number of contextual and methodological issues. These were: 'resistance among colleagues to innovative nursing practice; the difficulty of measuring well-being in patients whose physical condition is deteriorating; maintaining uniformity of practice within a diverse group of collaborating nurse researchers; and the tension between the nursing role and the necessity of an ethically demanding research design'.

These problems are associated with RCTs in general and with 'socially complex interventions', in particular. Lindsay (2004) describes socially complex interventions as those which are difficult to define and which are influenced by contextual factors that are difficult to control. The Medical Research Council (2000) illustrates the difference for simple and complex interventions as follows:

> If we were to consider a randomized controlled trial of a drug vs. a placebo as being at the simplest end of a spectrum, then we might see a comparison of a stroke unit to traditional care as being at the most complex end of the spectrum. The greater the difficulty in defining precisely what, exactly, are the 'active ingredients' of an intervention and how they relate to each other, the greater the likelihood that you are dealing with a complex intervention.

As explained earlier many, but not all, nursing interventions are complex and not easily 'packaged'. The *Framework for Development and Evaluation of RCTs for Complex Interventions to Improve Health* (Medical Research Council, 2000) is a useful document which provides guidance for individuals considering the evaluation of a complex intervention.

There are numerous examples of RCTs in nursing and midwifery practice. Some of these include:

- An evaluation of a training programme in techniques of self-control and communication skills to improve nurses' relationships with relatives of seriously ill patients (García de Lucio et al., 2000).

- Relaxation and music to reduce post-surgical pain (Good et al., 2001).

- A comparison of Amethocaine gel and placebo in the management of procedural pain in neonates (Moore, 2001).

- A comparison of the ability of foam swabs and toothbrushes to remove dental plaque (Pearson and Hutton, 2002).

- An evaluation of satisfaction with midwifery care (Harvey et al., 2002).

- Effect on hip fractures of increased use of hip protectors in nursing homes (Meyer et al., 2003).

Evaluating experiments

When evaluating a research study, the first task is to make sense of the information provided in the article or report. In the case of experimental studies, it is vital to look for the hypothesis (or hypotheses) or objectives and identify the independent and dependent variables. The next step is to find out how they are operationally defined. If the experimental hypothesis is that 'the use of an information booklet will lead to an increase in knowledge', readers must be clear about what the 'information booklet' consists of, how the participants 'use' it and how 'knowledge' is measured. Does a list of questions adequately measure participants' knowledge? In health research, the criteria for measuring outcomes can reflect professional prejudices. For example, if the hypothesis is 'dressing A is more effective than dressing B in the treatment of leg ulcers', the 'effectiveness' outcome can be measured by the time each type of dressing takes to heal the wound. However, other criteria, such as the side-effects of, or the degree of comfort of patients with, the dressing should also be part of the outcomes to be assessed. Cartwright (1988) goes further and states that:

> Measurements of morbidity and mortality are inadequate on their own. Assessments of treatment should also take account not only of physical side effects but of the social costs of attending for treatment, and the possible anxieties created.

The population taking part in experiments must be clearly defined: readers need to know what the inclusion criteria are. As DerSimonian et al. (1982) explain:

> If the selection criteria are not clearly stated, a reader is uncertain about who the subjects were and how they were selected. It is difficult to generalize the findings of such a trial to groups other than the subjects themselves.

A description of subjects in each group with reference to the relevant variables must be given. It is not enough to say that the groups are similar in important characteristics such as age, gender or educational background. Figures must be provided to allow readers to decide for themselves whether this is the case. Not all crude data can or should be made available. However, data on the profile of subjects in each group are important because any of their characteristics could be a confounding variable. An important piece of information often withheld is the illness condition of subjects in both groups. Without knowing how similar or different the groups are, it is difficult to decide with certainty that severity of illness is not a confounding factor.

As explained earlier, researchers often omit to give adequate information about the treatment of control groups. Readers need to know whether both groups received the same attention and care apart from the experimental drug or intervention. Could it be that in testing 'the effects of information giving on anxiety levels', the fact that those in the experimental group had someone to talk to was enough to reduce their anxiety? Did those in the control group receive the same amount of attention from the experimenters?

The allocation of subjects to experimental and control groups can in itself be biased. Many reviewers would simply not bother to read about an experiment if it were not randomised. When subjects are randomised, the precise method of allocation must be described for readers to decide whether there was a possibility that bias may have crept in.

Researchers must also explain clearly who were 'blind' in the experiment and how this was achieved. The difficulty in maintaining blindness has been discussed earlier. You must look for assurances from the researcher that adequate measures were taken to ensure blindness. For example, in a ward where some patients are given the experimental intervention and others the usual one, how can the experimenter be sure that the subjects did not talk to each other?

Those who left or were withdrawn from the experiment must be accounted for: it could be that the new intervention did not work for them. In any case, subject 'mortality' must be taken into account in the analysis and interpretation of data and should not be ignored.

The precise method of data analysis must also be described clearly and the findings stated unambiguously. To evaluate the validity and reliability of the findings, the factors identified in the previous section, such as history, instrumentation, selection and mortality effects, must be considered. Researchers must identify the limitations of their study. In practice, it is rare that experimenters do not suspect confounding variables of having interfered with the experiment. Therefore those who do not discuss the possible effects of confounders run the risk of taking their findings at face value. Finally, you must assess whether the findings, if valid and reliable, are applicable to your own clinical situation.

Systematic reviews of RCTs have revealed a number of deficiencies in the reporting of trials. Thornley and Adams (1998), in their review of 2000 trials on the Cochrane Schizophrenia Group's Register, found that 'the quality of reporting was poor and showed no sign of improvement over time'. Moher et al. (2001) commented that 'despite several decades of educational efforts, RCTs are still not being reported adequately'. The Consolidated Standards of Reporting Trials statement (CONSORT) was developed to help authors improve reporting by use of a checklist and flow diagram (see Moher et al., 2001).

A number of authors have also developed their own checklists for evaluating the quality of RCTs. These include Moher et al. (1995) and Sindhu et al. (1997).

SUMMARY

Summary and conclusion

In this chapter, we have explained the meaning of 'experiment' and identified the main characteristics of a true experiment as intervention, control and randomisation. Different types of design, such as between-subject, within-subject and single-case, have been highlighted, as have the main differences between true and quasi-experiments.

In nursing, the number of experiments remains low relative to other designs such as the survey or case study. Nonetheless, there are numerous examples of the valuable contribution of experiments to nursing practice.

We have shown that experiments have strengths and weaknesses, as do other approaches. The methodological problems and ethical implications can, to some extent, be managed. Together they do not merit the total rejection of the experiment as a research approach. Such an action would be tantamount to 'throwing out the baby with the bathwater' (Downs, 1988).

Quasi-experiments, RCTs and other research designs can all contribute towards the pool of nursing and human knowledge. The experiment does not deserve the mystique that often seems to surround it (McMahon, 1994), nor does it merit the indifference with which some researchers regard it.

References

Allen M, Knight C, Falk C and Strang V (1992) Effectiveness of a preoperative teaching programme for cataract patients. *Journal of Advanced Nursing*, 17:303–9.

Barnett A G, van der Pols J C and Dobson A J (2005) Regression to the mean: what it is and how to deal with it. *International Journal of Epidemiology*, 34, 1:215–20.

Beck S L (1989) The crossover design in clinical nursing research. *Nursing Research*, 38, 5:291–3.

Berg A, Hansson U W and Hallberg I R (1994) Nurses' creativity, tedium and burnout during 1 year of clinical supervision and implementation of individually planned nursing care: comparison between a ward for severely demented patients and a similar control ward. *Journal of Advanced Nursing*, 20:742–9.

Bithell C (1994) Single subject experimental design: a case for concern. *Physiotherapy*, 80, 2:85–7.

Bland J M (2004) Cluster randomised trials in the medical literature: two bibliometric surveys. *BMC Medical Research Methodology*, 4:21–7.

Bonell C (1999) Evidence-based nursing: a stereotyped view of quantitative and experimental research could work against professional autonomy and authority. *Journal of Advanced Nursing*, 30, 1:18–23.

Brennan P and Croft P (1994) Interpreting the results of observational research: chance is not such a fine thing. *British Medical Journal*, 309:727–30.

Britton A, McKee M, Black N, McPherson K, Sanderson C and Bain C (1999) Threats to applicability of randomising trials: exclusions and selective participation. *Journal of Health Services Research and Policy*, **2**:112–21.

Brooker C, Peters J, McCabe C and Short A J (1999) The views of nurses to the conduct of a randomized controlled trial of problem drinkers in an accident and emergency department. *International Journal of Nursing Studies*, **36**, 1:33–9.

Cartwright A (1988) *Health Surveys in Practice and in Potential* (London: King Edward's Hospital Fund for London).

Centre for Reviews and Dissemination (CRD) (2001) *Undertaking Systematic Reviews of Research on Effectiveness*, 2nd edn (University of York: CRD).

Closs S J and Cheater F M (1999) Evidence for nursing practice: a clarification of the issues. *Journal of Advanced Nursing*, **30**, 1:10–17.

Cochrane A L (1972) *Effectiveness and Efficiency: Random Reflections on Health Services* (London: The Nuffield Provincial Hospitals Trust).

Cook T D and Campbell D T (1979) *Quasi-Experimentation: Design and Analysis Issues in Field Settings* (Boston, MA: Houghton Mifflin).

Cross J and Tyson S F (2003) The effect of a slider shoe on hemiplegic gait. *Clinical Rehabilitation*, **17**:817–24.

Cullum N (1997) Identification and analysis of randomised controlled trials in nursing: a preliminary study. *Quality in Health Care*, **6**, 1:2–6.

Cupples M E and McKnight A (1994) Randomised controlled trial of health promotion in general practice for patients at high cardiovascular risk. *British Journal of Medicine*, **309**:993–6.

Dale A and Cornwell S (1994) The role of lavender oil in relieving perineal discomfort following childbirth: a blind randomized clinical trial. *Journal of Advanced Nursing*, **19**:89–96.

Dane F C (1990) *Research Methods* (Belmont, CA: Brooks/Cole).

Day L, Fildes B, Gordon I, Fitzharris M, Flamer H and Lord S (2002) Randomised factorial trial of falls prevention among older people living in their own homes. *British Medical Journal*, **325**:128–31.

Dennis M (1997) Commentary: why we didn't ask patients for their consent. *British Medical Journal*, **314**:1077.

DerSimonian R, Charette J L, McPeek B and Mosteller F (1982) Reporting methods in clinical trials. *New England Journal of Medicine*, **306**, 22:1332–7.

Downs F S (1988) Editorial: On babies and bathwater. *Nursing Research*, **37**, 1:3.

Dumas R (1987) Clinical trials in nursing. *Recent Advances in Nursing*, **17**:108–25.

Ellis K, Davies S and Laker S (2000) Attempting to set up a randomized controlled trial. *Nursing Standard*, **14**, 12:32–6.

Featherstone K and Donovan J L (1998) Random allocation or allocation at random? Patients' perspectives of participation in a randomized controlled trial. *British Medical Journal*, **317**:1177–80.

Fetter M S, Feetham S L, D'Apolito K et al. (1989) Randomized controlled trials: issues for researchers. *Nursing Research*, **38**, 2:117–20.

García de Lucio K, García López F J, Marín López M T, Mas Hesse B and Caamano Vaz M D (2000) Training programme in techniques of self-control and communication skills to improve nurses' relationships with relatives of seriously ill patients: a randomized controlled study. *Journal of Advanced Nursing*, **32**, 2:425–31.

Good M, Stanton-Hicks M, Grass J A, Anderson G C, Lai H-L, Roykulcharoen V and Adler P A (2001) Relaxation and music to reduce post-surgical pain. *Journal of Advanced Nursing*, **33**, 2:208–15.

Harvey S, Rach D, Stainton M C, Jarrell J and Brant R (2002) Evaluation of satisfaction with midwifery care. *Midwifery*, **18**, 4:260–7.

Homer C S E (2002) Using the Zelen design in randomized controlled trials: debates and controversies. *Journal of Advanced Nursing*, **38**, 2:200–207.

Kleijnen J, de Craen J M, Van Everdingen J, and Krol L (1994) Placebo effect in double-blind clinical trials: a review of interactions with medications. *Lancet*, **344**:1347–9.

Koh K, Ray R, Lee J, Nair A, Ho T and Ang P C (1994) Dementia in elderly patients: can the 3R Mental Stimulation Programme improve mental status? *Age and Ageing*, **23**:195–9.

Lindsay B (2004) Randomized controlled trials of socially complex nursing interventions: creating bias and unreliability? *Journal of Advanced Nursing*, **45**, 1:84–94.

Martin F, Ayewole A and Moloney A (1994) A randomized controlled trial of a high support hospital discharge team for elderly people. *Age and Ageing*, **23**:228–34.

McMahon R (1994) Trial and error: an experiment in practice. In: J Buckeldee and R McMahon, *The Research Experience in Nursing* (London: Chapman & Hall).

Medical Research Council (2000) *A Framework for Development and Evaluation of RCTs for Complex Interventions to Improve Health* (London: MRC).

Medical Research Council (2002) *Cluster Randomized Trials: Methodological and Ethical Considerations.* MRC Clinical Trials Series (London: MRC).

Meyer G, Warnke A, Bender R and Mühlhauser I (2003) Effect on hip fractures of increased use of hip protectors in nursing homes: a cluster randomised controlled trial. *British Medical Journal*, **326**:76.

Moher D, Jadad A R, Nichol G, Penman M, Tugwell P and Walsh S (1995) Assessing the quality of randomized controlled trials: an annotated bibliography of scales and checklists. *Controlled Clinical Trials*, **16**:62–73.

Moher D, Schultz K F and Altman D G (2001) The CONSORT statement: revised recommendations for improving the quality of reports of parallel-group randomized trials. *The Lancet*, **357**:1191–4.

Moore J (2001) No more tears: a randomized controlled double-blind trial of Amethocaine gel vs. placebo in the management of procedural pain in neonates. *Journal of Advanced Nursing*, **34**, 4:475–82.

Moore L, Campbell R, Whelan A, Mills N, Lupton P, Misselbrook E and Frohlich J (2002) Self help smoking cessation in pregnancy: cluster randomized controlled trial. *British Medical Journal*, **325**:1383–8.

Morton V and Torgerson D J (2003) Effect of regression to the mean on decision making in health care. *British Medical Journal*, **326**:1083–4.

Newell D J (1992) Randomised controlled trials in health care research. In: J Daly, I McDonald and E Willis (eds), *Researching Health Care* (London: Tavistock/Routledge).

Oldham J (1994) Experimental and quasi-experimental research designs. *Nurse Researcher*, 1, 4:26–36.

Passmore A P, Wilson Davies K W, Stoker C and Scott M E (1993) Chronic constipation in long-stay elderly patients: a comparison of lactulose and a senna–fibre combination. *British Medical Journal*, **307**:769–71.

Pearson L S and Hutton J L (2002) A controlled trial to compare the ability of foam swabs and toothbrushes to remove dental plaque. *Journal of Advanced Nursing*, **39**, 5:480–9.

Plant H, Bredin M, Krishnasamy M and Corner J (2000) Working with resistance, tension and objectivity: conducting a randomized controlled trial of a nursing intervention for breathlessness. *Nursing Times Research*, **5**, 6:426–36.

Pocock S (1983) *Clinical Trials: A Practical Approach* (Chichester: John Wiley & Sons).

Polit D and Hungler B (1983) *Nursing Research: Principles and Methods*, 2nd edn (Philadelphia: J B Lippincott).

Portsmouth K, Henderson K, Graham N, Price R, Cole J and Allen J (1994) Dietary calcium intake of 18-year old women: comparison with recommended daily intake and dietary energy intake. *Journal of Advanced Nursing*, **20**:1073–8.

Richards S C M and Scott D L (2002) Prescribed exercise in people with fibromyalgia: parallel group randomised controlled trial. *British Medical Journal*, **325**:185–7.

Riddoch J and Lennon S (1994) Single subject experimental design: one way forward. *Physiotherapy*, **80**, 4:215–18.

Robbins H, Hundley V and Osman L M (2003) Minor illness education for parents of young children. *Journal of Advanced Nursing*, **44**, 3:238–47.

Roland M and Togerson D J (1998) Understanding controlled trials. What are pragmatic trials? *British Medical Journal*, **316**:285.

Ross N (1999) Randomised block design is more powerful than minimisation. *British Medical Journal*, **318**:263.

Sagawa M, Oka M and Chaboyer W (2003) The utility of cognitive behavioural therapy on chronic patients' fluid intake: a preliminary examination. *International Journal of Nursing Studies*, **40**:367–73.

Selkowitz D M, Cameron M H, Mainzer A and Wolfe R (2002) Efficacy of pulsed low-intensity ultrasound in wound healing: a single-case design. *Osstomy Wound Management*, **48**, 4:40–50.

Shuldham C and Hiley C (1997) Randomised controlled trials in clinical practice: The continuing debate. *Nursing Times Research*, **2**, 2:128–34.

Silverman W A (1994) Patients' preferences and randomised trials. *Lancet*, **343**:1586.

Sim J (1991) Nursing research: is there an obligation on subjects to participate? *Journal of Advanced Nursing*, **16**, 11:1284–9.

Sindhu F, Carpenter L and Seers K (1997) Development of a tool to rate the quality assessment of randomized controlled trials using a Delphi technique. *Journal of Advanced Nursing*, **25**:1262–8.

Smith H W (1991) *Strategies of Social Research*, 3rd edn (St Louis, MO: Holt, Rinehart & Winston).

Thornley B and Adams C (1998) Content and quality of 2000 controlled trials in schizophrenia over 50 years. *British Medical Journal*, **317**:1181–4.

Torgerson D J and Roland M (1998) What is Zelen's design? *British Medical Journal*, **316**:606.

Webb C (2003) Research in Brief. An analysis of recent publications in JCN: sources, methods and topics. *Journal of Clinical Nursing*, **12**:931–4.

Webb C (2004) Editor's note: Analysis of papers published in JAN in 2002. *Journal of Advanced Nursing*, **45**, 3:229–31.

Weijer C, Chapior S H, Glass K C and Enkin M W (2000) Clinical equipoise and not the uncertainty principle is the moral underpinning of the randomized controlled trial. *British Medical Journal*, **321**:756–8.

Zelen M (1979) A new design for randomized controlled trials. *New England Journal of Medicine*, **300**:1242–5.

Zelen M (1990) Strategy and alternative designs for clinical trials: an update. *Statistics in Medicine*, **9**:645–56.

12 Samples and Sampling

Introduction

One of the important decisions in designing a study is what data to collect and from whom. When the study population is too large, as is often the case, researchers have to resort to strategies to obtain the same information from a smaller group of people. In this chapter, we will explore the meaning of samples, identify a number of sampling techniques and discuss their strengths and limitations. In particular, we will explore the use of samples in quantitative and qualitative research.

Samples and populations

One of the crucial tasks in designing a research project is to decide on the number and characteristics of the respondents who will be invited to take part in the study. It is not always possible to include the entire population in a study, not least because of the costs involved. Having more respondents means that researchers spend more time in collecting and analysing data, so the life span of the project itself is, therefore, increased. It is also easier to collect more, and in-depth, data from a smaller than a larger number of people. For these reasons, researchers sometimes select a proportion of the total number of potential respondents from whom to collect data. A proportion or subset of the population is known as the sample. A carefully selected sample can provide data representative of the population from which the sample is drawn.

A population can be defined as the total number of units from which data can potentially be collected. These units may be individuals, organisations, events or artefacts. In a study on the use of evidence by staff nurses in medical wards in the UK, all staff nurses (individuals) working in this type of ward in the UK constitute the population under study. If a study is to find out which types of dressing are used in surgical wards in a particular health district, the population is all surgical wards (organisations) in that district. All the dressings would also constitute a population of artefacts. In a study of psychiatric patients' aggressive behaviour at meal times over a period of three months in one hospital, all the meal times (events) during the three-month period make up the population. And in a historical study of how nurses were portrayed in newspapers in the nineteenth century, all the newspapers (artefacts) during this period make up the population. In layman's language, 'population' is mainly used to describe people, but in research terms it has a wider meaning. For the purpose of this chapter, the individuals, organisations, events and artefacts that make up a population will be referred to as 'units'. It is sometimes important to use the entire units of a population in a study. For example, the decennial Census of Population, undertaken by the Office of National Statistics, comprises data from all households in the UK.

In theory, all the units of a population (also called the theoretical population), could potentially take part in a study, but in practice this may not be possible for various reasons. A researcher asking questions of patients with Alzheimer's disease in a ward will quickly realise that not all patients are able to take part. She may decide to include only those who are at an early stage of the disease. Additionally, she may exclude those who are restless and aggressive. In stipulating the inclusion criteria (early stage of disease) and exclusion criteria (restlessness and aggressive behaviour), the researcher has defined the target population, that is, the population to be studied or, as it is commonly referred to, the study population.

The target population is, therefore, the group which a researcher aims to draw a sample from. This population or group is defined by taking into account how they can be accessed and who can realistically take place.

The units of a population are never totally homogeneous (i.e. sharing the same characteristics). Although all staff nurses in medical wards work in the same type of clinical setting, they are not a homogeneous group because they differ in such variables as age, gender, years of experience or qualifications. Depending on the research question and the resources, the researcher may want to include only full-time day staff nurses with three years' experience and may exclude those who are educated at graduate level. In practice, researchers must have good reasons for including and/or excluding units of population and must also clearly define these criteria. For example, 'patients in the early stages of Alzheimer's disease' needs to be operationally defined.

The target population, once defined, becomes the population of interest from whom the data can potentially be collected. In fact, the target population is a subset of the theoretical population. Sometimes all the units in the target population are included in the study, but more often a sample or subset of the target population is selected. When this happens, it is to the target population rather than the theoretical population that generalisations may be made.

In a study of 'postoperative pain', MacLellan (2004) used the following inclusion criteria to define her population: gynaecological, orthopaedic, urological and general surgical patients on the planned theatre lists of two selected hospitals. The exclusion criteria were: patients 'admitted to the intensive care unit or high dependency unit, confused, unable to use a 10-cm Visual Analogue Scale (VAS) or did not consent' (MacLellan, 2004). Therefore her findings are generalisable to those who match the characteristics of participants included in this study. To maximise the generalisability of research findings, researchers should, as much as possible, be as inclusive as possible.

Sample frame

A list of all the units of the target population provides the frame from which a sample (if required) is selected. Therefore the sample frame contains the same number of units as the target population. There are some ready-made sample frames. For example, if a researcher decides to explore the learning styles of current nursing undergraduates at one university, the sample frame would be a list of the names of all nursing undergraduates who are currently studying there. The researcher would simply cross out the names of those who did not meet the inclusion criteria. Examples of ready-made lists that may potentially be used as sample frames are the Nursing and Medical Council (NMC) register, the general practitioner's list of patients and the post-code address file. Sometimes two or three lists may be combined to form a sample frame. For example, in Woodcock et al.'s (1994) study of 'planned home and hospital births in Western Australia [WA] 1981–1987', the cohort of all WA planned, singleton home births 'was identified from the Midwives' Notification System, together with midwives' home birth records and Health Department of WA Transfer forms'. These three lists were combined to provide a sample frame from which samples were selected. There are some drawbacks in using existing registers or lists as they may be incomplete, biased or not up to date.

It is not always possible or desirable to construct sample frames. For studies on sensitive issues such as sexually transmitted diseases, drug addiction or crime, ready-made lists are, understandably, not available. Participants are often recruited by means of newspaper adverts and newsletters, from support groups or by word of mouth. Sample frames are necessary when the researcher seeks to draw representative samples and thereafter to generalise from the data. It is important to note, however, that in qualitative research the concept of generalisation has a different meaning than it does in quantitative research, and that sample frames are rarely used by qualitative researchers. This will be discussed later on in this chapter.

Selected and achieved samples

A sample is defined as a subset of the target population. When all the units of the target population cannot be studied, the researcher may decide to select a small proportion of this population from whom to collect data. The selection method or procedure is called sampling. The most common example of the use of samples is in the opinion polls taken prior to elections. A sample of potential voters is carefully selected whose views, the pollsters believe, would represent those of the rest of the voting population.

The units in the sample selected by the researcher are the ones invited to take part in the study. However, not everyone invited is available, willing or able to take part, although the researcher will have laid down inclusion and exclusion criteria. People change addresses and cannot be traced; others are too busy or are uninterested. Whatever the reasons, the selected sample, through non-participation or through non- or part-completion of questionnaires or other tools, loses some units and becomes the achieved sample. Although the achieved sample is normally smaller than the selected sample, some researchers may exceptionally decide to replace units in the original sample that did not take part by other units from the target population. Research Example 32 shows one instance of how a selected sample was reduced to an achieved sample.

Types of sample

There are two basic types of sample:

- probability
- non-probability.

In a probability sample, every unit in the target population has a more than zero chance (usually known in advance by the researcher) of being selected. For example, if a sample of 10 students is to be selected from a target population of 50, each student will have a 1 in 5 or 20 per cent chance of being selected. In probability samples, the chance of selection for each unit is known in advance.

The main characteristic of a probability sample is that it is randomly selected from the target population. The term 'random', in the layman's sense, usually means haphazard, as when an interviewer picks out people as they come out of a doctor's surgery. Those who look approachable to the interviewer or those who do not seem to be in a hurry may be chosen. Apart from being subjective, this method of sampling has no sample frame. Therefore the chances of all those attending surgery on that particular day, of being selected, is not known. In research terms, the random selection of units for a sample is carried out according to a specified objective method, such as giving each unit a number, putting all the numbers in a box and picking out blindly one number at a time until the required size of the sample is drawn (there are more 'scientific ways' to do this, as explained below). The aim, in quantitative research, is to select a sample representative of the target population.

Non-probability samples are made up of units whose chances of selection are not known in advance. In the example of people leaving a doctor's surgery, those who were available before the researcher arrived had a zero chance of selection, whereas the chances (of being selected) of those who were interviewed are not known, as the potential number of all those who could have been interviewed is also not known.

Qualitative researchers often use non-probability samples because, according

RESEARCH EXAMPLE 32

Complementary therapy practice: defining the role of advanced nurse practitioners
Patterson et al. (2003)

Sample frame
Selected sample
Achieved sample

Patterson et al. (2003) surveyed a sample of advanced nurse practitioners about their role and their learning needs relating to complementary therapy practice. These nurses were selected from the register of the College of Nurses of Ontario.

Comments:

1 The College of Nurses of Ontario kept a list of nurses 'who indicated that they were employed in direct patient care as a nurse practitioner, clinical nurse specialist or nurse educator during the year 2001'. This list constituted the *sample frame* from which random samples can be selected.

2 In 2001, there were 889 on this list and 738 met the inclusion criteria set by the researchers. A random sample of 402 was selected from this population for participation in this study. Thirteen people 'were ineligible because of retirement, being a student or they were no longer at the designated address'. The remaining 389 were therefore the *selected sample*.

3 Out of the selected sample, 215 returned 'usable questionnaires', giving a response rate of 55.3% ([215 ÷ 389] × 100). The *achieved sample* was therefore 215.
   The response rate is the percentage of the selected sample that actually takes part in the study. It is calculated as follows:

$$\text{Response rate} = \frac{\text{Achieved sample}}{\text{Selected sample}} \times 100$$

Example: If the achieved sample numbered 45 and the selected sample 60, the response rate is:

$$\frac{45}{60} \times 100 = 75\%$$

to them, the purpose of qualitative research is to contribute to an understanding of phenomena. They therefore choose the sample which can best provide the required data, whatever the sampling method is. In fact, qualitative researchers sometimes substitute the term 'sampling' by 'recruitment'. The use and nature of samples in qualitative research is further discussed in a later section.

If the purpose of the study is to examine relationships between variables and make generalisations then a probability sample is preferred. On the other hand, if the purpose is to explore phenomena in depth, researchers need to ensure that the sample has experience and/or views that can be useful in achieving this objective. The emphasis is less on representation and more on what they can contribute. Other factors that researchers take into consideration include the availability of, and access to, potential participants and the resources allocated to the study. In quantitative research, decisions about samples and sampling are not taken after the research question and the methods of data collection are known: all three must be considered at the same time as they depend on each other. Sampling also has implications for the analysis of data. For example, inferential statistics (see Chapter 16) are based on the assumption that random samples of populations have been used to generate data (Williamson, 2003). Watson (2004), for example, explained that inferential statistics 'can apply to a convenience sample but any claims should be attenuated by warnings about the extent to which the results may be generalised'.

In qualitative research, the researcher is a tool of data collection and analysis. As Walker (1985) explains, 'decisions regarding the composition of the sample for a qualitative study emerge from the objectives and are modified by considerations governing choice of method and the scope of the study'. According to the author, 'the rigorous sampling procedures used in quantitative research are inappropriate to the nature and scale of qualitative work'. Decisions about samples and the sampling method can be taken both prior to and during the data collection stage.

Types of probability sample

There are four types of probability sample:

- simple random
- stratified random
- systematic random
- cluster random.

Each of these sampling procedures requires a sample frame before a random selection can be drawn.

Simple random sample

The most common form of random sampling is one in which each unit in the sample frame is given a number; these are then put into the proverbial hat and numbers are drawn one at a time until the size of sample, specified in advance, is reached. Each unit has an equal chance of being selected. Simple random sampling is so called because once a number is given to each unit, it then takes only one step: picking numbers. Once a number is taken out of the hat, the chances of those remaining are altered from what they were at the start of the process. For example, if a researcher decides to draw a sample of 10 from a population of 50, the chance of selection of each unit at the start of the operation is 1 in 5. After 5 units have been selected, the chance of each of the 45 units remaining in the hat being selected is altered to 1 in 9.

Simple random sampling is mostly suitable for a population that is more or less homogeneous and from which any sample drawn is unlikely to be seriously biased. An example of a homogeneous sample can be found in a study of undergraduates by Ashley (1994). The sample, consisting of 125 students,

> was homogeneous with regard to age, race and gender. The sample ranged in age from 21 to 23 years. All respondents were female and 98% of the sample was white.

However, when the population has varied characteristics (i.e. is heterogeneous), it may be unwise to rely on simple random sampling to obtain a representative sample possessing the main variables being studied.

Stratified random sample

When the sample frame contains units that vary greatly in variables such as age, gender, education, experience or illness condition, it is possible that simple random sampling may not be the most appropriate form of sampling in order to achieve representation. If one or more of these variables are important for the study, it is wise not to trust the selection process to chance. There are reasons why variables should sometimes be assured of representation. For example, some illness conditions are more prevalent in one gender than another. Myocardial infarction is more common in men and breast cancer in women. Any sample of patients with either condition must be stratified if gender representation is important for the study. Stratified random sampling consists of separating the units in the sample frame in strata (layers) according to the variables the researcher believes are important for inclusion in the sample, and drawing a sample from each stratum using the simple random sampling method.

For example, in a study of student nurses' satisfaction with support from lecturers, if the sample frame of 150 students comprises the following: 75 year 1 students, 45 year 2 students and 30 year 3 students, the researcher must seek the views of students of each of these three groups if the findings are to be generalised to the target population. A simple random sample may by chance under- or overrepresent one or more of these groups, or may not even include any representative of one of the smaller groups. To ensure representation, the sample frame of 150 students is divided into its year-group composition before a proportionate sample from each group is drawn. The sampling method involves three steps as follows:

Step 1 Stratify the sample frame into its constituent group
 e.g. Year 1 students: 75 (50%)
   Year 2 students: 45 (30%)
   Year 3 students: 30 (20%)

Step 2 Decide on a sample size and the proportion for each stratum
 e.g. Total sample size required = 50
   Sample size of Year 1 = 50% of 50 = 25
   Sample size of Year 2 = 30% of 50 = 15
   Sample size of Year 3 = 20% of 50 = 10

Step 3 Draw a simple random sample of the required size from each stratum
 e.g. Year 1 students = 25 out of 75
   Year 2 students = 15 out of 45
   Year 3 students = 10 out of 30

In this example, a proportionate stratified random sample of each stratum was drawn. This means that each unit from each of the strata had the same chance of selection (1 in 3). However, if the size of the Year 3 sample is not large enough to represent the views of the students, the researcher may decide to increase the size of this sample in order to increase their representation. The sample then becomes a disproportionate stratified random sample.

If gender as a variable is also important for this study, the sample frame would have to be stratified into male students and female students before a proportionate or disproportionate random sample could be drawn from each stratum. The heterogeneity of the target population is not in itself the only reason for stratification. The decision to stratify depends on the research question and the variables of interest to the researcher. Research Example 33 examines a study where stratified random sampling was used.

Systematic random sample

Systematic samples are drawn by choosing units on a list at intervals prescribed by the researcher in advance. The most basic system is choosing every nth number on a list until the required sample size is reached. A researcher may decide to interview the occupants of every third house on a street to find out about their health beliefs, or a teacher may pick out every fifth student on the register to ask about their views on the organisation and delivery of the course.

For a systematic random sample to be drawn, there must be a sample frame and every unit on the frame must have a chance of being selected. If a systematic random sample of 10 is to be drawn from a sample frame of 50, every 5th

RESEARCH EXAMPLE 33

Information provided to patients undergoing
gastroscopy procedures   *Thompson et al. (2003)*

Stratified random sampling

The aim of this study was to investigate the information given by nurses to patients prior to a gastroscopy investigation. Eighteen acute hospitals (six major and 12 minor) offered this service. Since it was not possible to survey the total population of nurses involved in giving this information, it was important to select a sample which was representative of those working in the major and the minor hospitals.

A multi-stage sampling strategy was used. It was decided to carry out a stratified random sample of the hospitals first. Using a simple random selection procedure, three out of six major hospitals and six of the 12 minor hospitals were invited to take part in the study.

All registered nurses working in wards offering gastroscopy procedure in the selected hospitals were asked to complete a questionnaire.

Comments:

1   In this example, hospitals rather than individuals were stratified.

2   If a simple random sample of all 18 hospitals were carried out, it is possible, given the small numbers, that the final sample may not have been representative of both major and minor hospitals.

number (50 divided by 10) on the list is chosen. To avoid starting with number 1 each time, the researcher can pick a number at random between 1 and 5 and proceed to choose every fifth number from it. Say number 4 is picked at random as the starting number, every fifth number (9, 14, 19, 24, 29, 34, 39, 44, 49) will be selected until a sample size of 10 (including the starting number, 4) is obtained. One of the limitations of this type of sampling is that lists may have biases of their own. It is possible that every fifth name on a list is male and that they could by chance be selected, therefore creating a gender bias in the sample.

The sample frame could also have patterns or trends. For example, at weekends (especially on Friday and Saturday nights) people may attend Accident and Emergency (A&E) units for different accidents or injuries than during weekdays. A chronological list of patients, in this case, may contain what is known as a 'periodic' or 'cyclical' trend. A researcher using the A&E list of patients as a frame to draw a systematic random sample may, by chance, pick a disproportionate number of weekenders.

One way to offset this drawback is to rearrange the names on the list and

A methodology for sampling and accessing homeless individuals in Melbourne, 1995–96   *Reid et al. (1998)*

Systematic sampling

After constructing a list of accommodation places for homeless people, the researchers decided to use a systematic random technique to select approximately 400 participants. The sample frame consisted of 13,482 beds.

They explained that:

by drawing on the 13,482 listed beds and a randomly selected starting point, the calculated sampling interval of every 34th bed was applied to identify the bed's associated establishment.

Comment:

1   The figure 34 was obtained by dividing the sample frame by 400. This strategy produced a sample of 396 (13,482 divided by 34).

therefore break any periodic cycles it may contain. A systematic random sample will not be random unless the sampling frame is first put into random order. Research Example 34 illustrates the use of systematic sampling.

Cluster random sample

A cluster is defined in the *Oxford Dictionary* as 'a group of similar things'. Sometimes the units of a study population are already in the form of clusters. For example, each district has a number of hospitals. Each hospital is a cluster of health professionals, and within hospitals each ward is also a cluster of nurses. When the population already exists in clusters, it is sometimes more practical and cost-efficient to sample the clusters first and then sample the units from the selected clusters.

Suppose that the aim of our study is to find out the knowledge of, and attitude to, primary nursing among nurses in general hospitals in Wales. A simple random sampling will involve listing all staff nurses working in all the general hospitals in the country. When the sample frame is ready and a simple random sample of staff nurses is drawn, it is possible that some hospitals will be over-represented and others underrepresented. Researchers may have to travel to hospitals where two or three nurses have been selected. The whole exercise can be demanding, time-consuming and costly. A stratified random sample would ensure that each hospital is proportionately represented in the sample, but the cost of compiling a sample frame and travelling to all the hospitals can still be enormous. However, stratified random sampling is necessary if the purpose is to study differences between hospitals. Cluster random sampling, on the other hand, involves randomly sampling the hospitals before drawing a random sample of nurses from each of the selected hospitals or using the whole population of the randomly selected hospitals. In the above example, if there are 20 general hospitals, a cluster random sample of eight hospitals could be drawn. Thereafter, a simple random sample can be drawn from a list of nurses in the selected hospitals. This type of sampling is known as multi-stage, as it often involves more than one stage. In doing so, a more in-depth study can also be carried out with less cost. Cluster random sampling is appropriate when the clusters are more or less homogeneous and when the final number of clusters selected is not small. For example, choosing a random sample of two hospitals out of ten may decrease the viability of generalising the findings to the ten hospitals. Therefore cost alone should not be the deciding factor in choosing this type of sampling.

A combination of stratified and cluster sampling can also be used. In the above example, if psychiatric, mental handicap and geriatric as well as general hospitals were included in the study, these hospitals could be divided into strata representing each specialty before a cluster random sample of each stratum was drawn.

Cluster random sampling is also called multi-stage sampling because it can involve many stages. The use of cluster sampling is illustrated in Research Example 35. For a detailed and insightful example of multi-stage sampling involving cluster, stratified and simple random sampling see Marsland and Murrells (2000).

Types of non-probability sample

There are five types of non-probability sample, which can be divided into two broad and overlapping categories: purposive or judgemental, and convenience. The first involves judgement and choice on the part of the researcher, thereby giving her a degree of control over the composition of the sample. With convenience sampling, on the other hand, the researcher chooses according to who or what is available. In practice, this distinction is not rigid since both may involve a degree of judgement and convenience.

The five types of non-probability sample are:

- accidental

- purposive

- volunteer

- snowball

- quota

Innovation adoption behaviour among nurses

Coyle and Sokop (1990)

Cluster sampling

'Ten hospitals were randomly selected from the American Hospital Association listing of all medium-sized hospitals (250–500 beds) in North Carolina. Due to the mixed reports on the effect of organisational size on innovation adoption . . . only medium-sized hospitals were included in this study in order to control for this variable. Two hundred registered nurses, 20 from each institution, were randomly selected from lists provided by Directors of Nursing in each of the participating hospitals. To be included in the study, the nurses had to be employed full-time on the day, evening, or rotating night shift, with direct patient care responsibilities on adult medical-surgical or intensive care units.'

Comments:

1 The sample frame is the American Hospital Association (AHA) listing of all medium-sized hospitals. A cluster sampling of these hospitals was carried out. The researchers did not, however, state from how many hospitals the sample of ten was drawn.

2 The size of the selected sample of registered nurses was 200 (20 from each of the ten hospitals). If the same size of sample were to be drawn from more than ten hospitals, that is, from the total number of hospitals in the AHA list, it is clear that the number of nurses selected from each hospital could have been very small indeed.

3 To ensure representation of all ten hospitals, the authors carried out stratified random sampling to select 20 nurses from each hospital.

Accidental sampling

In accidental samples, only those available have a chance of being selected. Interviewing shoppers outside a supermarket on their health beliefs is one way to select an accidental sample. Only those visiting the supermarket at that time and on that day will have a chance of being selected. In this type of sampling, there is no sample frame.

There are occasions when accidental sampling is appropriate. For example, if a researcher wants to find out the patients' views on the information they receive on admission to hospital, she may decide to interview the first 50 consecutive patients following admission. She does not have a sample frame as she does not know who will be admitted. No one outside the first 50 patients will have a chance of selection. By accident, the sample may comprise mostly those with minor problems or of a particular social class.

Accidental sampling can have implications for the data. For example, waiting at street corners to interview people about satisfaction with health services in the area could mean that only pedestrians will be chosen. Those who have cars, and who may perhaps be more affluent, may be excluded. With accidental sampling, there is degree of subjectivity involved in the selection, as the researcher does not always choose everyone who happens to be available.

Purposive or purposeful sampling

This method of sampling, used mainly but not exclusively in qualitative research, involves the researcher deliberately choosing who to include in the study on the basis that those selected can provide the necessary data. Thus if she wants to investigate the leadership styles of hospital general managers, she can deliberately choose (hand-pick) managers with different styles in order to study the concept of leadership from different perspectives. For this, she may have to rely on her own judgement and/or that of those she believes can help her to make the choice. In this study, generalising the findings to the target population of managers is not the main concern of the researcher. Instead, she is seeking to contribute to the understanding of leadership styles. The sample is deliberately chosen by the researcher on the basis that these are the best available people to provide data on the issues being researched.

In choosing a purposive sample, the researcher must be guided by her research question and not be tempted to choose samples out of convenience or leave it to others to make the selection. The use of purposive samples in qualitative research is discussed further in this chapter. Research Example 36 shows the use of purposive sampling.

Volunteer sampling

Perhaps the weakest form of sampling is one in which people volunteer to take part and are therefore self-selected. It is a sample of convenience over which the researcher has little control, instead being dependent on the sample volunteering to take part. There are two categories of volunteer. Firstly, there are those who offer to take part in a study before coming into contact with the researcher or her associates. An example of this is when people respond to a notice board or newspaper advert asking for subjects to take part in a study (see Gagliardi [2003] for an example of a recruitment advertisement for volunteers). The researcher exerts little or no influence on the prospective subject except perhaps when financial or other inducements are offered. The second type of volunteer is those who are part of a captive population, either as patients in a hospital or students on a course. It is more difficult to know whether these groups really volunteer and whether their actions are what van Wissen and Siebers (1993)

The assumption of caregiving: grandmothers raising the children of the crack cocaine epidemic

Roe et al. (1994)

Purposive, volunteer and snowball sampling

The community advisory group played a central role in the construction of a rich and varied sample. Initial sampling identified differences in caregiving experience based on age, number of dependent grandchildren, sources of financial support, marital status and social support. Later sampling enabled comparisons based on factors such as employment, health status and additional caregiving responsibilities.

  Potential respondents were identified through health and social service providers, a dense network of community contacts, an invitational flyer, and snowball referrals from study participants. The latter two strategies were particularly effective in finding women who were without telephones, were not well connected to health and social services, and were in other ways likely to be overlooked by more traditional sampling methods.

Comments:

1   This is an example of the use of flexible sampling methods, which is common in qualitative research.

2   The use of purposive or judgemental sampling is indicated by the involvement of the community advisory group in sample selection. A judgement had to be made by the researchers and the group on who to select.

3   The 'invitational flyer' was used to recruit volunteers to the project.

4   Snowball sampling was resorted to in order to recruit women who were 'likely to be overlooked by the more traditional sampling methods', which depend greatly on the existence of lists or records.

term 'uncoerced voluntary participation'. How 'voluntary' this type of participation is in reality is the question that the researcher and the readers of the subsequent report or article must ask. There are a number of reasons why a captive population may 'volunteer' to take part in a study:

● moral obligation – they may feel that the research will be of benefit to other patients;

● gratitude – in return for the care they receive;

- fear of reprisals – if they refuse they think they may be punished;

- fear of being labelled as uncooperative;

- the need to conform.

For these reasons, the validity of the data could be seriously questioned, especially if, in addition, the volunteer may not trust the confidentiality and anonymity of the data.

Volunteering is itself an act of cooperation and reflects the personality of those more likely to volunteer. They may be conformists and traditional in outlook and could thus bias the sample. Those who are self-selected may show more interest and motivation than those who do not. Therefore volunteer samples are limited because we know little or nothing of those who do not take part in the study. Research Example 36 (above) shows how volunteers were recruited in one study.

Snowball sampling

In simple terms, this means that a respondent refers someone they know to the study, who in turn refers someone they know, until the researcher has an adequate sample. Sometimes it is difficult for the researcher to identify people who could take part in a study because of the sensitivity of the topic or because the researcher may not have ready access to a sample. For a sample of drug takers or petty criminals, the researcher may depend on initial contacts to direct them to others who may be willing to take part. However, snowball sampling is not used exclusively when sensitive topics are being researched or when potential participants are scarce. In qualitative research, the number of units in the sample is often not decided in advance. As the fieldwork progresses, the researcher may come across other potentially useful participants and enlist them as she goes along. One of the major drawbacks of snowball samples is that participants may refer people of similar backgrounds and outlook to themselves. Walker (1985) warns against the indiscriminate use of snowball sampling:

> Interviewers must not recruit their friends; nor as a rule are they allowed to 'snowball', i.e. to use people already recruited as a source of other people to approach as this would lead to groups in which participants know each other and are likely to have similar views.

Ehlers et al. (2001) acknowledge the difficulties in obtaining a sample frame for their study of the 'well-being of gays, lesbians and bisexuals (GLBs) in Botswana'. They explain how they obtained their sample using the snowball technique:

The consultants hand-picked GLB respondents and handed at least two questionnaires to each one. In this way each known GLB could complete one
questionnaire and hand another questionnaire to another GLB known to
him/her. This process of 'snow-ball' sampling was continued until 100 questionnaires had been handed out. The respondents, comprising the hidden
GLB population in Botswana, could not be reached in any other way.

The use of snowball sampling is shown in Research Example 36.

Quota sampling

Quota sampling involves elements of purposive and stratified sampling without random selection. In this type of sampling, the researcher recognises the
need for different groups in the sample to be adequately represented. In a
survey of students' views on the resources and support they receive in a nursing department of a university, there are a number of groups that should be
represented in the sample. These could include full-time and part-time
students, students on all the courses offered, school leavers and mature
students, and males and females. Thus the researcher may allocate 20 to each
group. Depending on the aim of the research, proportionate or non-propor-
tionate samples can be used. In accidental sampling, it is left to chance who is
included in the sample. In quota sampling, the researcher allocates places in
advance.

Quota sampling involves two stages. In the first stage, the quota allocation is
decided. For example, in a study of nurses' attitude to primary nursing, 20
places could be allocated to each of the following grades of nurses – C, D, E, F
and G – making a total of 100 nurses. Or the researcher could allocate the 100
places according to the proportion of each grade. The second stage involves
selecting the sample. If there is a sample frame of nurses and a random sample
of 20 in each grade is drawn, the quota sampling becomes a stratified random
sampling, or after deciding on quotas, the researcher can purposefully choose 20
nurses whom she believes will provide the data for the project. She can also wait
at the exit of the nurses' canteen and interview those who are available until the
quota for each of the grades is met.

In quota sampling, the overriding concern of the researcher is to have various elements represented. However, the sampling procedure remains a non-
probability one because there is no recourse to random selection. In the above
study, while the researcher is interested to find out the views of nurses in each
grade, these nurses would not necessarily be representative of the rest of the
nurses in the hospital mainly because no random sampling was effected. The
study by Roe and May (1999), outlined in Research Example 37, makes use of
quota sampling to achieve its objectives.

It is not unusual for a researcher to use a mixture of sampling methods.
Research Example 36 shows three types of sampling in the same study.

Incontinence and sexuality: findings from a qualitative perspective
Roe and May (1999)

Quota sampling

As the author explains:

> the objectives were to explore the impact of incontinence on an individual's sexuality and to identify the impact of health interventions for the management of incontinence on sexuality.

Comments:

1 This paper reports the qualitative findings of a larger project which evaluated the health interventions by primary health care teams and continence advisory services on patient outcomes related to incontinence.

2 The researchers explored the impact of effective as well as ineffective interventions. Therefore it was important that their sample reflected this choice. As they explain:

> A quota sample of subjects whose incontinence was regarded as being either successfully managed ($n = 14$) or unsuccessfully managed ($n = 12$) by continence advisers, community nurses and health visitors for the NHS Trusts were interviewed.

3 By using a quota sampling method (rather than leaving it to chance) the researchers ensured that the views of both groups were taken into account.

Sampling in quantitative research

It is generally believed that, in quantitative research, the samples are large and probability sampling is frequent, while qualitative researchers use small, non-probability samples. Although this is a fair description as far as sample size is concerned, it is not unusual to observe from research journals that many quantitative researchers use convenience samples and some qualitative ones resort to random selection. Convenience samples are probably the most frequently used of all types of sample in both types of research. Webb (2003) reviewed all papers published in 2001 and 2002 in the *Journal of Clinical Nursing*. She concluded that the vast majority of quantitative and qualitative studies used convenience samples. When Webb (2004) did a similar exercise for all 256 papers published in the *Journal of Advanced Nursing* throughout 2002, she found that 'virtually all the empirical studies were based on convenience samples'. Cowman and Conroy (2004) explain that in real-life research sample frames are rarely available, and as a result 'non-random samples are therefore the rule rather than the exception'.

In quantitative research, the data from randomly selected samples are generalised to the target population and sometimes beyond, to similar populations and settings. The purpose of research is not only to study the specific but to draw general principles and conclusions in order to apply them to similar situations outside the particular population and setting being studied.

Sampling in qualitative research

Qualitative researchers believe that the phenomena they study are culture specific and time-bound, and that their findings are a result of the interaction between the researcher and the researched. This means that although the same phenomena may exist in other cultures, they are often manifested and experienced differently in different cultures or settings. Also since the findings were obtained at a specific point in time (i.e. time-bound), the study cannot be replicated and the findings are not necessarily generalisable to other settings. Therefore sampling for the purpose of generalising to other populations and settings is normally not the prime reason for researchers in the qualitative tradition, although, as Schofield (1993) pointed out, 'a consensus appears to be emerging that for qualitative researchers generalisability is best thought of as a matter of the "fit" between the situation studied and others to which one might be interested in applying the concepts and conclusions of that study'.

Stake's (1978) notion of 'naturalistic generalisation', which involves the use of the findings of one study in order to understand similar situations, is a useful one. For the findings of qualitative research to have wider implications than for the specific population and setting they emerged from, there is a need to study the 'typical' instead of the 'unusual' (Schofield, 1993).

There is a great deal of overlap and confusion in the way researchers describe their sampling strategies in qualitative research. Terms such as 'purposive' and 'theoretical' sampling are often used interchangeably (Coyne, 1997). There is a need to understand the differences and similarities between them and the purpose for which they can be used.

In a broad sense all qualitative sampling methods can be described as 'selective' since they involve the subjective judgement of the researcher in the selection process. Beyond this, there are different types of selective samples including, among others, purposive and theoretical sampling. A cursory examination of qualitative and mix-method studies in the literature shows at least four different ways in which researchers sample their participants.

In some studies the researcher selects among accessible and consenting participants those who can, in her judgement, contribute most towards understanding the phenomenon under investigation. The emphasis is on obtaining different perspectives from participants so that the phenomenon can be revealed in all its dimensions and facets. It is helpful therefore to select those who can offer insights into the phenomenon by virtue of having some experience or views about it. Particular attention is paid to those who hold different, conflicting or contradictory views, even if those individuals are not representative of the population or group to which they belong. Demographic characteristics such as gender, age, occupation, status or education are often taken into account, as people with different attributes may have different views. This type of sample can be called purposive since participants are selected on purpose because they have enough experience and abilities to answer the research question. One can say that all samples are purposive because researchers always choose people who can answer the question (e.g. they would ask mothers about the experience of giving birth, not fathers). The difference between this and purposive sampling in qualitative research is that in the latter the researcher chooses on purpose those who have different characteristics and different contributions to make, while in the former this is left to chance.

Purposive samples are frequently used in phenomenological studies. The size of sample and the individuals selected are decided upon at the start of the study. It is possible to increase the size of the sample if not enough data are forthcoming, or stop sampling if the same data are being repeated.

Larsson et al. (2003) describe how they selected their sample in their phenomenological study of 'lived experiences of eating problems for patients with head and neck cancer during radiotherapy':

> The informants were undergoing radiotherapy for head and neck cancer at two oncology clinics in Sweden. The inclusion criterion was that informants were expected to experience eating problems because of side-effects of radiotherapy. In order to achieve a broad description as possible of the phenomenon under study, they were chosen to represent different categories of gender, age and civil status.

Another frequently used procedure in qualitative research is 'theoretical sampling'. The term comes from Glaser and Strauss (1967) and is mainly used in grounded theory studies. Strauss and Corbin (1998) define it as

> data gathering by concepts derived from the evolving theory and based on the concept of 'making comparisons', whose purpose is to go to places, people or events that will maximise opportunities to discover variations among concepts . . .

The essential feature of theoretical sampling is that the researcher does not know, in advance, who to interview or observe. As data are analysed, the emerging ideas (which need to be further explored) guide the researcher in her choice of other people (or documents or events) to collect data from. In McCaughan's

(2002) study of 'information needs and information seeking behaviour of newly diagnosed cancer patients', one of the emerging ideas from data collected at the beginning of the study was patients' frequent use of lay sources. It was important that she followed up these sources (faith healer, hairdresser etc.) in order to understand the behaviour of these patients. Prior to the study, McCaughan (2002) did not intend to include these lay sources in her sample nor did she anticipate that she might have to.

As can be seen from the above example, data collected and analysed at the beginning of a grounded theory study guide further selection of participants. Researchers using a grounded theory approach therefore need an initial sample to start with. They normally resort to a small purposive sample and thereafter use theoretical sampling. This tends to cause problems when they apply for funding, because they cannot state in advance all the sources of data which they will eventually use.

In ethnographic studies, the concept of samples and sampling have different meanings from these two types (purposive and theoretical) described above. This is mainly because ethnographic studies involve spending prolonged periods in particular settings. The number of people with whom the researcher comes into contact and the varying contributions which they make are not easily quantified or even described. The term 'key informants' refers to people whom the ethnographer relies upon for providing information and insights, and access to other people, events and artefacts (such as documents or other evidence). Everyone in the setting and any other source of information (within practical, legal and ethical limits) are potentially useful in providing data. Researchers have to convey this in their publications, as well as the reason for selecting the setting where the study is carried out.

Finally, in mix-methods studies, researchers may want to confirm the findings of a questionnaire by means of qualitative interviews. They may select a random sample of respondents in order to obtain representative views. However, if the purpose of selecting a representative (random) sample in this case is to generalise to the target population, one should remember that generalisability depends not only on random selection but on other factors such as predetermined, objective, structured and standardised methods of data collection and analysis.

To some extent, overlap and confusion in the use and description of qualitative sampling methods are inevitable because the different techniques share some of the same characteristics, such as subjective judgement in selecting participants, flexibility to increase the sample to learn more about a phenomenon or to stop when no new ideas are emerging. There is also scope to interview or observe the same participant on more than one occasion. However, one should also understand the differences between different types of sampling and the purpose, process and implications of using them. Coyne (1997) explains that 'distinctions between sampling strategies may be helpful for the neophyte researcher, but conforming to those arbitrary distinctions may not be helpful for the purpose of the qualitative study'. It is less important for researchers to name the type of sampling used correctly than to explain precisely how the sample was selected, the reasons for their decisions and the implications for the findings. For further discussions of sampling in qualitative research see Coyne (1997) and Thompson (1999).

Critiquing samples and sampling

Although qualitative researchers may not claim that their data are generalisable to other settings, it is important for them to describe their samples and sampling method adequately for the reader to assess whether they are useful to other settings. Smith (1994) analysed all research articles published in the *Journal of Advanced Nursing*, the *International Journal of Nursing Studies*, the *Journal of Clinical Nursing* and the *British Medical Journal* in 1992. She found that there was insufficient information about how samples were accessed and what the sampling techniques were. More recently, Webb (2003, 2004), in a similar exercise, found a lack of information on the type and purpose of sampling and no information, in quantitative studies, on power calculation or justification for the size of sample used.

The components of a study (including the units of analysis, concepts generated, population characteristics and settings) must be sufficiently well described and defined in order for other researchers to use the results of the study as a basis for comparison (Goetz and LeCompte, 1984).

In quantitative research, the purpose of sampling is to collect valid and reliable data from a subset of the population that would be representative of the whole population. These findings are often expected to be generalisable to other similar populations and settings. The representativeness of the sample and the generalisability of findings depend on at least four factors: the size and the characteristics of the sample, the method of sampling, the setting where the study was carried out and the response rate.

Sample size

Small samples in quantitative research are also unlikely to yield results of significance. In fact, academic journals may refuse publication of quantitative research projects in which small samples have been used, except if little research exists on the topic. Clearly a sample size of 10 out of a student population of 300 is unlikely to be representative, even if the sample is one of probability. The degree of representativeness will increase with a sample of 50 and above.

Power calculation is carried out in order to determine the size of sample required in order that statistical analysis can be used to confirm or reject correlation or causal relationships between variables. The size of sample depends on the magnitude or extent of anticipated changes. If the change is estimated to be large then a smaller sample is required than if change is small. For example, if in a study assessing the effects of an educational programme on knowledge scores of participants researchers expect an increase of 20 points (on a scale of 0 to 100), then a small sample can detect these changes. On the other hand, if a drug is being tested on its effectiveness in reducing temperature by 0.5 of a degree, than a larger sample is required in order to ascertain that this change is statistically significant.

If a sample is too small, it may fail to detect that the experimental (new) intervention is more effective than the conventional one. In this case it is the small sample size which may be responsible for showing no difference, when in fact there may be one. Why not use a large sample? Large samples are costly and time-consuming. It is also unethical to recruit more participants than necessary in a study.

It is beyond the scope of this book to explain how sample sizes are calculated. Computer software have been developed for this purpose. A simple on-line search will reveal many useful web-sites to explain and perform power calculation.

In appraising a quantitative study, you should expect a justification of the sample size. Where correlational relationships are investigated, a statement of how the sample size was calculated should be provided.

Equally important is the degree of 'fit' between the sample and the population from which it is drawn. This means that the sample must be similar in characteristics to the population. For example, if in a study of stress among hospital nurses the composition of the target population is staff nurses 50 per cent, health care assistants 30 per cent, and clinical managers 20 per cent, the sample must more or less reflect a similar proportion of these three groups. Certain variables, such as gender or age, may be more important in one study than in others; therefore the samples must reflect the target population in these key variables. The more homogeneous the target population, the more representative the sample is likely to be. Samples for heterogeneous populations need to be large and carefully selected. Stratified random sampling is often the answer.

In general, qualitative studies use small samples, but it is a misconception to think that 'numbers are unimportant in ensuring the adequacy of a sampling strategy' (Sandelowski, 1995). However, size is not the starting point. It is the purpose for which the sample is required which should decide how many respondents are recruited. In in-depth studies, the sample is unlikely to be large. There have been cases where a sample of two or three respondents has been studied. It is possible, although unlikely, that such a sample size could yield a range of different perspectives if this is what the researcher is seeking. On the other hand, if researchers carry out qualitative interviews with 100 respondents, it is possible that saturation of data could be reached very quickly. The time and effort required to interview all of them could be better spent in more in-depth interviews with, for example, 50 of them, with the option of interviewing some of the same respondents more than once. The more varied the population from whom the data are required, the larger the sample size should be.

In quantitative studies, the focus is on how particular views or beliefs are distributed in a population. In qualitative studies, researchers are interested in the range of their experiences in order to obtain as complete an understanding of the phenomenon as possible. If these experiences are suspected to vary greatly in a population or if the population that possesses these experiences themselves vary in terms of demographic variables such as age, race, gender or social class, it makes sense that the sample should take this into account.

The flexible and enquiring nature of qualitative research makes hard and fast rules inappropriate. According to Sandelowski (1995), researchers have to make their own judgements. She explains that:

> Numbers have a place in ensuring that a sample is fully adequate to support particular qualitative enterprises. A good principle to follow is: An adequate sample size in qualitative research is one that permits – by virtue of not being too large – the deep, case-oriented analysis that is a hallmark of all qualitative inquiry, and that results in – by virtue of not being too small – a new and richly textured understanding of experience.

In considering the feasibility of applying the findings of a study to your own practice, you must assess how similar or different the studied sample is to 'your' population. For example, it may not be appropriate to apply the findings of a study on stroke patients with an average age of 50 to a group of patients with an average age of 65. Tornquist et al. (1993) explain what the reader must look for in samples:

> To evaluate methods, ask these questions about the study: who was in the study sample? Were these individuals unique in some way, or were they typical of people for whom the intervention or study results should apply? Examine carefully the sample characteristics that are most important for deciding on the applicability of the results to others. The key characteristics depend on the topic selected.

Sampling method

Although probability samples are likely to be more representative than non-probability samples, representativeness is not necessarily assured with random selection. The decision on which form of random sampling to use depends on, among other things, the availability of lists and the composition of the population and the research questions. Whatever the sampling methods, these must be described in enough detail for you to decide whether the sample has any bias. Just stating that a random or a convenience sample was drawn, without explaining how, is not helpful. It is important for researchers to say who selected the sample. Often this is left to managers and practitioners, resulting in researchers having little control over who is included in the study.

The setting

To generalise findings from research in one setting to another requires careful consideration of how similar or different they are. The findings of a study of support to informal carers of people with dementia in the USA may not be applicable to carers in the UK. Statutory voluntary services as well as social networks are likely to be different in the two countries. Far from rejecting the results, they could serve as a basis for comparisons, thereby enhancing one's understanding of support for carers in general. The setting in which data are collected can also introduce bias into the findings. Researchers must provide you with adequate details of the context in which research is carried out. The responses from a 'captive' population of patients (in hospital, receiving care) may not be the same as when they are interviewed in their own homes. The social and cultural factors in the environment in which research takes place must be taken into consideration.

Response rate

Another aspect of sampling that you need to monitor is the response rate. The lower the response rate, the less representative the achieved sample is likely to be of the target population.

Those who do not respond may have characteristics different from those who do. In a study of attitudes to homosexuality, it is possible that non-respondents are not interested in the topic or that they are homophobic and are so 'disgusted' that they do not take part. Some people may see non-responding as a form of protest.

It is difficult to define an acceptable response rate. Researchers usually compare their response rates with the 'norm' in similar studies. What is more important is for researchers to attempt to explain non-responses and their possible implications for the data. Research Example 32 (see p. 260) shows how a response rate is calculated.

SUMMARY

Summary and conclusion

In this chapter, we have looked at some of the common terminologies used in relation to samples and sampling. The uses, strengths and limitations of the main sampling methods in nursing research have been discussed. Samples are the sources of research data and as such must be carefully selected and soundly justified. Researchers must provide readers with adequate information on the composition of the target population and sample, as well as the sampling method, to enable them to evaluate the representativeness of the sample, the usefulness and possible generalisability of the findings.

References

Ashley J (1994) Study groups: are they effective in preparing students for NCLEX-RN? *Journal of Nursing Education*, **33**, 8:357–64.

Cowman S and Conroy R M (2004) A response to: misrepresenting random sampling? A systematic review of research papers by G R Williamson (*Journal of Advanced Nursing*, 2003, **44**:278–88). *Journal of Advanced Nursing*, **46**, 2:221–3.

Coyle L A and Sokop A G (1990) Innovation adoption behavior among nurses. *Nursing Research*, **39**, 3:176–80.

Coyne I T (1997) Sampling in qualitative research. Purposeful and theoretical sampling; merging or clear boundaries? *Journal of Advanced Nursing*, **26**:623–30.

Ehlers V J, Zuyderduin A and Oosthuizen M J (2001) The well-being of gays, lesbians and bisexuals in Botswana. *Journal of Advanced Nursing*, **35**, 6:848–56.

Gagliardi B A (2003) The experience of sexuality for individuals living with multiple sclerosis. *Journal of Clinical Nursing*, **12**:571–8.

Glaser B and Strauss A (1967) *The Discovery of Grounded Theory: Strategies for Qualitative Research* (Chicago, IL: Aldine).

Goetz J P and LeCompte M D (1984) *Ethnography and Qualitative Design in Educational Research* (Orlando, FL: Academic Press).

Larsson M, Hedelin B and Athlin E (2003) Lived experiences of eating problems for patients with head and neck cancer during radiotherapy. *Journal of Clinical Nursing*, **12**:562–70.

MacLellan K (2004) Postoperative pain: strategy for improving patient perspectives. *Journal of Advanced Nursing*, **46**, 2:179–85.

Marsland L and Murrells T (2000) Sampling for a longitudinal study of the careers of nurses qualifying from the English pre-registration Project 2000 diploma course. *Journal of Advanced Nursing*, **31**, 4:935–43.

McCaughan E (2002) Information needs and information seeking behaviour of newly diagnosed cancer patients. Unpublished thesis. Coleraine, University of Ulster.

Patterson C, Kaczorowski J, Arthur H, Smith K and Mills D A (2003) Complementary therapy practice: defining the role of advanced nurse practitioners. *Journal of Clinical Nursing*, **12**, 6:816–23.

Reid G, Speed B, Miller P, Cooke F and Crofts N (1998) A methodology for sampling and accessing homeless individuals in Melbourne, 1995–96. *Australian and New Zealand Journal of Public Health*, **22**, 5:568–72.

Roe B and May C (1999) Incontinence and sexuality: findings from a qualitative perspective. *Journal of Advanced Nursing*, **30**, 3:573–9.

Roe K M, Minkler M, and Barnwell R S (1994) The assumption of caregiving: grandmothers raising the children of the crack cocaine epidemic. *Qualitative Health Research*, **4**, 3:281–303.

Sandelowski M (1995) Sample size in qualitative research. *Research in Nursing and Health*, **18**:179–83.

Schofield J W (1993) Increasing the generalisability of qualitative research. In: M Hammersley (ed.), *Social Research: Philosophy, Politics and Practice* (London: Sage).

Smith L N (1994) An analysis and reflections on the quality of nursing research in 1992. *Journal of Advanced Nursing*, 3:385–93.

Stake R E (1978) The case-study in social inquiry. *Educational Researcher*, 7:5–8.

Strauss A and Corbin J (1998) *Basics of Qualitative Research: Techniques and Procedures for Developing Grounded Theory*, 2nd edn (London: Sage).

Thompson C (1999) Qualitative research into nurse decision making: factors for consideration in theoretical sampling. *Qualitative Health Research*, **9**, 6:815–28.

Thompson K, Melby V, Parahoo K, Ridley T and Humphreys W G (2003) Information provided to patients undergoing gastroscopy procedures. *Journal of Clinical Nursing*, **12**, 6:899–911.

Tornquist E M, Funk S G, Champagne M T and Wiese R A (1993) Advice on reading research: overcoming the barriers. *Applied Nursing Research*, **6**, 4:177–83.

Walker R (ed.) (1985) *Applied Qualitative Research* (Aldershot: Gower).

Watson R (2004) A response to: misrepresenting random sampling? A systematic review of research papers by G R Williamson (*Journal of Advanced Nursing*, 2003, 44:278–88). *Journal of Advanced Nursing*, **46**, 2:220–1.

Webb C (2003) Research in Brief. An analysis of recent publications in JCN: sources, methods and topics. *Journal of Clinical Nursing*, **12**:931–4.

Webb C (2004) Editor's note: Analysis of papers published in JAN in 2002. *Journal of Advanced Nursing*, **45**, 3:229–31.

Williamson G R (2003) Misrepresenting random sampling? A systematic review of research papers. *Journal of Advanced Nursing*, **44**:278–88.

van Wissen K A and Siebers R W L (1993) Nurses' attitudes and concerns pertaining to HIV and AIDS. *Journal of Advanced Nursing*, **18**:912–17.

Woodcock H C, Read A W, Bower C, Stanley, F J and Moore D J (1994) A matched cohort study of planned home and hospital births in Western Australia 1981–1987. *Midwifery*, **10**:125–35.

13 Questionnaires

> **OPENING THOUGHT**
>
> When you don't know the answer, question the question.
> Anonymous

Introduction

This chapter will take a close look at the questionnaire as a method of data collection in nursing research, in particular its value and limitations and the advantages and disadvantages of different modes of questionnaire administration. The strategies that researchers can use to ensure and enhance the validity and reliability of questionnaires are examined, and some of the ethical implications of this popular method of data collection are explored and discussed.

Use of questionnaires in nursing

The questionnaire is by far the most common method of data collection in social and health research. However, it is not useful for research purposes only. We have all, at some time or other, been asked questions or to fill in a form, for example when attending a general practitioner's surgery or an accident and emergency department. Nurses have a number of forms to complete as part of their work. The hospital admission form itself is a questionnaire seeking information such as the name, date of birth, next of kin, previous admission, family medical history and any previous illness of the patient. Clinical specialties may have their own forms asking specific questions. For example, a 'pre-operative screening chart' in one hospital asked questions about 'allergies, general health (hypertension, diabetes, cardiac disease), skin problems, dental problems and social habits'. Below is an extract from a 'clinical' questionnaire administered to patients at a fracture clinic.

Q5	Any past illnesses?	☐ Yes	☐ No
Q6	Do you have blackouts or faint easily?	☐ Yes	☐ No
Q7	Do you get breathless easily, i.e. asthma?	☐ Yes	☐ No
Q12	Do you have transport to and from hospital?	☐ Yes	☐ No
Q13	Do you live alone?	☐ Yes	☐ No
Q14	Do you smoke?	☐ Yes	☐ No

Most of these forms or questionnaires that nurses administer to clients serve two main purposes: diagnostic and record-keeping. The information gathered provides the basis for any subsequent diagnosis and treatment. It is useful for assessing clients' needs and helps in the formulation of care plans. Other general information is routinely kept by health centres and hospitals for administrative, accounting and planning purposes. It provides indicators of admissions, discharges, morbidity, mortality, resource allocation, uptake of services, deployment of personnel, and so on.

These questionnaires were not designed primarily for the collection of research data, although patients' notes, care plans and other records are valuable sources of data for researchers conducting retrospective studies. Many of these questionnaires would not withstand a rigorous validity and reliability test, but they are usually useful for the purpose they serve, that is they provide the necessary information on which clinical and policy decisions can be made. There are, of course, ethical and legal issues involved in the use of information from patients' notes for research purposes.

Stone (1993) sums up the use of questionnaires by pointing out that they are not the exclusive preserve of academics and that they have many uses, including screening, audit, administration and public relations, as well as their more familiar role in research.

What is a questionnaire?

A questionnaire can be described as a method that seeks written or verbal responses from people to a written set of questions or statements. It is a research method when it is designed and administered solely for the purpose of collecting data as part of a research study. It is a quantitative approach since it is predetermined (constructed in advance), standardised (the same questions in the same order are asked of all the respondents) and structured (respondents are mainly required to choose from the list of responses offered by the researcher).

Questionnaires can be used in descriptive, correlational and experimental studies. In descriptive studies, they may not only provide data that facilitate understanding of the phenomena being investigated, but can also generate data from which concepts and hypotheses can be formulated. Thus they contribute to the production of knowledge inductively.

In correlational studies, questionnaires can provide data to support or reject hypotheses and thereby contribute deductively to the production of knowledge. In a study by Sarmiento et al. (2004) on nurse educators' workplace empowerment, burnout and job satisfaction, three hypotheses were tested by means of the following four questionnaires/scales: the Conditions of Work Effectiveness Questionnaire, the Job Activities Scale, the Maslach Burnout Inventory Educator Survey and the Global Job Satisfaction Questionnaire.

In Harvey et al.'s (2002) randomised controlled trial comparing two models of maternity care, the outcomes were measured by the Labour and Delivery Satisfaction Index, the Attitudes about Labour and Delivery Experience Questionnaire and the Six Simple Questions Questionnaire.

The questionnaire is, however, most frequently used in survey designs. In fact, the term 'questionnaire' is often used interchangeably with 'survey'. A distinction needs to be made between them. A survey is a research design that can comprise one or more methods of data collection. Questionnaires can be used on their own or in conjunction with interviews and/or observations. For a survey on the dental health of schoolchildren, data can be collected by asking questions (by means of either questionnaires or interviews) and by observing the presence or absence of dental caries in these schoolchildren. Some surveys can be carried out almost entirely by observations, as in the case of a 'survey on food intake', when the food intake is observed, weighed and analysed.

Questionnaires in nursing research

The little evidence which is available suggests that the questionnaire is the most widely used method of data collection in nursing research. Smith (1994) carried out a meta-analysis of articles in four journals published in 1992 (the *Journal of Advanced Nursing*, the *International Journal of Nursing Studies*, the *Journal of Clinical Nursing* and the *British Medical Journal*). She reported that both professional groups (nurses and doctors) used a variety of research methods. Those writing in the *British Medical Journal* were 'far more likely to employ the use of records, often involving large data bases and to use laboratory-based tests', while nurses were 'more likely to employ self-design questionnaires and interview' (Smith, 1994). The total number of articles with questionnaires was 86, compared with 46 for interviews and 20 for observations.

In Webb's (2003) analysis of all papers published in the *Journal of Clinical Nursing* in 2001 and 2002, she found that questionnaires were most frequently used by researchers (37.8 per cent) followed by 'in-depth/unstructured interviews' (15.6 per cent). Webb (2004) also analysed all papers published in the *Journal of Advanced Nursing* in 2002. In 50 studies (29.1 per cent) interviews were used alone compared with 45 (26.2 per cent) studies which used questionnaires alone. The internet has opened up vast opportunities for collecting data by specially designed web-sites and/or by electronic mail (see O'Connor and Madge [2003] for an example of a web-based survey). One advantage of this method over the more common 'pen and paper' survey is that data can be analysed more readily and large populations can be accessed.

The questionnaire is potentially the quickest and cheapest – and a relatively confidential and frequently anonymous – method of collecting large amounts of information from a large number of people scattered over wide geographical areas. They are efficient in providing data on the attributes of clients and staff, and are employed in the evaluation of practice and policy and in the assessment of the needs of clients and staff. They have also been increasingly used in the measurement of concepts and constructs as varied as, for example, empathy, burn-out, social support, pain, coping, hope, stress and quality of life. There are, of course, other methods that are equally, if not better, suited to the study of these phenomena. Researchers must always choose the most appropriate data collection method or methods in order to answer the research question, while taking into account the use to which the findings will be put and the resources available, including funding and time.

Questionnaires have been used mainly to collect information on facts, attitudes, knowledge, beliefs, opinions, perceptions, expectations, experiences and the behaviour of clients and staff. The most common factual data collected by questionnaires are demographic ones, such as age, gender, occupation, social class and qualifications. These are very useful for constructing profiles of clients and staff and in exploring their correlation with other attributes, such as personality, attitudes or expectations. Other facts related to practice include physiological measures, such as temperature, pulse, respiration or blood pressure, and other occurrences, such as the amount of fluid intake, attendance at outpatient departments and frequency of bowel movements.

The attitudes, knowledge and beliefs of clients are studied because they can influence, among other factors, how people regard their health and illness, how and which services they use, how compliant they are with nursing and medical treatment and advice, and what actions they take to promote their health. The attitudes, knowledge and beliefs of health professionals can also influence their practice. For example, their knowledge of, and attitudes to, research may determine whether and how they utilise research.

The opinions, perceptions, expectations and experiences of clients and practitioners are legitimate areas of inquiry because nursing is about meeting the needs of the client. The self-report of the client and the objective assessment of the nurse can combine to give an expert service sensitive to individual needs.

Although behaviour is best studied by observation, it is sometimes not feasible or practical to do so, as in the case of sexual practices and behaviours of dubious legal or moral status. Past behaviour, unless captured on film, cannot be studied by observation, nor can behavioural intentions. The questionnaire, on the other hand, can ask respondents to report on past, actual and potential behaviours, as perceived by them.

All the above phenomena that are commonly studied by means of questionnaires are important in helping professionals to better organise and deliver care and treatment in institutions and in the community. The data produced can also be useful in promoting health, preventing illness and disability and contributing to effective rehabilitation. Figure 13.1 gives some examples of the use of questionnaires in nursing research.

- Lindqvist et al. (2004)   **Coping strategies of people with kidney transplants**

  The authors devised a questionnaire designed to collect demographic data (gender, age, place of residence etc.) and to measure the perceived effectiveness in coping with the disease. The second questionnaire used was the Jalowiec Coping Scale. 'The results may be used to inform nurses about coping styles that patients have found effective in handling their situation' (Lindqvist et al., 2004).

- Shaker et al. (2004)   **Infant feeding attitudes of expectant parents: breastfeeding and formula feeding**

  In this study the Iowa Feeding Attitude Scale was used to assess each parent's infant feeding attitudes. Data on demographic factors were also collected. According to the authors, 'an understanding of parental knowledge and attitudes towards infant feeding is necessary to inform the design of effective breastfeeding promotion intervention'.

- McDonnell et al. (2003)   **Acute Pain Teams in England: current provision and their role in post-operative pain management**

  The aim of the study was to provide an accurate picture of the current level of Acute Pain Team provision in all acute English hospitals. A questionnaire, with some of the questions from other surveys, was developed by the authors. This study demonstrates the use of questionnaires in providing data which can be potentially useful in informing health policy and the delivery of services.

Figure 13.1   Examples of phenomena studied with the use of questionnaires

Question formats

Researchers have developed a range of question formats to collect valid and reliable data efficiently and to analyse them quickly. These are strategies designed to facilitate respondents in providing the necessary and relevant information in a short time and in a relatively painless way. The choice of question format depends mainly on the type of data that researchers want to collect. If they set out to elucidate from respondents which factors affect their job dissatisfaction, they could ask a type of question that is open enough to allow them to formulate their own responses. On the other hand, if researchers want to compare the degree to which staff are satisfied with their job, they may offer respondents a number of categories to choose from, such as 'very satisfied', 'satisfied', 'neither satisfied nor dissatisfied', 'dissatisfied' and 'very dissatisfied'. Common question formats in questionnaires include: closed, open-ended, vignettes and rating scales.

Closed questions

Common formats of closed questions include:

- two-way questions

- checklists

- multiple-choice questions

- ranking questions.

Two-way questions, as the term suggests, offer a choice between two responses, as shown below:

Male ☐   Female ☐   (please tick one box)

A true/false or an agree/disagree as well as a yes/no option can also be offered, as in the following example:

	Please tick one box	
The reliability of an instrument is the degree to which it measures what it is expected to measure.	*True* ☐	*False* ☐
A knowledge of nursing theories is essential for the practice of nursing.	*Agree* ☐	*Disagree* ☐
Do you think that every nurse should learn how to do research?	*Yes* ☐	*No* ☐

Checklists provide respondents with a list of responses from which to select. They can 'tick' as many items or statements as they think are applicable. The following example of a checklist question comes from McKenna et al.'s (2004) study of barriers to evidence-based practice in primary care:

15. **Please tick the source(s) of information that you use to inform your practice on a day-to-day basis** (tick as many as apply).

Media	☐	Evidence-based circulars	☐
Colleagues	☐	Official clinical guidelines	☐
Conferences	☐	Protocols	☐
Central Services Agency	☐	Courses	☐
Journals	☐	Drug representatives	☐
Own judgement	☐	Other	☐

Sometimes the checklist is not exhaustive, and respondents are asked to add to the list. In the above example McKenna et al. (2004) provide this opportunity.

Multiple choice is another format used in questionnaires. This offers respondents a list of responses, normally in the form of statements, from which they can select the one most applicable to them:

Please tick one journal which you read most frequently.
Midwifery ☐
Journal of Advanced Nursing ☐
Scandinavian Journal of Caring Sciences ☐
Qualitative Health Research ☐
Journal of Clinical Nursing ☐
Journal of Community Nursing ☐
Nurse Education Today ☐
Nurse Researcher ☐

Sometimes researchers want to know how respondents prioritise their needs, whom they consult most or least for health advice or what interventions they find most or least useful. To obtain rapid answers, they ask respondents to rank from a list of responses. The following is an example of a *ranking question* on schoolchildren's knowledge of, and attitudes to, mental illness:

Where did you get information on mental illness from?
Please rank the items below by putting 1 to 6 in the boxes provided
(1 = *most information*, 6 = *least information*)
School teacher ☐
Television ☐
Books ☐
Magazines ☐
Parents ☐
Friends ☐

Closed questions are asked when researchers consider that they know all the potential answers and only require respondents to select the one or ones that apply to them. Such questions are appropriate for demographic data and in cases where there are a more or less fixed number of alternatives. For example, a researcher can ask a closed question such as that shown below, when medication can only be given via these three routes:

By which route do you normally administer medication X? Please tick one box.
Orally ☐
Intramuscularly ☐
Intravenously ☐

Closed questions yield data that allow for comparison between respondents as all the responses are in the same format. They can be precoded, thereby making analysis a relatively easy task. The main problem with closed questions is that the researcher may omit an important response and thereby obtain a result different from that had the response been included. For example, if in the above ranking question the researcher omitted 'magazines' from the list, the school-children in the survey would rank what is on offer and therefore provide different data to those obtained if 'magazines' had been included. Another example of forced choice is when a respondent is asked to rank in order from 1 to 6, when in reality he or she may want to rank two items at number 1. Researchers constructing closed questions must make sure that all possible choices are included, bearing in mind that respondents may be confused if they have to choose from too many categories.

The list of responses offered by the researcher may give the respondents an idea of what is normal. For example, by asking respondents to choose from a list of journals that nurses read, they may think that nurses normally read these journals, and that perhaps they should indicate that they do so as well. Therefore, checklists and multiple choices may unwittingly reveal to respondents what the norm is and thereby encourage them to give socially desirable answers.

These limitations can be offset to a large extent by careful and skilful construction of the questionnaire, by paying particular attention to the categories offered to respondents and by including questions in appropriate formats.

Open-ended questions

When researchers do not have all the answers and/or want to obtain respondents' views, they can formulate an open-ended question, as in the example below.

Please indicate below the main factors that contribute to your job satisfaction.

....

....

....

....

It is also possible to ask an open-ended ranking question in a different way:

Please list, in order of importance, 4 factors that contribute to your job satisfaction (1 = *most important*, 4 = *least important*).

1 ....

2 ....

3 ....

4 ....

Open-ended questions give respondents the opportunity to frame their answers in their own words. Questionnaires are designed to collect data quickly and in a relatively painless way. Thus too many open-ended questions will require more time and effort from participants, who may decide to skip these questions or provide superficial answers. There can be a large number of missing answers to open-ended questions which can cast doubt on the generalisability of the findings. Nonetheless, researchers often find that the most interesting data come from these type of questions.

Open-ended questions give respondents the opportunity to participate in, and interact with, the questionnaire in a way in which closed questions do not. An open-ended question must be clear and unambiguous, or different respondents will interpret it differently. For example, in a questionnaire on job satisfaction, the researcher who wants to know the types of clinical area where respondents work (that is medical, surgical or care of the elderly) may ask 'which type of ward do you work in?' The answers could be 'a 25-bedded ward', 'a mixed ward', 'a care of the elderly ward', 'an open ward' or 'a chaotic ward'. There is always the possibility with open-ended questions that the researcher understands the question differently from some respondents. The responses given above would not be useful to the researcher, as they do not answer the question in the way and form in which she wants it.

Responses to open-ended questions can also vary in length. Some respondents continue their answers on the back of the questionnaire, whereas others give a response in a few words. The space provided for responses is sometimes an indication of how long the researcher expects them to be. However, some respondents have larger handwriting than others. A bigger problem may be in deciphering what is written and in making sense of what is said. Open-ended questions can generate large amounts of data. In a study by Wahlberg et al. (2003) respondents were asked one open-ended question: 'What problems have you experienced with telephone advice?'. This generated 154 statements, which were later reduced to 24 'problem categories'. Analysis of responses from these questions can be time-consuming and difficult since responses are rarely made using the same terminologies, unlike the case in closed questions. The analysis of quantitative data is further discussed in Chapter 16.

Open-ended questions do not make a questionnaire a qualitative method, as some people believe. As I have explained elsewhere (Parahoo, 1993):

> questionnaire data are treated at face value; there is no opportunity to unravel the real meaning of each individual response. What people say and what they mean can be different, and several interviews with the same person are sometimes necessary to collect meaningful data.

Open-ended questions are valuable in that they give respondents some freedom in expressing themselves rather than their being constrained by the 'strait-jacket' style of closed questions.

To help respondents to provide answers to open-ended questions in a format which is more standardised, researchers can be more specific about the information required. In the example below, McKenna et al. (2004) use a semi-closed format to collect data in a more structured format (than the open-ended one). Data analysis will also be easier to perform.

Please supply brief details of the research study (*Please do not include filling out questionnaires, taking part in interviews etc. in this section*)

Research area	Your role in the research	Year carried out
1.		
2.		
If others, please continue on the back of this questionnaire		

Both closed and open-ended questions have their place in questionnaires. Researchers must use them judiciously and appropriately, and as much as possible use the strength of one to offset the limitation of the other.

Vignettes

Another imaginative strategy which can be used in questionnaires is asking people to respond to questions by providing them with short descriptions of a situation or event which closely resemble a real situation. Gould (1996) describes vignettes as:

> Simulations of real events which can be used in research studies to elicit subjects' knowledge, attitudes or opinions according to how they state they would behave in the hypothetical situation depicted.

This method is used in teaching and in examinations as well. For example, Chau et al. (2001) evaluated the effects of using videotaped vignettes in promoting nursing students' critical thinking abilities in managing different clinical situations. In examinations students are given a brief description of an 'event' or 'case', and their knowledge is tested by focused questions. In research, vignettes have been used to study a number of phenomena (see e.g. McKinlay et al., 2001; Gould et al., 2001; Hellzén et al., 2003). McKinlay et al. (2001) provide an example of a vignette in a study of 'nurses' behavioural intentions towards self-poisoning patients':

> Nurse A believes that the majority of self-poisoning patients are less of a priority in his/her work area and considers their reason for admission to hospital as self-inflicted. It is his/her view that patients with real illnesses may suffer as she/he has less time to spend with them as a result of spending time with self-poisoning

patients. In his/her opinion most admissions are 'attention seeking'. She/he believes that ideally all patients should be treated equally, but in reality other patients are the main priority and self-poisoning patients tend to come second.

One or more vignettes can be used in the same study. Sometimes researchers give different versions of the same vignette in order to compare responses. For example in McKinlay et al.'s (2001) study, there is another vignette depicting a 'positive behavioural intentional style' of another nurse.

Questions to vignettes can be open-ended or more structured. In a study by Hellzén et al. (2003), there is a questionnaire consisting of 13 pairs of categorical statements from which nurses were asked to choose 'the standpoint describing the way they should think and act towards the resident in the vignette by scoring their decisions on a two-degree scale'.

The advantages of using vignettes are that the problems associated with 'real life' observations such as observer's effect, access to participants and ethical issues are avoided, while at the same time providing opportunities to collect data from large number of participants (Gould, 1996). The main disadvantage is that 'similations' are not real-life situations. Therefore the generalisabilty of findings is limited. Although vignettes provides more 'context' than closed and open-ended questions, they are still uni-dimensional in that they cannot depict all types of pressures that nurses find themselves in real-life situations.

Rating scales

You may have come across a questionnaire in a popular magazine or newspaper in which readers are asked to 'tick' the appropriate boxes and add up their scores to find out how 'sexy', 'romantic' or 'intelligent' they are. If you have indulged in such an activity, you have in effect filled in a rating scale. If you have not, here is an extract from a scale in the *Daily Mail* (17 July 1995) entitled 'Are you hot on gossip?'

1. After the party I like talking about how others there looked
   AGREE   A . . .   ☐   DISAGREE   B . . .   ☐
6. I usually skip the gossip columns in newspapers
   AGREE   B . . .   ☐   DISAGREE   A . . .   ☐
10. The saying 'There is no smoke without fire' is often wrong
    AGREE   B . . .   ☐   DISAGREE   A . . .   ☐

There were ten items in all and readers were asked to add up their number of As and Bs. Those who scored eight or more As were described as:

You are so interested in gossip that you often prefer rumour and speculation about others than the hard truth.

If their score was two As or fewer, they were described as:

You probably prefer your own company to groups, and also realise that there are usually more mundane explanations for the events which grip and promote gossips.

While this may be light-hearted fun, the same principles apply to the construction of rating scales used in research and clinical practice.

Rating scales are sometimes referred to as questionnaires. There are, however, crucial differences between the two, especially with regard to their structure, design and purpose. Questionnaires, on the whole, contain a set of questions mostly in closed and open-ended formats. Responses to each of the questions are treated on their own and analysed separately, although researchers seek to correlate and cross-tabulate variables. Together, responses from all the questions provide an answer to the research question or hypotheses. Rating scales are made up of statements or items that respondents are required to rate. Each rated statement is given a score and the total score, as shown in the 'gossip scale', is given an interpretation.

Researchers designing questionnaires carefully select questions that reflect attributes of the concept or aspects of an issue or topic being studied. For example, for a questionnaire on job satisfaction, a researcher will make sure that the main components of job satisfaction, such as autonomy, pay, working environment, promotion prospects and good working relationships, are represented in the questionnaire. A rating scale is normally constructed by collecting a large number of statements on the phenomenon being rated and, through an elaborate process, whittling them down to a smaller number that can be administered to respondents.

There are different types of rating scales and different techniques for developing them. Although the process may differ, they all have to undergo the following steps:

1. *Develop a large number (pool) of items* or statements to indicate the strength of feeling of respondents towards the concept or issue being measured. This is done by searching the literature and/or asking people (by means of individual interviews, focus groups or questionnaires). Examples of statements relating to research utilisation in clinical practice are: 'Using research is a waste of practitioners' time', 'using research does not always improve practice' or 'research utilisation contributes a great deal towards enhancing practice'.

2. *Reduce the pool of items* to a manageable number. This is done with or without the help of a panel of experts or other respondents. Normally statements representing extreme views are eliminated.

3. *Carry out tests* to ensure the validity and reliability of the provisional scale by administering it to a sample of respondents. Usually tests include factorial analysis and Cronbach's alpha (see Chapter 16).

4. *Modify the scale* as a result of these tests and repeat the tests as appropriate, until the researcher is satisfied that the scale can consistently measure what it is supposed to measure.

A number of tools such as the Likert scale, the semantic differential scale and the visual analogue scales are frequently used to measure phenomena of interest to nurses and other health professionals. These are discussed below.

Likert scale

A Likert scale is an instrument used to measure attitudes, beliefs, opinions, values and views (Sechrist and Pravikoff, 2001). The scale comprises a set of statements (some positive and some negative) about the concept being measured and respondents are asked to choose from an odd number of responses (usually five), including a neutral one. Typical responses are 'strongly agree', 'agree', 'neither agree nor disagree', 'disagree' and 'strongly disagree'. Scores for each item range from 1 to 5 (5 for positive and 1 for negative statements). The scale is structured such that negative items are mixed to prevent respondents getting in a 'rhythm' of 'ticking' boxes in the same column. The total scores represent the strength of particular attitudes or views.

This type of scale was named after Likert (1932) who developed it to measure attitudes. It is a useful tool to gauge attitudes among groups of people in a relatively short time and cheaply, although if the tool is developed from scratch it can be expensive. Its limitation is mainly related to the total scores, which can be the sum of a combination of scores of individual items, therefore not particularly reflecting the strength of agreement with individual ones.

There is a difference between a Likert scale and a Likert-type scale. A Likert scale is developed systematically (similar to the process for a rating scale described above) and evaluated rigorously for validity and reliability. Likert-type or pseudo-Likert scale involves the formulation of items or statements which the researcher believes represent the concept being measured, without going through the necessary steps to generate and validate items. Usually the score of each item is reported individually. On the other hand, a Likert scale, rigorously developed, should provide a total score. In appraising a scale, readers should look for evidence of how it was constructed and its reliability scores. In a study of 'exercise among blue-collar workers', Blue et al. (2001) explain how they developed Likert scales to measure a number of concepts such as 'behavioural beliefs', 'subjective norm' and 'perceived behavioural control'. They interviewed 21 blue-collar workers to generate items or statements for the scale. These items were put to a panel of six judges who were 'experts in exercise research' and in developing these types of scales. Statistical tests were carried out to assess the validity and the reliability of those tools.

Semantic differential scale

The semantic differential (SD) scale originally developed by Osgood et al. (1957) is another technique or method that has been developed to measure an attitude or feeling towards a concept or phenomenon. It can be described as a set of opposite adjectives which respondents select from, to represent how they 'feel' about a particular item. Usually the item can be a statement, a word or a picture, and it is placed at the top of the scale. Respondents are asked to 'tick' or put an 'X' on a line which can range from five to nine gradings. Below is an example of an SD scale in a study of 'predictors of psychological distress in chronic pain patients' by Walker and Sofaer (1998):

> For each word pair below, please tick the box which represents how you feel MOST OFTEN these days:
>
> In control ☐☐☐☐☐ Helpless
> Worried ☐☐☐☐☐ Untroubled
> Calm ☐☐☐☐☐ Irritable

Only three pairs of adjectives are presented here although the scale itself consists of 12 items. These can vary, as can the number of gradings. In Blue et al.'s (2001) study of exercise among blue-collar workers, 'attitude toward physical activity' was measured by six bi-polar adjectives (pleasant/unpleasant, interesting/boring, good/bad, useful/useless, valuable/worthless, and helpful/harmful) on a seven-point scale.

An SD scale has three components: a stem, steps and anchors. In the scale used in Walker and Sofaer's (1998) study, the stem is 'how respondents feel'; it can also be expressed as a statement. The steps are the five gradations to choose from. The anchors are the adjectives on each side of the lines (e.g. in control/helpless). Respondents are instructed to put a 'X' in the space provided as quickly as possible. Normally they are advised not to reflect or think rationally, but to give their immediate reactions, as it is their attitudes, feelings and emotions that are being measured. Such scales are used with the assumption that 'meanings often can be or are usually communicated by adjectives' (Waltz et al., 1991). The total score obtained by each respondent is an indication of the strength of their attitudes or feelings. These scores can then be subjected to statistical analysis.

According to Bowles (1986), the semantic differential model 'is a highly acceptable and frequently used measure of attitude and it lends itself to statistical techniques for validation purposes'. Henerson et al. (1987), on the other hand, find that the 'semantic differential yields only general impressions without information about their source' and are therefore 'not often worth the effort expended'.

Visual analogue scales

Another attitude-measuring instrument, similar to the semantic differential format, is the visual analogue scale (VAS). The main difference between the two is that with the SD technique respondents have a series of steps or graduations (from 5 to 9) to choose from. On the other hand, with the VAS, the response is recorded on a line representing a continuum between two points or anchors, thus allowing more freedom to respondents to put their 'X' in any position on the line. Cline et al. (1992) give a clear description of the VAS:

> Operationally, the VAS is a vertical or horizontal line, 100 mm in length, anchored by terms that represent the extremes of the subjective phenomenon the researcher wishes to measure. Subjects are asked to indicate the intensity of a sensation by placing a line across the VAS at a point that represents the intensity of the sensation at that moment in time. Responses are scored by measuring the distance between from the lowest anchor point to the subject's mark across the line.

An example of horizontal and vertical VAS is given in Figure 13.2. The line can be of different lengths although the popular length is 100 mm. The vertical VAS is also preferred because it is more 'directly analogous to the "more" (high, top) and "less" (low, bottom) ends of the continuum of degree or intensity commonly measured by the VAS', and because it 'eliminates difficulty with problems in left–right discrimination and adds to the sensitivity of the scale without altering its validity' (Waltz et al., 1991). However, this is not always the case.

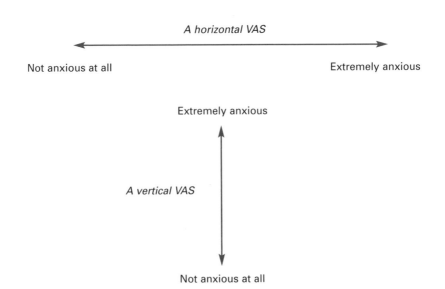

Figure 13.2 A horizontal and a vertical visual analogue scale (VAS)

In a study of the 'relationships of dyspnoea, physical activity and fatigue in patients with chronic obstructive pulmonary disease' Woo (2000) used a vertical VAS (VVAS) to measure dyspnoea. He explains that the scale consisted of a 100 mm vertical line with anchors of 'no shortness of breath' at the bottom and 'shortness of breath as bad as can be' at the top. Although Woo (2000) does not give a reason for choosing the vertical rather than the horizontal VAS, he points out that 'evidence of the validity of the VVAS has been indicated by its positive correlation with the horizontal VAS'.

Another example of the VAS (horizontal) is from a study by Hennessy and Hicks (2003) of the 'ideal attributes of Chief Nurses in Europe'. As they explain:

> The 16 attributes were randomly presented in the second round questionnaire, with a visual analogue scale attached to each. In accordance with convention, the visual analogue was an unmarked 10 cm line with the left hand pole labelled 'not at all important' and the right hand pole labelled 'extremely important'. Each attribute had a number of exemplars to illustrate the nature of the quality under consideration. Respondents were asked to consider these qualities in relation to the ideal Chief Nurse, and then to make a mark along the visual analogue scale to indicate the importance of each quality.

The VAS has been particularly useful in measuring different types of pain including acute pain (Bijur et al., 2001), menstrual pain (Larroy, 2002) and postnatal nipple pain (Duffy et al., 1997).

The advantage of the VAS is that it is easy to administer and simple for participants to understand (Cline et al., 1992). The language is uncomplicated, and the scale takes little time to complete. It can also chart changes over time in the feelings or attitudes being measured. Its disadvantage is that people with visual impairment or psychomotor disability may find it difficult to make their mark on the line. The concept of a line measuring feelings may not be as easily understood by some respondents as it is by researchers.

The VAS has been found to be sufficiently reliable (Bijur et al., 2001) but as Crichton explains, it is a highly subjective form of assessment which is more useful when charting change within individuals than when comparing across a group of individuals at one time point (Crichton, 2001). Larroy (2002) compared the VAS with numeric scales (i.e. respondents are asked to rate their pain on a scale of 1 to 10). The author found a high degree of correlation between the two but recommends the numeric scale for use in epidemiological and prevalence studies as they are 'easier and more convenient to use than the VAS' (Larroy, 2002). She also reported that while the VAS can be very precise, some participants had great difficulty understanding the principles behind it.

Advantages and disadvantages of questionnaires

These depend partly on the mode of questionnaire administration. Questionnaires can be self- or researcher administered. A self-administered questionnaire is one in which respondents write their responses on the questionnaire without the researcher helping in any way. Normally the latter is not present, but there are cases when the researcher is in the same room or in the vicinity. The questionnaire can be delivered personally or posted, hence the term 'postal questionnaire'. Alternatively, the researcher can read the questions and record the responses on the questionnaire. This can be either 'face-to-face' or over the telephone. This type of 'face-to-face' encounter is more like a structured interview (described in Chapter 14).

Questionnaires can also be administered to a group of people, for example students in a classroom. Telephone surveys are becoming increasingly popular in the social and health sciences, and questioning by telephone is extensively used in market research. An example of a telephone survey in nursing research is Jinks et al.'s (2003) study of 'public health roles of health visitors and school nurses'.

The main advantage of questionnaires is that they can reach large numbers of people over wide geographical areas and collect data at a lower cost than can other methods such as interviews and observations. Because they are structured and predetermined and cannot as a rule be varied, both in their wording and in the order in which they are answered, they have a fair degree of reliability. The data collected from all respondents are in the same form, and comparisons can be made between them without great difficulty. Closed questions and rating scales can be precoded and can thereafter be easily and quickly analysed, especially if computer packages, which are becoming increasingly more efficient, are used. Self-administered questionnaires have the advantage of keeping the respondents anonymous except in cases where the researcher deliberately uses a code to identify non-responders for follow-up purposes. They also allow respondents to answer in their own time and at their own convenience. They can have the time to check records, especially when they answer factual questions.

One of the major advantages of self-administered questionnaires is the absence of interviewer effect. Dockrell and Joffe (1992) analysed data from their study of young people and HIV/AIDS and concluded that, while face-to-face interviews gave them insight into the behaviour of the respondents, the latter were often uncomfortable in discussing their sexual activities. According to them, the questionnaire, with fixed choices, might be more appropriate and could lead to a more accurate reporting of such activities (Dockrell and Joffe, 1992). In the case of telephone questionnaires, the interviewer effect can be less than in 'face-to-face' encounters, due to the physical absence of the person asking the questions.

Finally, the questionnaire designer can improve the instrument by piloting it many times before administering it to respondents, thereby increasing its validity and reliability. It can also be useful for other researchers to borrow and adapt for use in their studies.

The main disadvantage with the self-administered questionnaire is that there is no opportunity to ask respondents to elaborate, expand, clarify or illustrate their answers. Respondents themselves have no opportunity to ask for clarification. They may understand questions differently from researchers, thereby not inspiring confidence in the validity of questionnaires. Developing and testing a questionnaire can be time-consuming and costly. It can also be a laborious process involving a number of stages and drafts.

Questionnaires tell us little about the context in which respondents formulate their responses. In interviews, researchers can read the body language and take it as a cue to probe further, if appropriate. As Nay-Brock (1984) explains, it is difficult 'to take into account any reluctance or evasiveness on the part of the respondent because the non-verbal responses of the respondents cannot be observed'. The data collected from questionnaires are sometimes superficial and can only be taken at face value (Parahoo, 1993). They are devoid of the context which gives rise to them and, although they may attempt to measure important contextual variables, they typically separate the measured behaviour from its particular historical, social and cultural contexts (Mechanic, 1989).

Questionnaires do not suit everyone, in particular those who have difficulty in reading and comprehension and in articulating written responses. This may lead some respondents to confer with others or ask them to complete the questionnaires. The implications of this for knowledge and attitude questions are obvious.

Another serious problem with questionnaires is low response rates. There are a variety of reasons why people may not respond to questionnaires. 'Respondent burden' is the discomfort put on them by making use of their effort and time in completing questionnaires or taking part in research generally. Health professionals (as participants in research studies) can be prone to question fatigue. With increasing demands on their time and increasing emphasis on the need for research it can be difficult for them to find time to reply to questionnaires. Various strategies can be used to increase response rates, including making respondents feel that their responses are valuable and ensuring that the questionnaire is easy to respond to, not too lengthy, and well structured and presented. Other methods of data collection such as interviews and observations can also impose a burden on participants.

Some of the above disadvantages are inherent in the method, in that the questionnaire is by its very nature limited to collecting certain types of data, but many of the other disadvantages can be overcome through skilful construction. The questionnaire's popularity as a method of data collection suggests that, to many people, the advantages outweigh the disadvantages. In Chapter 3 some of the limitations of questionnaires were also discussed.

Validity and reliability of questionnaires

For questionnaires to be of use to practitioners and policy makers, they have to produce valid and reliable data. The validity of a questionnaire is the extent to which it addresses the research question, objectives or hypotheses set by the researcher. For example, if a questionnaire is designed to assess patient satisfaction, it must 'assess' rather than 'explore' patient satisfaction with nursing care; all the questions, together, must also reflect fully the concepts of 'patient satisfaction' and 'nursing care'. It can happen that the questionnaire only addresses physical care and ignores other aspects, such as psychological, social and spiritual care. Therefore such a questionnaire can hardly be said to assess satisfaction with 'nursing care'. Two questions can be asked when assessing the validity of a questionnaire:

1. Does the questionnaire answer the research question?

2. Do the questions adequately represent the different attributes of the concepts or the different aspects of the issues being studied?

The reliability of a questionnaire refers to the consistency with which respondents understand, and respond to, all the questions. For example, if a question such as, 'What type of accommodation do you live in?' is put to respondents, would all of them interpret the terms 'type', 'accommodation' and 'live' in the same way? Do all respondents use the terms 'house', 'flat' and 'studio' in the same sense? Some may reply that they live in 'comfortable' or 'cheap' or 'council' accommodation. Others may 'live' in more than one accommodation. It is clear, therefore, that responses to this question will not be consistent if respondents interpret it differently. Two questions that can be asked when assessing the reliability of a questionnaire are:

1. Are the questions or statements clear and unambiguous enough for a respondent to understand and to respond to them in the same way each time they are presented to him (except where respondents have different answers to give), and for the respondent to understand them in the same way as others do?

2. Do all respondents interpret the instructions given by the researcher in the same way?

A questionnaire can be reliable without being valid, but it cannot be valid if it is not reliable. In the above example of a questionnaire assessing patients' satisfaction with nursing care, if the questions and instructions are interpreted in the same way by all respondents but the questionnaire content does not represent all the different aspects of nursing care, the questionnaire is reliable but not valid. If some respondents interpret the questions differently from others, their responses are not reliable and cannot also be taken as a valid assessment of 'patients' satisfaction with nursing care' as a result of the confusion over the meaning of some questions. Therefore reliability is a necessary but not a sufficient condition for validity.

Earlier in this chapter, we looked at the type of phenomena, such as facts, knowledge and attitudes, that nursing research questionnaires describe or measure. However, they present a number of difficulties to researchers. In theory, facts are believed to be the easiest type of data that questionnaires can collect; in practice, it may be quite different. Yet, people can also be 'economical with the truth' for various reasons; facts can be 'coloured' to make responses more socially desirable. For example, some people who cannot afford two meals a day may not want the world to know about it. Lydeard (1991) explains that 'prestige bias, social desirability, ego, or practical/ethical standards, all are different names for the same phenomenon, i.e. responders are modest/social drinkers that rarely smoke, brush their teeth with alarming frequency and never allow their children to watch dubious television programmes'.

Answers can also be exaggerated to protest or support particular causes. The context in which questionnaires are administered can affect the reliability and validity of the data. Researchers in the health field often have to deal with captive populations such as patients in a ward or clinic. Robinson (1996) gives the following example from the National Birthday Trust's (NBT) study of pain relief in labour (Chamberlain et al., 1993) to show that 'questions answered before discharge are answered differently from the same questions asked later'. In the NBT's study, '70% of women questioned after delivery said they had been free to choose their method of pain relief', but when questioned 6 weeks after delivery, this had 'fallen to 55%' (cited in Robinson, 1996).

Memory distortion, memory gaps and selective memory can all be responsible for inaccuracies in self-reporting. Memory distortion can happen when, for example, a past event is seen to be worse or better than it was because the 'passing of time' has put a different perception to it. Memory gaps simply refer to the forgetfulness of events of little significance to respondents, especially if they happened a long time ago. With selective memory, respondents choose to remember certain events, for example joyful ones, and repress others that are painful.

Events and activities that require respondents or researchers to make an assessment, as in the case of the 'amount of fluid intake' or the 'frequency of bowel movements', can be under- or overreported as these involve a subjective judgement. These difficulties in and limitations of collecting reliable factual information must be borne in mind when evaluating data. They do not in themselves undermine the usefulness of questionnaires in the collection of such data. By systematic development and rigorous testing, the reliability of questionnaires and scales can be greatly enhanced.

Measuring attitudes is a complex and challenging task. According to Henerson et al. (1987), 'an attitude is not something we can examine and measure in the same way we can examine the cells of a person's skin or measure the rate of her heartbeat'. They illustrate the complexity of attitudes with the example of racial prejudice:

> when we attempt to measure an attitude such as racial prejudice, we find it is blurred by peer group pressures, the desire to please, ambivalence, inconsistency, lack of self awareness.

It is sometimes surprising to find that questionnaires are designed to measure a particular attitude using only two or three questions. This shows a lack of understanding of the complexities of measuring and assessing such concepts.

Measuring respondents' knowledge by questionnaire is a less challenging task than is measuring attitudes. However, there are particular problems that can threaten the reliability and validity of the responses. For example, self-administered questionnaires, as explained earlier, give opportunities for respondents to confer with others or consult other sources. Mulliner et al. (1995) pointed out in their study 'exploring midwives' education in, knowledge of and attitudes to nutrition in pregnancy' that it was 'considered unrealistic to expect midwives to respond to a postal questionnaire attempting to assess their nutritional knowledge'.

For interviewer-administered questionnaires, researchers often make an appointment with respondents and disclose in advance the remit of the questionnaire, thereby possibly giving them the opportunity to 'brush up' on the topic. Assessing the knowledge of health professionals, no matter what method is used, can be threatening to them even when the promise of confidentiality is offered. The response rate may understandably be low, and the number of partially completed questionnaires is often high. It is difficult to ascertain whether a non-response to a question means that the respondent did not know the answer, did not understand the question or simply chose to ignore it.

People often give an opinion when asked even if they have little or no knowledge of the topic or have not thought seriously about it. Multiple-choice and checklist questions offer the opportunity for guesswork. Many of the questions asked in a questionnaire can only be answered conditionally.

Studying behaviour and behavioural intention with the use of questionnaires can also be particularly difficult. Earlier, we mentioned some of the problems with self-reporting, including memory distortion, memory gaps and selective memory. Behavioural intention is the 'nut' that policy makers, planners and opinion pollsters would dearly like to 'crack'.

Sparrow (1993) conducted recall interviews to find out why opinion polls failed to predict a Conservative victory in the 1992 UK general election. His study revealed that some people who told interviewers they would vote for a particular party decided on the last day to vote differently, and that there was 'a group of people who were unwilling to say who they would vote for in the original poll, but gave details of their voting behaviour in the recall interviews'.

The reliability of questionnaires depends largely on question wording and questionnaire structure. Lydeard (1991) explains that 'it is difficult enough to obtain a relatively unbiased answer even from a willing, alert individual who has correctly understood the question but the task becomes virtually impossible if hampered by poor question wording'.

The importance of question wording is illustrated in an example in Robinson (1996). As she explains:

> When the General Household Survey was collecting data on chronic illness, they asked 'Do you suffer from any disability?' The response rate was far lower than researchers expected. Next time they asked 'Do you HAVE any disability?' and got a more accurate response. Many people had disabilities, but did not consider they suffered from them or perhaps were unwilling to say that they did.

Some of the threats to reliability come from questions that are ambiguous, double-barrelled, leading, double-negative and hypothetical. Question order and the length of the questionnaire can also affect responses.

Fowler (1992) took seven questions from questionnaires used in national health surveys, and subjected them to a 'special pretest procedure' and found that they contained poorly defined terms. When they were clarified and administered, they yielded significantly different results. Terms like 'often', 'sometimes' or 'happy' can mean different things to different people. Schaeffer (1991) gives this interesting illustration:

> In the movie *Annie Hall*, there is a scene with a split screen. On one side Alvie Singer talks to his psychiatrist; on the other side Annie Hall talks to hers. Alvie's therapist asks him, 'How often do you sleep together?' and Alvie replies, 'Hardly ever, maybe three times a week'. Annie's therapist asks her, 'Do you have sex often?' Annie replies, 'Constantly, I'd say three times a week.'

As the author says, the fact that frequency can be reported in different ways is a source of concern for researchers. Below are examples of the types of question that can affect the reliability and validity of questionnaire data.

Double-barrelled:

Traditional nurses are more realistic and concise in formulating care plans than degree nurses:

Agree ☐   Disagree ☐

Leading:

In the UK 30 000 people die each year from smoking-related diseases. Indicate your reaction to this statement by marking an X on the line below.

Very concerned ◄————————————► Apathetic

Double-negative:

Are you not taking the sleeping tablets as prescribed?

Yes ☐   No ☐

Hypothetical:

Would you like free dental care?

Yes ☐   No ☐

Lengthy and uninteresting questionnaires not only affect response rates, but can also lead respondents to take them lightly. Self-administered questionnaires that are time-consuming to complete may cause fatigue and lack of concentration, especially to people who are not accustomed to reading and writing. The order of the questions, the way in which they are grouped and their sensitivity (or lack of it) can all affect responses. Mechanic (1989) points out that 'we have many relevant methodological studies, and some solutions, to such problems as acquiescence, social desirability effects, format biases, recall difficulties, and many more, but the complexity of these issues means that in the average study most of these cautions are acknowledged but ignored'.

The reliability and validity of questionnaires can be greatly enhanced by careful preparation and skilful construction, paying particular attention to the needs and circumstances of potential respondents and anticipating how they would react. One thing to remember is that, despite all the efforts made to construct and administer a reliable and valid questionnaire, there will always be some respondents who will interpret terms or questions differently. Large samples can, to some extent, accommodate minor individual inconsistencies. There are a number of strategies that researchers can use in order to reduce bias and ambiguities and ensure the validity and reliability of questionnaires.

Assessing validity

There are a variety of validity tests that can be applied, the main ones described here being content validity, criterion-related validity and construct validity.

Content validity

This type of validity refers to the degree to which the questions or items in the questionnaire adequately represent the phenomenon being studied. If the questionnaire sets out to measure staff nurses' nutritional knowledge in relation to the care of diabetic patients, a content validity test would ensure that there are enough relevant questions covering all the major aspects of the nutritional knowledge that nurses are required to have for nursing this particular group of patients. Content validity also ensures that irrelevant questions are not asked.

Content validity can be illustrated by the example of a teacher setting questions on an examination paper for a particular module. All the questions together must address the whole content of the module.

To assess content validity, the questionnaire is submitted to a panel of judges with experience and knowledge of the topic, who can make suggestions for the adequacy and relevance of the questions. Redsell et al. (2004) assessed the face and content validity of the Consultation Assessment and Improvement Instrument (CAIIN) for primary care nurses. They carried out focus group interviews with nurses and assessed the use of the instrument by scrutinising '18 video recordings of seven nurses in consultation with real patients' (Redsell et al., 2004). Appropriate changes to the CAIIN were made as a result of this exercise.

Another common method of validating the content of questionnaires is by calculating the Content Validity Index (CVI). This is achieved by asking a group of experts to rate the relevance of items in the questionnaire (for example, by choosing between responses such as 'not relevant', 'somewhat relevant', 'quite relevant', and 'very relevant') and by calculating the degree of agreement or disagreement between them on individual items (Wynd et al., 2003). Mastaglia et al. (2003) explain how content validity could be ensured when developing an instrument. They provide a checklist for experts to rate questionnaire items in terms of clarity, content validity and internal consistency.

There is no statistical test for content validity, although an index of content validity can be calculated based on the degree of agreement of the panel members.

Content validity is sometimes referred to as 'face validity' (Smith, 1991). Redsell et al. (2004) offer the following distinction between the two terms:

Face validity: the extent to which the assessment instrument subjectively appears to be measuring what it is supposed to measure.

Content validity: the extent to which the instrument includes a representative sample of the content of a construct.

In effect, face validity involves giving the questionnaire to anyone, not necessarily an expert on the subject, who can 'on the face of it', assess whether the questions reflect the phenomenon being studied. Greater or lesser weight may be given to face validity depending on how it was accessed. Methods range from giving the questionnaire to colleagues to have a cursory review of items to asking a number of participants in a survey to comment on the tool. Jenkinson et al. (1996) used questionnaires and interviews to assess the face validity and internal reliability of the Short Form 36 Health Survey Questionnaire. They found out that several questions were perceived by respondents 'as inappropriate or difficult to answer'. Face and content validity are the ones most frequently reported in the literature.

Criterion-related validity

Another way to find out about the validity of a questionnaire is to compare its findings with data collected on the same phenomenon by other methods, such as another questionnaire or clinical observations. The data from these other sources become the criteria with which data from the present questionnaire can be compared. If the data are similar, the questionnaire can be said to have criterion-related validity. There are two types of criterion-related validity: concurrent and predictive.

Concurrent validity refers to other current criteria (hence concurrent) with which comparisons can be made. For example, for a questionnaire measuring pain to have concurrent validity, the data from the questionnaire must correspond to other data, such as nurses' observations relating to requests for painkillers and other behaviours. If the questionnaire is able to distinguish those who have pain from those who do not, data from other sources, including nurses' observations, must tell a similar story about the same patients. If this happens, the questionnaire can be said to have concurrent validity.

Predictive validity refers to data available in the future that will confirm whether or not data from the present questionnaire are valid. For example, a questionnaire that can distinguish between those who have positive and those who have negative attitudes towards people with a learning disability will have predictive validity if their future behaviours are consistent with the findings of the questionnaire. The difference between predictive and concurrent validity, then, is the difference in the timing of obtaining measurements on a criterion (Polit and Hungler, 1995).

Dijkstra et al. (1998) evaluated the 'criterion-related validity' of the 'nursing-care dependency (NCD) scale'. They compared the NCD scale with a number of other scales and concluded that 'the NCD was able to purposefully distinguish diagnostic groups of demented patients when an external criterion was used'.

Construct validity

This is the most difficult type of validity for a questionnaire to achieve. It refers to how well a questionnaire or scale measures a particular construct. Examples of constructs are self-esteem, burn-out, social support and empathy. Each of these constructs is difficult to define, let alone measure. Researchers have to resort to the theoretical and research literature before they can break down each construct into attributes, which can thereafter form the items or questions on a scale. The construct validity of an instrument is its ability to measure the intended construct. It should be able to discriminate or differentiate between similar constructs. Crichton (2000) gives this useful example:

suppose we have an instrument that is claimed to measure 'health'. We would then expect that those who are ill, of lower social class and frequent visitors to their GP to gain scores indicating worse health than individuals who are well, in a higher social class and infrequently visit their GP. Thus validation of the instrument involves ensuring that it can discriminate between these groups.

It is difficult for a newly constructed questionnaire to achieve construct validity as it has to be tested in a multitude of settings and with different populations over a number of years. For examples of studies testing the construct validity of scales see Dijkstra et al. (1999) and Vlaminck et al. (2001).

Assessing reliability

A number of reliability tests have been devised to find out the consistency with which questionnaires collect data. Among the well-known ones are test–retest, alternate-form and split-half.

Test–retest

The test–retest simply involves administering the questionnaire on two occasions and comparing the responses. For example, an 'attitude towards mental illness' questionnaire can be administered to a group of chemistry students. The same questionnaire can then be readministered to the same group three weeks later. The second set of responses from each individual should not differ unless something has happened to change their attitudes. If a group of student nurses were given the same questionnaire on two occasions and had visited a psychiatric hospital in the interval between the two administrations, a difference in results could be explained. If nothing has happened in the period between the two administrations that might change their attitudes, the scores must be the same; the questionnaire thus passes the test–retest and can be said to be reliable.

Bohannon et al. (2004) assessed the test–retest reliability of the short form health survey (SF-12) with 31 patients who experienced an ischemic stroke 3–12 months previously. The SF-12 was administered twice by telephone at mean intervals of 16.2 days between tests. 'Scores differed less than 1.5 points and the study supported the test–retest reliability of the SF-12 administered by telephone to post-stroke patients' (Bohannon et al., 2004).

Alternate-form test

The alternate-form reliability test (also known as equivalence) is carried out by asking the questions in two different forms. Sometimes the order of the categories can be altered. For example, if we take a question from Fretwell's (1982)

'Rating Questionnaires for Learners', we can carry out an alternate-form reliability test by changing the order of her original categories A into a new form B as shown below:

A Original version	B New version
a. I learnt little on this ward	(d) I learnt very much on this ward
b. I learnt quite a lot on this ward	(c) I learnt a lot on this ward
c. I learnt a lot on this ward	(b) I learnt quite a lot on this ward
d. I learnt very much on this ward	(a) I learnt little on this ward

Another way of testing alternate forms of reliability is to substitute the wording of the question by equivalent terms without altering the meaning of the question. Litwin (1995) offers the following example, in which version A can be changed to version B.

Version A
During the past week, how often did you usually empty your bladder?

1 to 2 times per day 1
3 to 4 times per day 2
5 to 8 times per day 3
12 times per day 4
More than 12 times per day 5

Version B
During the past week, how often did you usually empty your bladder?

Every 12 to 24 hours 1
Every 6 to 8 hours 2
Every 3 to 5 hours 3
Every 2 hours 4
More than every 2 hours 5

Split-half test

This test involves dividing or splitting the instrument into two equal halves and finding out whether or not their scores are similar. For example, for an attitude rating scale with ten statements, the researcher will take the total score of the first five and compare it with the score of the last five. If the scores are similar, the statements or test items are said to be homogeneous. No item has a greater value than any other in assessing an attitude. This means that all the items are designed to make the respondent react consistently in the same way if they possess a particular attitude. If this happens, the test shows high internal consistency.

The split-half test can only be carried out with questionnaires that measure a concept or phenomenon, and applies only to instruments for which there is a total score. Most questionnaires that set out to describe or explore particular phenomena do not fall into this category.

There are other tests for validity and reliability; only those most frequently reported in the literature are described here.

To sum up, the validity of an instrument is established mainly by comparing its responses or scores with the scores of other sources (other research instruments, clinical observations or other records). On the other hand, the reliability of an instrument is tested mainly by comparing its own responses or scores (on different occasions, with different wordings or structure, and between items).

Pilot testing the questionnaire

Even before validity and reliability tests are carried out, researchers can refine their questionnaires by administering them to a small group of people similar in characteristics to the intended respondents. Those who have done so have been amazed at the types of error, not just typographical, that can be detected. The first and most efficient way to find out the quality of a questionnaire is to test or 'pilot' it. The responses will give the researcher a fair idea of whether all the respondents understand the questions in the same way, whether the format of the questions is the most suitable for this population, whether they understand the instructions and how relevant the questions are. She can also find out whether the length of the questionnaire and its structure are likely to affect responses. Researchers who take the opportunity to consider respondents' views on the above aspects of the questionnaire, listen to the problems encountered by them, and seek to resolve some of the doubts they (the researchers) have about their questionnaires, are likely to learn a lot about the strengths and weaknesses of their tools. Researchers are professionals whose 'language' and culture can be different from those of the potential participants in their study. It is important for them to realise that their questionnaires reflect their value positions and may create a different impression on respondents from the one they anticipate.

Critiquing questionnaires

Many authors of reports or articles do not give a detailed description of the questionnaires for readers to assess their validity and reliability. Only on rare occasions are questionnaires included as an appendix; often only a brief description of the number of items is given. Other information that is frequently missing includes pilot testing, validity and reliability tests, reminders or follow-ups to increase response rates and information about non-responders.

When assessing the use of a questionnaire in a research study, you must look at how the questionnaire was developed, if this is the case. Did the researcher formulate the items only from her own experience and/or the literature? Content validity is likely to be enhanced if efforts were made to consult the literature or other instruments for relevant items to be included. If a questionnaire is borrowed and adapted, does the author comment on how the validity and reliability of the original instrument has been affected? You should also determine whether the questionnaire was piloted, with whom, how and with what results. More than one round of piloting is an indication that serious attempts have been made to refine it. You must also find out other measures taken to enhance validity and reliability. How were face or content validity ensured? Was the questionnaire given to one or more 'experts' to comment and make suggestions? Construct validity, especially in studies that use existing, well-established tools, is sometimes reported. For most self-designed questionnaires, it is not fair to expect the author(s) to comment on concurrent, predictive or construct validity, as the data to establish these are not always readily available.

It is sometimes possible to evaluate the wording or formats of questions only when these appear in the article or report. When the questionnaire is available, you can assess its content validity, how appropriate or effective the question formats are, and the possibility of biases in the wording. The structure of the questionnaire must facilitate rather than hinder respondents in providing answers. The questionnaire as a whole must make sense and the questions should not jump from one topic to another and back again. You can find out whether the instructions are clear and whether the length and presentation are likely to encourage respondents to complete it.

One of the main sources of bias in studies using questionnaires is low response rate. This happens when the characteristics and attributes of non-responders are different from responders. Volunteer and accidental samples, in particular, can be different from those who did not volunteer. Such bias can be taken into account and corrected, to some extent, by statistical means. However, the nature and extent of non-respondent bias 'can only be made by collecting data directly from non-respondents' (Lynn, 2003). In a survey of 'general practitioners and their views of the NHS changes', Armstrong and Ashworth (2000) compared responders and non-responders. They found that the latter 'differed significantly from responders in many of their views'. When appraising the validity of findings in surveys, you should look for information on the characteristics of those who did not respond. However, finding out about non-responders can be costly and difficult since they can continue to refuse to respond.

Your task in assessing a questionnaire is to find out how valid and reliable it is in answering the research questions. However, it is important to remember that it is easier to critique a questionnaire than to construct one. Perhaps for this reason alone, researchers rarely attach their questionnaires to their articles.

Ethical aspects of questionnaires

The self-administered questionnaire is one of the few methods of data collection that can potentially keep respondents anonymous. This can be an advantage because it gives them the opportunity of making their views known without being identified, unless of course, each questionnaire is numbered or coded for the purpose of sending reminders to those who have not replied. One way to maintain anonymity and increase response rates is to send a reminder to all participants regardless of who replied (which can be costly), but bias may be introduced if a respondent replies twice and this is overlooked by the researcher.

Confidentiality and privacy, as with other methods of data collection, must also be respected. However, both confidentiality and respect for privacy are easier to promise than to fulfil. Despite the best efforts and intentions of researchers, there are ways in which respondents can be identified by others or identify themselves. Privacy must mean what it says, that is the questionnaire must be administered to the respondent alone and in a private place. Robinson (1996) relates how, as a patient, 'in the local gynaecology ward, lying in one of those small bays', she overheard a 'private' conversation. As she describes:

> A white coated woman approached the patient in the opposite bed and asked if she would mind answering a few questions. The captive patient of course agreed. To my horror I recognized the intimate questions as part of the cancer epidemiology questionnaire I had approved at the Ethics Committee. We had not specified the interviews should be private, because it had never occurred to us that the researcher would do anything else.

Researchers are expected to obtain informed consent from respondents. However, because the questionnaire seems to be less intrusive than the interview or observation and less interventionist than the experiment, there is a tendency to think that it can cause no harm. Often, obtaining approval from an ethical committee is not thought to be necessary. Questionnaires, however, can be intrusive by asking people embarrassing and sensitive questions, and can invade privacy. They can open 'old wounds' with no one at hand to offer support. The following three consecutive questions taken from a real questionnaire on cervical screening exemplify the potential of questionnaires to do harm:

		Yes	No
Q9	Do you have any history of sexually transmitted disease?	☐	☐
Q10	Have you been sexually abused in the past?	☐	☐
Q11	Does your family have a history of cervical cancer?	☐	☐

Apart from being highly personal, these questions can trigger memories of traumatic experiences. The potential harm of these types of question is awesome. A respondent who has been sexually abused in the past can rightly ask why the researcher wants to know this and why she should tell anyone about it. This questionnaire may not be typical of questionnaires in general, but it shows that researchers can ignore, or be unaware of, the sensitive nature of their questions.

The questionnaire, by psychologically assaulting respondents, can itself be an instrument of abuse.

Sheikh et al. (2001) explained the moral issues raised when research conducted at a distance uncovers information about participants which indicates that they may be at increased risk of harm. Their study on the psychological morbidity among general practice managers raised a number of ethical and research dilemmas. They were concerned that 17 per cent of managers had 'scores indicative of depression, with 5 per cent of responders reporting that they entertained suicidal ideas' (Sheikh et al., 2001).

Evans et al. (2002) expressed concern that the 'likely impact of questionnaires upon patients is not often considered and therefore, the balance of benefit and harm not fully explored'. In their study of breast cancer among women, some respondents asked questions, for example, about risks of getting cancer and risks related to treatment. Evans et al. (2002) pointed out that debriefing opportunities are not readily available when questionnaires are used to collect data. Sheikh et al. (2001) suggest that a warning might be added 'at the top of the questionnaire pointing out that the questions asked might bring to the surface distress which the participants might wish to discuss in the context of a confidential helpline'.

Questionnaires can make people feel guilty about their lifestyles, for example by asking them questions about healthy living. They can identify their lack of knowledge on particular topics. Knowledge questions can be threatening to health professionals as the data may fall into the hands of their employers. One can ask also whether it is ethically right for people to participate in studies and not be told what the findings are, as would be the case for most research studies. The latter are published in journals of which lay people are unaware, and which professionals themselves may not read. Robinson (1996), writing about the ethical implications of questionnaire design and administration, concluded that 'badly designed research is per se unethical and should not be done at all' and that 'at best it wastes patients' time and at worst it can do outright harm'.

SUMMARY

Summary and conclusion

The questionnaire is the most popular method of data collection in health and social research. Like other methods, it has a number of advantages and disadvantages. It is suitable mainly for collecting data on facts, knowledge, attitudes, beliefs and opinions when it is carefully prepared, constructed and administered. It is clear also that questionnaire data must not be taken at face value. Readers must assess the validity and reliability of the instrument where possible, and researchers must provide evidence of validity and reliability checks they have carried out. If used wisely and sensitively, the questionnaire has the potential to provide valuable data on which policy and practice decisions can be made.

References

Armstrong D and Ashworth M (2000) When questionnaire response rates do matter: a survey of general practitioners and their views of the NHS changes. *British Journal of General Practice*, 50:479–80.

Bijur P E, Silver W and Gallagher E J (2001) Reliability of the visual analog scale for measurement of acute pain. *Academic Emergency Medicine*, 8, 12:1153–7.

Blue C L, Wilbur J and Marston-Scott M C (2001) Exercise among blue-collar workers: application of the theory of planned behavior. *Research in Nursing and Health*, 24:481–93.

Bohannon R W, Maljanian R and Landes M (2004) Test–retest reliability of short form (SF)-12 component scores of patients with stroke. *International Journal of Rehabilitation Research*, 27, 2:149–50.

Bowles C (1986) Measure of attitude toward menopause using the Semantic Differential Model. *Nursing Research*, 35, 2:81–5.

Chamberlain C, Wraight A and Steer P (eds) (1993) *Pain and Its Relief in Childbirth* (Edinburgh: Churchill Livingstone).

Chau J P C, Chang A M, Lee I F K, Ip W Y, Lee D T F and Wootton Y (2001) Effects of using videotaped vignettes on enhancing students' critical thinking ability in a baccalaureate nursing programme. *Journal of Advanced Nursing*, 36, 1:112–19.

Cline ME, Herman J, Shaw E R and Morton R D (1992) Standardization of the Visual Analogue Scale. *Nursing Research*, 41, 6:378–80.

Crichton N (2001) Information point: Visual Analogue Scale. *Journal of Clinical Nursing*, 10:706.

Dijkstra A, Buist G and Dassen T (1998) A criterion-related validity study of the nursing-care dependency (NCD) scale. *International Journal of Nursing Studies*, 35:163–70.

Dijkstra A, Buist G, Moorer P and Dassen T (1999) Construct validity of the Nursing Care Dependency Scale. *Journal and Clinical Nursing*, 8:380–8.

Dockrell J and Joffe H (1992) Methodological issues involved in the study of young people and HIV/AIDS: a social psychological view. *Health Education Research*, 7:509–16.

Duffy E P, Percival P and Kershaw E (1997) Positive effects of an antenatal group teaching session on postnatal nipple pain, nipple trauma and breastfeeding rates. *Midwifery*, 13, 4:189–96.

Evans M, Robling M, Maggs Rapport F, Houston H, Kinnersley P and Wilkinson C (2002) It doesn't cost anything just to ask, does it? The ethics of questionnaire-based research. *Journal of Medical Ethics*, 28, 1:41–4.

Fowler F J Jr. (1992) How unclear terms affect survey data. *Public Opinion Quarterly*, 56:218–31.

Fretwell J E (1982) *Ward Teaching and Learning* (London: Royal College of Nursing).

Gould D (1996) Using vignettes to collect data for nursing research studies: how valid are the findings? *Journal of Clinical Nursing*, 5, 4:207–12.

Gould D, Kelly D, Goldstone G and Gammon J (2001) Examining the validity of pressure ulcer risk assessment scales: developing and using illustrated patient simulations to collect data. *Journal of Clinical Nursing*, 10:697–706.

Harvey S, Rach D, Stainton M C, Jarrell J and Brant R (2002) Evaluation of satisfaction with midwifery care. *Midwifery*, 18:260–7.

Hellzén O, Kristiansen L and Norbergh K G (2003) Nurses' attitudes towards older residents with long-term schizophrenia. *Journal of Advanced Nursing*, 43, 6:616–22.

Henerson M E, Morris L L and Fitz-Gibbon C T (1987) *How to Measure Attitudes* (Newbury Park, CA: Sage).

Hennessy D and Hicks C (2003) The ideal attributes of chief nurses in Europe: a Delphi study. *Journal of Advanced Nursing*, 43, 5:441–8.

Jenkinson C O, Peto V and Coulter A (1996) Making sense of ambiguity: evaluation of internal reliability and face validity of the SF 37 questionnaire in women presenting with menorrhagia. *Quality in Health Care*, **5**, 1:9–12.

Jinks A, Smith M and Ashdown-Lambert J (2003) The public health roles of health visitors and school nurses. *British Journal of Community Nursing*, **8**, 11:496–501.

Larroy C (2002) Comparing visual-analog and numeric scales for assessing menstrual pain. *Behavioral Medicine*, **27**, 4:179–81.

Likert (1932) *A Technique for the Measurement of Attitudes* (New York: Columbia University Press).

Linqvist R, Carlsson M and Sjöden P O (2004) Coping strategies of people with kidney transplants. *Journal of Advanced Nursing*, **45**, 1:47–52.

Litwin M S (1995) *How to Measure Survey Reliability and Validity* (Newbury Park, CA: Sage).

Lydeard S (1991) The questionnaire as a research tool. *Family Practice*, **8**, 1:84–91.

Lynn P (2003) PEDAKSI: Methodology for collecting data about survey non-respondents. *Quality and Quantity*, **37**:239–61.

Martin C R and Thompson D R (2002) The hospital anxiety and depression scale in patients undergoing peritoneal dialysis: internal and test–retest reliability. *Clinical Effectiveness in Nursing*, **6**:78–80.

Mastaglia B, Toye C and Kristjanson L J (2003) Ensuring content validity in instrument development: challenges and innovative approaches. *Contemporary Nurse*, **14**:281–91.

McDonnell A, Nicholl J and Read S M (2003) Acute Pain Teams in England: current provision and their role in postoperative pain management. *Journal of Clinical Nursing*, **12**, 3:387–93.

McKenna H P, Ashton S and Keeney S (2004) Barriers to evidence-based practice in primary care. *Journal of Advanced Nursing*, **45**, 2:178–89.

McKinlay A, Couston M and Cowans S (2001) Nurses' behavioural intentions towards self-poisoning patients: a theory of reasoned action, comparison of attitudes and subjective norms as predictive variables. *Journal of Advanced Nursing*, **34**, 1:107–16.

Mechanic D (1989) Medical sociology: some tensions among theory, method and substance. *Journal of Health and Social Behaviour*, **30**:147–60.

Mulliner C M, Spiby H and Fraser R B (1995) A study exploring midwives' education in, knowledge of and attitudes to nutrition in pregnancy. *Midwifery*, **11**, 1:37–41.

Nay-Brock R M (1984) A comparison of the questionnaire and interviewing techniques in the collection of sociological data. *Australian Journal of Advanced Nursing*, **2**, 1:14–23.

O'Connor H and Madge G (2003) Focus groups in cyberspace: using the Internet for qualitative research. *Qualitative Market Research: An International Journal*, **6**, 2:133–43.

Osgood C E, Suci G J and Tannenbaum P H (1957) *The Measurement of Meaning* (Chicago: University of Illinois Press).

Parahoo K (1993) Questionnaire: use, value and limitations. *Nurse Researcher*, **1**, 2:4–15.

Polit D F and Hungler B P (1995) *Nursing Research: Principles and Methods*, 5th edn (Philadelphia: J B Lippincott).

Redsell S A, Lennon M, Hastings A M and Fraser R C (2004) Devising and establishing the face and content validity of explicit criteria of consultation competence for UK secondary care nurses. *Nurse Education Today*, **24**, 180–7.

Robinson J (1996) It's only a questionnaire . . . ethics in social science research. *British Journal of Midwifery*, **4**, 1:41–4.

Sarmiento T P, Laschinger H K S and Iwasiw C (2004) Nurse Educators' workplace empowerment, burnout, and job satisfaction: testing Kanter's theory. *Journal of Advanced Nursing*, **46**, 2:134–43.

Schaeffer N C (1991) Hardly ever or constantly? Group comparisons using vague quantifiers. *Public Opinion Quarterly*, **55**:395–423.

Sechrist K and Pravikoff D (2001) *Semantic Differential Scale: Cinahl Information Systems* (California: Cinahl).

Shaker I, Scott J A and Reid M (2004) Infant feeding attitudes of expectant parents: breastfeeding and formula feeding. *Journal of Advanced Nursing*, 45, 3:260–8.

Sheikh A, Hurwitz B and Parker B (2001) Ethical and research dilemmas arising from a questionnaire study of psychological morbidity among general practice managers. *British Journal of General Practice*, 51:32–5.

Smith H W (1991) *Strategies of Social Research*, 3rd edn (St Louis, MO: University of Missouri).

Smith L N (1994) An analysis and reflections on the quality of nursing research in 1992. *Journal of Advanced Nursing*, 19:385–93.

Sparrow N (1993) Improving polling techniques following the 1992 General Election. *Journal of Market Research Society*, 35, 1:79–89.

Stone D H (1993) Design a questionnaire. *British Medical Journal*, 307:1264–6.

Vlaminck H, Maes B, Jacobs A, Reyntjens S and Evers G (2001) The Dialysis Diet and Fluid Non-Adherence Questionnaire: validity testing of a self-report instrument for clinical practice. *Journal of Clinical Nursing*, 10, 5:707–14.

Wahlberg A C, Cedersund E and Wredling R (2003) Telephone nurses' experience of problems with telephone advice in Sweden. *Journal of Clinical Nursing*, 12:37–45.

Walker J M and Sofaer B (1998) Predictors of psychological distress in chronic pain patients. *Journal of Advanced Nursing*, 27:320–6.

Waltz C F, Strickland O L and Lenz E R (1991) *Measurement in Nursing Research*, 2nd edn (Philadelphia: F A Davis).

Webb C (2003) Research in Brief. An analysis of recent publications in JCN: sources, methods and topics. *Journal of Clinical Nursing*, 12:931–4.

Webb C (2004) Editor's note: Analysis of papers published in JAN in 2002. *Journal of Advanced Nursing*, 45, 3:229–31.

Woo K (2000) A pilot study to examine the relationships of dyspnoea, physical activity and fatigue in patients with chronic obstructive pulmonary disease. *Journal of Clinical Nursing*, 9:526–33.

Wynd C A, Schmidt B and Schaefer M A (2003) Two quantitative approaches for estimating content validity. *Western Journal of Nursing Research*, 25, 5:508–18.

14 Interviews

It is the province of knowledge to speak and it is the privilege of wisdom to listen.

Oliver Wendell Holmes

Introduction

The beliefs, attitudes, experiences and perception of clients and staff are important for the organisation, delivery and evaluation of care and treatment. The interview has an important part to play in collecting data to inform the decisions and actions of health professionals, as well as in providing insights into how clients access and use health services and their experience of them.

This chapter will discuss the use of interviews in clinical practice and in research, the different forms of research interviews and their advantages and disadvantages. It will also explore the ethical implications, as well as the validity and reliability, of different forms of interviewing. Finally, what you should look for when critiquing studies that use interviews will be suggested.

Interviews in clinical practice

In our everyday life, we engage in interactions that involve asking, and being asked, questions. We can say that we all are 'interviewers' and 'interviewees'. Verbal communication is the most effective means available to humans with which to convey our feelings, experiences, views and intentions. However, we do not normally call these verbal interactions interviews; most of the time they are merely casual conversations. Some of us have been interviewed for a job or a place on a course or watched others being interviewed on television. These interviews are different from casual conversations in that they have (or should have) a clearer agenda, often prepared in advance and with a specific purpose, and are limited in duration. Health professionals, too, carry out interviews for the purpose of obtaining information from clients that can be used to assess, plan, implement and evaluate care and treatment. Nurse–client interactions involve both formal interviewing and casual conversations throughout the time that the client is in contact with the professional. With clinical interviews, the aim is not only to obtain valuable information, but also to build trust between the professional and the client. Thus a therapeutic relationship is initiated and developed.

Nurse training programmes tend to put a lot of emphasis on communication skills, in particular how to talk with, and listen to, patients. In Chapter 1, we explained that some knowledge of, and skills in, research methods can help to sharpen nurses' ability to ask questions, listen and observe.

Research interviews

A research interview, on the other hand, is a verbal interaction between one or more researchers and one or more respondents for the purpose of collecting valid and reliable data to answer particular research questions. In the clinical interview, the client is the raison d'être of the interview, while in a research interview, the interest in the respondent is as far as the interview goes. In some types of interview, the degree of interaction is greater than in others, but the researcher's aim is not to develop therapeutic relationships. The purpose of clinical interviews is to collect data to enhance the health of the client; the data collected in research interviews serve to satisfy the researcher's curiosity and, if the findings are valid and reliable, they may ultimately be used to enhance client care.

Research interviews can be face-to-face (in the same room or by video-conferencing), via the internet and by telephone. Face-to-face interviews (individual or focus groups) will be discussed throughout this chapter. Although the internet is a medium frequently used to access available information, it also promises to be a useful tool for researchers to obtain data from respondents from different parts of the country or of the world, in a simple way and at low costs (Scholl et al., 2002). While these advantages are obvious, the problems with on-line collection of data are only beginning to emerge. According to O'Connor and Madge (2003) the suitability of cyberspace as a venue for more qualitative on-line research, for example, in-depth interviewing, has received little attention.

Telephone interviews, on the other hand, have a long history. In the United States, it is the most dominant form of interviewing (Holbrook et al., 2003). Like on-line interviewing, it is less expensive and time-consuming than face-to-face interviewing. Its main disadvantage is that only those who are accessible via telephones can be interviewed. It is also difficult to ascertain who one is really speaking with. Response rates can also be lower than in face-to-face interviews. Holbrook et al. compared telephone interviews with face-to-face ones. They found telephone respondents to be 'less cooperative and engaged in the interview, and were more likely to express dissatisfaction with the length of the interview than were face-to-face respondents, despite the fact that the telephone interviews were completed more quickly than face-to-face interviews' (Holbrook et al., 2003).

Garbett and McCormack (2001) carried out telephone interviews in their study of 'practitioners' views of practice development'. They concluded that although the telephone interview approach proved fruitful in the context of limited resources, 'the brevity of the conversations meant that deeper exploration of ideas was difficult'.

Whatever the form of interviews, they can collect data inductively and deductively. They are used in surveys, case studies and experiments. The type of data collected also depends on how interviews are structured and the degree of control which researchers or participants have over their content and process. Wengraf (2001) identifies four types of interviews (on a continuum): 'unstructured', 'lightly structured', 'heavily structured', and 'fully structured'. Corbin and Morse (2003) describe three 'modes' of interviewing: 'unstructured', 'semi structured' and 'quantitative/closed-ended'. There seems to be consensus in the literature that two types of interviews – 'structured' and 'unstructured' – are at the opposite ends of a spectrum. In between these positions are 'semi-structured' interviews, so called because researchers keep some control over the content and process of the interview. As we shall see later, the degree of researchers' control in semi-structured interviews can vary widely.

In structured interviews the questions are structured, predetermined and standardised. They tend to collect quantifiable data. Unstructured interviews, on the other hand, are used mainly in qualitative studies to explore phenomena. The term 'unstructured' can be misleading, since in practice no research interview can be totally unstructured. Therefore, in this chapter the term 'qualitative interview' will be used to describe interviews in which researchers ask broad questions and invite participants to express their feelings, opinions and perceptions on particular issues, events or experiences. The three types of interviews, structured, qualitative and semi-structured, will be described below.

Structured interviews

In the previous chapter, it was pointed out that questionnaires can be administered by researchers in person. This, in effect, is a structured interview. It involves the researcher asking all the questions as they are formulated in the questionnaire. Neither the wording nor the sequence of the questions can be altered. The questionnaire, in this case, is normally referred to as a standardised 'interview schedule'.

The presence of the researcher can be beneficial in many ways. If the researcher wants to prevent respondents from consulting other sources in answering the questionnaire, as is the case with knowledge questions, she can administer it in person. Unwittingly face-to-face structured interviews can help to boost the response rate as participants may feel 'obliged' to take part. The presence of the researcher may act as a pressure for them to participate. The main reason for the interviewer's presence, however, is to offer clarification and support, if needed. Sometimes respondents provide incomplete or inadequate responses or 'skip' questions altogether. Their non-verbal behaviour may also communicate their confusion or lack of understanding of certain questions. In such cases, the task of the researcher is to clarify terms without changing the meaning of the questions. For example in a study of 'health and memory in people over 50' by Neadley et al. (1995), the interviewer was allowed to substitute the word 'nerves' for 'anxiety and depression' in the question 'have you ever suffered from anxiety/depression?' in case people did not understand them.

To obtain complete and accurate responses, the interviewer can ask 'such non-directive probes as: 'In what way?', 'How do you mean?', 'Could you say a bit more?' (Cartwright, 1986). As can be seen from these probes, the interviewer does not seek in-depth information but encourages the respondent to think more seriously about the questions and provide more detail (where necessary) in the responses. Her task is to make sure that the respondent understands the question and that she, in turn, understands the answer. Another reason for structured interviews is for the interviewer to help those who have difficulty in reading questions or formulating written responses. By asking the questions and recording the answers, the interviewer also facilitates the research process since the meaning of what is said can be clarified on the spot and she does not have to decipher handwriting other than her own. In some cases, the interviewer codes the responses as they are offered.

The fewer the number of interventions by the interviewer, the more structured the interview. Consistency in asking the questions as they appear on the schedule and in making the same information available to all respondents are the hallmarks of structured interviews. The aim is to achieve standardisation.

As the purpose of the structured interview is to collect data from a predetermined and structured questionnaire, and the interviewer's role is to administer the questionnaire in the same way to all respondents without any alterations, the structured interview is a quantitative method of data collection. According to Waltz et al. (1991), 'the structured interview is used most appropriately when identical information is needed from all respondents, when comparisons are to be made across respondents who are relatively homogeneous in background and experience, and when large or geographically dispersed samples are used'. Structured interviews are particularly suitable for those who are ill, frail or too young to complete questionnaires. However, self-administered questionnaires may be more appropriate for data of an embarrassing or private nature, since the structured interview negates one of the main strengths of questionnaires – the potential for respondents to remain anonymous.

Structured interviews, like structured questionnaires, are often employed in the collection of data on knowledge, attitudes, beliefs, opinions, practice and service provision. For example, Fitzgerald et al. (2003) used a structured interview consisting of 33 items to identify patterns in nursing practice in a large metropolitan hospital. As they explain:

> The questions posed were fixed (e.g. 'who evaluated the patient care?'). The respondent was then allowed to answer without prompting. The facilitator had a list of most likely responses that could be filled in with ease. For example, 'who evaluated the patients care? – (a) team leader, (b) nurse assigned to the patient, (c) CNC, (d) senior nurse, (e) RNs only, (f) other describe'.

Validity and reliability of structured interviews

Since the questionnaire is the tool of data collection in structured interviews, it is subject to the same validity and reliability threats as the questionnaire. Equally, the same tests of validity and reliability can be carried out. The main advantage of the structured interview over the self-administered questionnaire is the opportunity provided to respondents to seek clarification. By helping them, where necessary, to understand the question, they are more able to give appropriate and relevant answers, thereby enhancing the validity of the instrument. In structured interviews, it is also possible for the researcher to observe non-verbal signs that alert her to occasions when respondents experience difficulties with the questionnaire.

Since all the questions are (ideally) asked in the same way, structured interviews have a high degree of reliability, but interviewers may have difficulty in ensuring that the amount and type of clarification they give to respondents is more or less uniform. When more than one interviewer is used in the same study, it is possible that some are more able than others to extract information from respondents. Since structured interviews seek to achieve a high degree of standardisation, these issues are pertinent to the reliability of the tool and can, to some extent, be resolved through interviewer training.

The presence of the interviewer can, on the other hand, introduce a number of biases. Respondents may be more inclined to give socially desirable answers or at least mould their responses to fit the occasion. Personal characteristics of interviewers, such as gender, age, race, clothing, language and accent, can all affect the responses; there are numerous examples in the sociological literature of how personal characteristics can interfere with the collection of valid and reliable data (see for example Hyman, 1954; Sudman and Bradburn, 1974; Cartwright, 1986). According to Davis (1980), even the manner in which respondents are greeted can cause 'unintended variations in responses'. As she explains, 'a difference in some set with the chummy "Hi" as opposed to the slightly more formal "Hello" to the even more formal "How do you do?" creates a different interactional climate'. Research Example 38 describes the use of structured interviews in one study.

Use of herbal therapies by older, community-dwelling women
Gözüm and Ünsal (2004)

A structured interview

The aim of this study was 'to determine the prevalence of herbal therapy use among women over 65 years who live independently in the community, and to compare the socio-demographic characteristics and health status of older women who use herbal therapies and those who do not'.

An interview schedule was developed for data collection. Face-to-face structured interviews were carried out with a random sample of 385 'older participants' at five primary health care centres in Turkey.

Comments:

1   The interview schedule was similar to a questionnaire. It contained questions on perceived health status, use of herbal therapy and sociodemographic factors. These standardised questions helped the researchers to determine the prevalence of herbal therapy use and how it correlated with demographic factors.

2   The interview schedule was highly structured. For example, perceived health status was measured by a visual analogue scale 'that ranged from one (poor) to five (excellent)'. Other examples include 'Please tell me (yes or no) have you used herbal therapy in the past 12 months?' and 'Who introduced you to the herbal therapies (family member or friend, media, health care professionals or others)?' This type of interview is designed to collect data on predetermined questions of interest to researchers. The questions were highly structured to allow comparison of data.

3   The interview schedule was prepared, tested for face validity and piloted prior to administration (as is the case for self-administered questionnaires).

Qualitative interviews

A number of terms have been used to describe qualitative interviews. Among the most common are 'unstructured', 'in-depth', 'depth', 'informal', 'non-directive', 'focused' and 'open'. Sometimes a combination of these has been offered, such as 'in-depth focused' (Reid et al., 2003), 'unstructured formal' (Hogston, 1995), 'non-directive' (Vandendorpe, 2000), 'focused non-directive' (Green and Holloway, 1997) and even 'in-depth semi-structured' (Nolan et al.,

1995). Others, such as Hanson (1994), describe their method simply as 'qualitative interviews'. The array of terms reflects both the various ways in which qualitative interviews are carried out and the liberal use of terminologies in describing these methods.

The term 'unstructured' has become synonymous with 'qualitative'. Yet, as Jones (1985) points out, 'there is no such thing as a totally unstructured interview' and 'the term is over-used and often carelessly used'. To avoid confusion, it would be more helpful if researchers simply described their methods as qualitative (if this is the case) and explained in detail their assumptions, purposes and process.

'Qualitative interview' is a broad term used to denote a family of interviews that share the common purpose of studying phenomena from the perspective of the respondent. In its most unstructured form, the qualitative interview resembles 'everyday conversations for the purpose of collecting and validating data' (Chenitz, 1986). However, not all qualitative interviews are completely unstructured, as everyday conversations are supposed to be. The degree of structure and control, as well as the process of interviewing, vary from interview to interview.

Structure and control

With structured interviews, the researcher must ask everyone the same questions in the same manner. A researcher wishing to explore, by means of a qualitative interview, a phenomenon such as students' experience of preparing for examinations may not have a list of questions or topics but may decide to let them talk about their experiences. This type of interview is known as 'non-directive' as the interviewer does not 'direct' interviewees to topics but allows them free expression. The task of the interviewer, in this case, is to facilitate the flow of information with as little interruption as possible. As topics are brought up by the students, the interviewer may focus on some rather than others. Often new topics or new perspectives on the same topics are introduced as the interviews progress. Interviewers choose to have little control over the agenda in non-directive interviews. Bennett (1991) carried out 'unstructured non-directive' interviews with 'adolescent girls about their experience of witnessing marital violence'. As she explains:

> Although spontaneous descriptions were encouraged, when a participant had difficulty getting started, a prompt . . . was used: for example, 'Describe a typical day in your home'. For the most part, however, questions were used only to clarify or to encourage further description.

Completely unstructured interviews are difficult to manage. Some researchers introduce a degree of structure by selecting a number of areas within a topic to 'focus' the interview on. Waltz et al. (1991) describe the 'focused interview' as beginning:

with a rather loose agenda, for example, a list of topics to be covered. However, the interviewer may move freely from one topic area to another and allow the respondent's cues to help determine the flow of the interview. Although the interviewer may work from a list of topics to be covered, the way in which questions are phrased and the order in which they are asked are left to the discretion of the interviewer and may be changed to fit the characteristics of each respondent.

This degree of control that interviewers have in focused interviews should not turn the interaction into a rigid question and answer session (as is the case in structured interviews) but should be as near as possible to normal conversations. The list of topics provides a guide to researchers on what they want respondents to talk about. It is not intended in any way to achieve uniformity or to prevent respondents from taking the initiative to let their perspectives be known. For example, Brown and Williams (1995) explain, in their study of 'women's experiences of rheumatoid arthritis', that:

> a topic guide was developed from the existing literature in order to provide a basis from which interviews could proceed. Utilising nursing skills of listening and encouraging, the researcher allowed the women to introduce anything they felt to be important. The women's role as experts in knowing about rheumatoid arthritis was explicitly emphasized throughout the interviews.

Focused interviews also vary according to how 'loose' the lists of topics are. They can be broad or fairly specific, as an extract from the list of topics in a study by Kyngäs (2003) on 'patient education from the perspectives of adolescents' shows:

- everyday life with a chronic disease;

- experiences of being a patient at a hospital or visiting an outpatient department for follow-up;

- experiences about patient education; and

- social support.

Sometimes the extent of focus varies between interviews in the same study. Walker et al. (1995) carried out 'in-depth focused interviews to explore women's experiences regarding all aspects of their care during labour and delivery'. As they explain:

> Initial interviews were broadly focused to encourage respondents to recount experiences of personal relevance in relation to their maternity care. Audiotapes of the interviews were listened to, notes made and used to focus later interviews in order to elaborate fully upon all aspects of experience . . .

The qualitative interview process

The process of qualitative interviews can also vary. As explained above, some researchers 'allow' respondents to talk without too many interruptions and facilitate the process by listening and probing as appropriate. In this type of interview, the researcher does not reveal her own values and experience. Other interviewers share their experiences with respondents and find that their 'disclosures' help to build a trust between themselves and the respondents in the same way that happens in everyday interactions. Not only do some people feel they have to divulge a little bit of themselves in order for others to be more forthcoming with their own disclosures, but also this type of 'give and take' brings people closer when they know that both of them have some experience of the same phenomenon. Wilde (1992) comments that 'sharing part of one's personal life would seem to have an effect on the subject's view of the researcher, who becomes, in the subject's eyes, less of a professional and more of a human being'.

Perry et al. (2004) discuss the issue of 'involvement-detachment' in their study of the 'life experiences of young lesbian, gay, and bisexual people'. They point out that 'interviews by definition, are interdependent relationships that involve interaction between the researcher and the participant' and that 'the nature and quality of the communication is in no small measure 'influenced by the nature and quality of the relationship developed during the interview'.

The degree to which interviewers adopt passive roles in qualitative interviews can also vary. Gray (1994) describes how she had to adopt passive and active roles during her interviews on 'the effects of supernumerary status and mentorship on student nurses':

> I had to be flexible and able to alternate between an active and passive role depending on the nature of the interview and the amount of probing required to encourage the respondent to share information. Not to have this flexibility would result in either adopting a rigidly passive role (which would allow the respondents to focus on irrelevant material) or a role which allows the pace of the interview to gallop away uninhibitedly.

These real-life experiences of interviewers show that the interviewer–interviewee interaction in qualitative interviews differs from situation to situation, so researchers have to be flexible in their approaches. With structured interviews, although not all respondents take the same amount of time to answer all the questions, the duration of the interview is guided by the number of questions and would not normally vary greatly between interviews in the same study. This is not the case with qualitative interviews. The latter are time-consuming because of the in-depth nature of the information required and the diminished control of the researcher over the interview agenda. They vary in length in the same study, because each interaction between the interviewer and interviewee is unique. They could last between 30 minutes and 2 hours. It is unlikely that any phenomenon could be explored in depth in less than half an hour. On the other hand, a two-hour interview would tire researchers and respondents and cast doubt on their ability to concentrate on the task at hand.

In her study of 'women living with fibromyalgia', Schaefer (1995) reported that in-depth interviews lasted from 1 to 2.5 hours. This shows that qualitative interviews in the same study can vary greatly in length. The freedom and opportunity for respondents to talk and the difficulty that researchers face in keeping them 'on track' often make qualitative interviews last longer than they should.

In quantitative research, once a structured interview has been carried out, the researcher cannot go back to the respondents to ask for clarifications or to verify whether what was said was correctly understood by the interviewer. In qualitative research, the opportunity to go back to respondents exists and is often grasped. The reason for this is to continue the previous conversation, to find out whether people feel or think differently about the phenomenon on a different day, and mainly to validate their responses.

Therefore, each unstructured interview is different in process from the next. The researcher's role can vary from a passive one to one in which the sharing of experiences between interviewer and respondent is a key strategy in obtaining data. The duration of interviews within the same study can vary, and researchers have the freedom to interview the same respondents more than once if they so wish.

The content of qualitative interviews

Even with a list of topics, it is unlikely that every interview in the same study will cover strictly the same content. The aim of qualitative interviews is to know all possible ways in which respondents view or experience phenomena. As new perspectives are uncovered and new insights gained, the interviewer finds that earlier interviews are different in content from later ones. Qualitative interviews build on one another. The researcher accumulates perspective and experiences until a broad understanding of the phenomenon is obtained. And when saturation of data is reached (that is no new data emerge), the researcher may stop interviewing even if she had intended to do more interviews.

Researchers comment that their own skills improve as they do more interviews in the same study. Buckeldee (1994) relates her own experience:

Transcribing and preliminary coding of early interviews helped in several ways. First it gave me feedback about my interviewing skills (or lack of them at times!) which proved invaluable. It also helped to identify areas requiring further exploration which in turn helped to direct later interviews. Furthermore as the interviews progressed, my own confidence and skill in conducting interviews increased and was verified in later transcripts of interviews.

To sum up this section, we find that while the structure, process and content of structured interviews are characterised by consistency and standardisation, the key features of qualitative interviews are, in contrast, flexibility and versatility. These are reflected in the diversity of ways in which qualitative interviews are conducted.

Rigour of qualitative interviews

The concepts of reliability and validity belong to quantitative research and as such have been criticised as having little relevance to qualitative studies. This does not mean that qualitative researchers are less rigorous in the way they collect, analyse and interpret data. As already described, the term 'reliability' refers to the degree of consistency with which the instrument produces the same results if administered in the same circumstances. In qualitative interviews, no structured, predetermined or standardised tools are used. In their most structured form, qualitative interviews consist of a list of topics about which respondents are asked to talk. The qualitative interviewer is also a 'tool' of data collection. She sifts and analyses data in her mind during the interview, as well as transcribes and makes sense of the data thereafter. Each interview in the same study is a unique interaction and is not replicable. The same researcher would conduct the interview differently were it to happen again, and another researcher would also have conducted the interview differently. In contrast, structured interviews can be replicated and the data can be examined for consistency. In the quantitative sense, it can be said that the reliability of qualitative data is difficult to establish. However, to qualitative researchers, reliability is secondary to getting to the core of the phenomena they investigate. As Deutscher (1966) explains:

> We concentrate on consistency without much concern with what it is we are being consistent about or whether we are consistently right or wrong. As a consequence we have been learning a great deal about how to pursue an incorrect cause with a maximum of precision.

Some qualitative researchers reject the concepts of reliability and validity and offer instead such terms as 'accuracy', 'truth' and 'credibility'. To ensure rigour, they adopt a number of strategies, including reflexivity and validation of data by the interviewees themselves.

Reflexivity is the continuous process of reflection by the researcher on her own values, preconceptions, behaviour or presence and those of the respondents, which can affect the interpretation of responses. According to Holloway and Fulbrook (2001), 'interviewers should be aware of their own mind set regarding the research topic, particularly when interview questions are being developed, because personal knowledge and experience inevitably shape them'. A researcher may also reflect on how the data she collects can be influenced by how she is perceived by the respondent. Larsson et al. (2003) describe how they tried to practise reflexivity in their study of the lived experiences of eating problems among patients with head and neck cancer:

> To ensure credibility, our own perspectives on having eating problems related to radiation therapy were identified and as far as possible 'set aside' prior to and throughout the data collection and data analysis. This was carried out through our self-awareness and critical reflection on our preconceptions of the phenomenon under study.

Reflexivity by the researcher is, however, not enough nor easy to carry out. It is not always possible to stand back and examine the effect of one's preconceptions, especially if one is not always aware of what they are. This is why some researchers return to interviewees to find out whether or not they agree with the data. This data validation process by respondents is useful in providing the opportunity for clarification and for the researcher to recognise her own prejudices, if this is the case. In his study of 'nurses' perceptions of quality nursing care', Hogston (1995), after coding and categorising the data, returned to five of the informants to confirm that 'the interpretation was in keeping with what the informants meant'.

Another way to validate the data is to ask other researchers to examine all or part of the transcripts. The common practice of tape-recording interviews and transcribing the data verbatim (word for word) allows others to have an insight into what transpired between the researcher and the respondents and to compare their perception of it with that of the researcher. In her study of 'adolescent girls' experience of witnessing marital violence', Bennett (1991) describes how she sought help to verify her theories:

> An individual with research and clinical experience in family violence read all transcriptions, individual-level descriptions, condensed and transformed meaning-unit statements and the general-level description for the purpose of consensual validation.

Qualitative researchers recognise the subjective component in the interviewing process and seek to utilise it in order to obtain meaningful data. Some believe that building trust between researcher and respondent is crucial in getting access to the latter's perception of the phenomenon. To do so, the interviewer has to bend and mould the interview method to suit the phenomenon. For example, some interviewers, as explained earlier, may share their experiences in order to encourage respondents to 'open up'. This inevitably makes the interview a very subjective and unique experience. To achieve a degree of objectivity, it is therefore necessary to resort to some of the strategies mentioned above. While the same interviews cannot be repeated, other researchers can in time study the same phenomenon in a different setting with the same or different methods and the data can be compared.

Finally, in some cases, the hypotheses and theories developed out of qualitative interviews can be further tested by quantitative approaches. See Research Example 39 for an example of qualitative interviews in one study.

RESEARCH EXAMPLE 39

Living with a terminal illness: patients' priorities

Carter et al. (2004)

A qualitative interview

Carter et al. (2004) carried out a qualitative study 'exploring what people living with terminal illness considered were the areas of priority in their lives'. They deliberately chose an 'a non-directive interview style' in order to obtain patients' perceptions as opposed to researchers' perceptions. They explained that 'themes were collated after the interview rather than decided on beforehand'.

Comments:

1 The researchers were interested in participants' own perceptions. They were asked 'to identify the most important consequences of living with their illness, including any worthwhile experiences'. When requesting expansion or clarification, the interviewer 'referred to the participant's own description of an impact'.

2 The interviews in this study lasted between 30 and 60 minutes. This variance in duration of qualitative interviews is quite common, as the researcher does not have a predetermined set of questions, but relies on participants to share their experience. The participants in this study were also experiencing a terminal illness. This may account for the short duration (30 minutes) of some of the interviews as some may have experienced tiredness.

3 Two independent reviewers checked the validity of the analysis process and outcome.

4 This is one example of a qualitative interview. Reading accounts of other interviews will help you get an idea of the variety of this method of data collection.

Semi-structured interviews

Sechrist and Pravikoff (2002) describe a semi-structured interview as a:

> verbal questioning of study participants using a combination of preset questions and follow-up probes. For example, researchers interested in post-operative pain control experiences may interview hospitalized patients using a preset list of questions but allowing opportunity for the participant to explain their answers by asking them to amplify responses.

According to Barriball and While (1994), the semi-structured interview provides 'the opportunities to change the words but not the meaning of questions' because it 'acknowledges that not every word has the same meaning to every respondent and not every respondent uses the same vocabulary'. Validity is enhanced because respondents can be helped to understand the questions and interviewers can ask for clarifications and probe for further responses, if necessary.

The tool of data collection in semi-structured interviews is called an interview schedule. It differs from an interview guide in focused interviews in that the latter has broad areas or questions but allows the researcher the freedom to ask additional questions. The interview schedule in a semi-structured interview is in fact a questionnaire consisting of a list of preformulated questions, which can neither be omitted nor added to. However, in semi-structured interviews respondents can formulate responses in their own words and are not faced by multiple-choice answers to choose from.

Semi-structured interviews have elements of quantitative and qualitative research. They are similar to structured interviews in that the number and types of question are the same for all respondents, although the actual wordings may be varied for the purpose of making sure that respondents understand the question. As with structured interviews, they emphasise the notion of standardisation, that is respondents must be subjected to the same questions with minimal variations. In a semi-structured interview, the researcher is allowed some flexibility to 'probe'. The *Oxford Dictionary* describes 'probe' as 'penetrating investigation'. The use of probes in semi-structured interviews is limited to seeking clarification and obtaining more complete answers rather than to uncovering new perspectives. It is a cautious use of probes to ensure that the respondent is not 'led' nor influenced in any way by the interviewer. In contrast, as we have seen earlier, in qualitative interviews the researcher often uses subjectivity to obtain rich and meaningful data.

In semi-structured interviews, the researcher is very much in control of the interview process, and the predetermined questions provide the structure to the interview. In qualitative interviews, the degree of control and structure on the part of the interviewer is minimal to allow topics and perspectives to emerge. The researcher does not know in advance all the questions to ask and is very much guided by what respondents say. The researcher has to decide during the interview what questions to ask and how to formulate them.

Some semi-structured interviews have a mixture of closed and open-ended questions, while others may have only open-ended ones. This use of closed questions ensures a high degree of standardisation since all the responses fall within the categories offered by the researcher. Open-ended questions can be specific or broad. Specific open-ended questions, such as, 'Can you list the items of food which you have stopped consuming since you have started to take medication X?' or 'Please give as many reasons as possible as to why you do not take medication Y?', limit the range of responses. On the other hand, broad open-ended questions such as, 'Can you describe your feelings when you were first told that you have diabetes?' can prompt respondents to 'open up' and make it difficult for the researcher not only to probe cautiously and objectively, but also to offer the same amount and depth of probing to all respondents. Therefore, one can see how some semi-structured interviews are closer to quantitative and others to qualitative interviews. By trying to keep standardisation and yet be flexible, the researcher uses a mixture of quantitative and qualitative methods, which purists may frown upon.

Researchers conducting semi-structured interviews must recognise the tension between trying to have both standardisation and flexibility. Many qualitative researchers label their interviews as semi-structured when in fact they are focused qualitative interviews (which have a list of broad questions to guide the interaction rather than constrain it).

In practice, it is questionable whether in semi-structured interviews researchers ask exactly the same number of questions of all respondents and try to maintain the same degree of objectivity with all of them. If this does happen, the semi-structured interview can be said to fit more into the quantitative approach. If the researcher departs from the list of questions she comes with and starts probing deeply, the interview can be said to be focused and thus qualitative. The degree of standardisation or flexibility can provide clues to how quantitative or qualitative a semi-structured interview is.

Semi-structured interviews are popular precisely because they can provide quantitative- and qualitative-type responses that allow comparisons between respondents in the same study and can be applicable to other similar settings. They are useful in the study of sensitive topics and in increasing response rates. As with other methods, researchers must have a good rationale for using semi-structured interviews.

In their study of 'the perceptions and needs of continuing professional education among nurses', Barriball and While (1994) explain why they chose semi-structured interviews:

Semi-structured interviews were selected as the means of data collection because of two primary considerations. First, they are well suited for the exploration of the perceptions and opinions of respondents regarding complex and sometimes sensitive issues and enable probing for more information and clarification of answers. Second, the varied professional, educational and personal histories of the sample group precluded the use of a standardised schedule.

The validity of responses in semi-structured interviews is enhanced by the presence of the researcher, who can clarify the questions and seek clarification from the respondents. Because semi-structured interviews share elements of quantitative and qualitative interviews, they are subject to some of the same validity and reliability threats described earlier in this chapter. For an example of a semi-structured interview, see Research Example 40.

Focus groups

A focus group can be described as an interaction between one or more researchers and more than one respondent for the purpose of collecting research data. Kitzinger (1995) explains that 'the idea behind the focus group method is that group processes can help people to explore and clarify their views in ways that would be less easily accessible in a one to one interview'. The knowledge gain from focus groups is thus the outcome of this interchange and discussion of ideas. Interaction, the main ingredient of focus groups, takes place between the researcher (sometimes called a moderator) and participants, and between participants themselves. In selecting a focus group instead of individual interviews to explore participants' experience of a particular phenomenon, researchers want, specifically, to give them opportunities to share and discuss their ideas. It is an efficient way to obtain a broad understanding of phenomena from a variety of perspectives.

Focus groups, on their own, or in combination with other methods, is a common feature in health and nursing research. However, when Webb and Kevern (2001) searched and reviewed articles, in the CINAHL database, reporting focus groups in nursing, from 1990 to 1999, they found that out of 124 articles there were only 16 empirical papers using this method. Most were related to non-research-based work such as service development, health promotion, curriculum development or teaching. This shows that the popularity of focus groups in nursing research is more apparent than real. However, to develop practice, to brainstorm, to reach consensus, it remains a potent strategy.

Focus groups are frequently used in evaluation research, perhaps because different stakeholders can be brought together to give their views, and to clarify conflicting perceptions.

The process of focus groups consists mainly of the interviewer asking a broad question and inviting participants to volunteer answers, which in turn generates further questions. Sometimes, if the purpose is to evaluate a service or a programme, the interviewer may have a list of aspects or issues she wants them to focus on. Kitzinger and Barbour (1999) see the role of the interviewer as

Emotional experiences, empathy and burnout among staff caring for demented patients at a collective living unit and a nursing home
Kuremyr et al. (1994)

A semi-structured interview

The aim of this study was to describe the staff's emotional experiences when caring for elderly demented patients and to estimate their experiences of burnout and empathy in a collective living unit and a nursing home.

The data collection methods were 'the empathy construct rating scale, the burnout measure', and a semi-structured interview. An interview 'form' containing 60 questions was used.

Questions focused on four areas:

1. The staff. For example: Do you feel emotionally exhausted? Do you feel worthless? 2. The patient. For example: How would you describe the demented patient you have the best contact with? What are the patient's main problems? 3. The staff–patient relationship. On a scale of 1 to 5, for example: How strong is your emotional bond to the patient you have the best contact with? What are your feelings in situations when you have close contact with the patient? 4. The staff's occupational situation. For example: Do you get feedback from your work? If you feel emotionally exhausted and/or have feelings of burnout, what kind of support do you want? (Kuremyr et al., 1994)

Comments:

1   The prepared form or list of 60 questions was administered to all respondents, thereby imposing a high degree of 'researcher control' and standardisation in the interviewing process. However, some of the questions were open-ended and allowed respondents to answer in their own words. By not providing a list of answers for respondents to choose from (as is the case with structured interviews) and by seeking to listen to the respondents' own views, one can say that the researchers were collecting qualitative data. This is, however, different from a qualitative interview, in which respondents are allowed to speak freely and introduce new ideas which the researcher explores further. The researcher is in control of the content and the process of the interview.

2   In this study, the researchers know enough about the phenomena (emotional experiences, empathy and burn-out) to know what questions to ask. For example, one of questions they ask is 'do you feel worthless?' This assumes that they know that this is one of the feelings which staff can experience while 'caring for demented patients'.

encouraging participants 'to talk to one another: asking questions, exchanging anecdotes, and commenting on each others' experiences and points of view'.

The purpose of focus group interviews differs from that of individual interviews. When researchers want different perspectives on a phenomenon, they can gather people who can offer such insight in one or two sessions. They provide examples for instant comparisons (of perceptions and experiences) and spontaneous comments and reflections which can contribute to in-depth understanding of the phenomenon being studied. Purposive sampling may be used to group people known to have different views on the topic. However, researchers sometimes have to rely on volunteers, which may bias the findings.

Focus group interviews can follow or lead into individual interviews. Issues raised during these interviews can be pursued in more detail in the privacy of individual interviews. Alternatively, focus group interviews can be conducted in order to validate data previously collected in individual interviews. In the latter, respondents are asked their views or perceptions, free from group pressure. The interviewer can concentrate on one individual at a time and pursue the topic in greater depth. In focus group interviews, it is only possible to deal with general, and not personal, issues. For example, in a group interview the researcher studying burn-out may be able to find out what the respondents think generally of 'burn-out' and may be interested in finding out whether people agree or disagree with its meaning. It is not possible to assess each individual's level of 'burn-out'. The researcher can also answer general questions or attend to the concerns that participants may have in taking part in the study, thus allaying their anxieties.

Focus group interviews provide opportunities to brainstorm, perhaps for the purpose of generating items for a questionnaire. They can also be used to check question wording and formats, and provide opportunities to 'pilot test' an instrument. When focus group interviews are to be followed by individual interviews, the former can help to familiarise the interviewer with prospective or potential interviewees.

The major advantage of focus group interviews is that valuable data can be obtained quickly and cheaply. Some people are also more comfortable in voicing their opinions in the company of friends and colleagues than on their own, with an interviewer. Focus group interviews provide the opportunity for participants to reflect on, and react to, the opinions of others, with which they may disagree or of which they are unaware. Apart from the range of opinions that can potentially be obtained, underlying conflicts are often revealed that would otherwise have remained unknown to the researcher. Even when there is no heated discussion or disagreement, the sharing of experiences can provide valuable insight into phenomena.

Bloor et al. (2001) contend that 'focus groups have a much larger part to play as an ancillary method, alongside and complementing other methods' and that 'they are rarely an alternative to depth interviewing or surveys'. Sim (1998) explains that 'measuring strength of opinion from focus group data is problematic' and that 'the indicators used to measure attitudes in orthodox survey research are largely inapplicable to the context of focus groups'. One must also be cautious when generalising from focus groups to the target population. The groups are rarely large enough or randomly selected to be representative of larger group. As a result of drop-outs (which is frequent) the original group composition and group dynamics intended by the researcher can be drastically altered.

In quantitative terms, the findings from focus groups are not, in themselves, generalisable. Consensus reached by participants is often a function of group dynamics, in particular group pressure, rather than reflecting what each individual thinks or believes. For example, simply because seven out of ten participants agreed that a service was beneficial does not mean that they would give the same answers in a private, face-to-face interview or in response to a questionnaire. The purpose of focus group interviews is to identify all the different views, no matter how little or how much they are supported in the group. These views can, thereafter, be tested more generally in a survey.

One of the major disadvantages of focus group interviews is that dominant personalities or factions can monopolise the discussion and express their views at the expense of others. Interactions can be both productive and inhibitive. Experiences and views of some can trigger reactions in others, thereby producing rich and varied perspectives with which to view phenomena. Group dynamics and, in particular, the personalities and status of some individuals can inhibit others in participating fully and freely in the discussions. Some group members may be shy, unassertive or unable to articulate their views, so this type of interview requires group management as well as interviewing skills. The larger the group, the more difficult the task to manage it. Even if the interviewer is skilled, it is possible that the contribution of those who are frightened to voice their opinions will not be fully maximised.

Focus group interviews are also not suitable for the study of sensitive and personal issues and behaviours that do not conform to the norm. Klapowitz (2000), who compared data from focus groups with those from individual interviews, found that individual interviews were 18 times more likely to raise socially sensitive discussion topics than focus groups.

Recording data can also present difficulties. Taking notes when many people are talking at the same time is not feasible. Tape-recorders may only record those who are near to them, although video-recordings can be more effective as they are not only able to capture what is said, but can also reveal the group dynamics. Analysis of data from focus group interviews can also be daunting.

The process of focus group interviews varies, among other things, according to the number of participants, the skill of the researcher and the purpose of the interviews. If the purpose is to brainstorm, the process may be more flexible, with opportunities for spontaneous contribution. If the purpose is to seek respondents' views on a number of specific issues or if the researcher wants to validate findings from individual interviews, the agenda will dictate a more directive approach.

Focus group interviews are not replicable. The reliability and validity of the findings are difficult to ascertain on their own but can be compared with the findings of individual interviews or other methods, if used in the same study. Researchers have to reflect on the motives or reasons for what was said and by whom. They must also realise the potential effect of group pressure on the type of data they collect. The behaviour of participants in focus groups and in individual interviews can differ. There are examples in the literature of men showing more macho behaviours when in company of other men than when interviewed individually (Kitzinger, 1994; Wright, 1994) The interest in the behaviour of people when in groups is not new. Hume, in his *Treatise of Human Nature* in 1739, wrote:

> Everyone has observed how much more dogs are animated when they hunt in a pack, than when they pursue their game apart. We might, perhaps, be at a loss to explain this phenomenon, if we had not experience of a similar in ourselves.   (Hume, 1969)

For recent examples of focus groups see Friedman and Hoffman-Goetz (2003) and Tsiboukli and Wolff (2003). Research Example 41 illustrates the use of focus group interviews in a Swedish study. For discussions of focus group interviews see Sim (1998), Webb and Kevern (2001) and McLafferty (2004).

Nominal group technique

One design which combines some aspects of focus group interviews and the Delphi technique (see Chapter 10) is the nominal group technique (NGT). Van de Ven and Delbecq (1972) defined the NGT as

> a structured meeting which seeks to provide an orderly procedure for obtaining qualitative information from target groups who are most associated with a problem area.

The purpose of the NGT is to seek the views of group participants on a particular topic and to seek a consensus or agreement by asking them to rank or rate their responses. For example, participants may be asked their views on how to ensure the efficiency of a particular service. Each participant's views would be noted and followed by voting rounds and discussions until the selected views are finally ranked in order of importance.

The NGT differs from the focus group interview in that the format of the NGT is more structured. This is because the aim is to produce a ranked list of views or items. Each participant in a study using the NGT is asked to contribute his or her views to the discussion. In focus group group interviews, some participants may be more vocal than others, and some may not

RESEARCH EXAMPLE 41

Exploring views of Swedish district nurses' prescribing – a focus group study in primary health care

Wilhelmsson and Foldevi (2003)

Focus group interviews

The aim of this study was to gain deeper understanding of the different opinions among district nurses (DNs) and general practitioners (GPs) about district nurse prescribing and to explore the impact of the reform on primary care.

Comments:

1   Focus group interviews were ideally suited to the aim of this study. As the authors explain the purpose was 'not to generalize but to say something about underlying values that direct the discussion'.

2   Six group interviews were carried out (4 with DNs and 2 with GPs). Groups comprised members of the same occupation 'in order to achieve intimacy and mutual understanding between members so that an exchange of information could be facilitated'. Sometimes mixing professionals can also be illuminating. In particular, interprofessional understanding (or misunderstanding) of each other's roles and motives can be revealed'.

3   A list of questions was prepared prior to the interview. This is helpful when data from each group are compared.

4   Conducting focus group interviews requires training in order to facilitate discussion among group members. As the authors explain, 'the first interview in this study gave less information than the rest, probably because of inexperience'.

participate at all. The researcher (or group facilitator) also uses group dynamics to encourage discussions which can be loosely structured. The NGT, on the other hand, uses discussion in order to seek agreement, not to encourage disagreements.

The NGT differs from the Delphi technique (DT) in that it brings participants face-to-face while with the DT participants do not meet, and are surveyed at a distance. The purpose of the NGT is very similar to that of the DT. Therefore it is understandable that both techniques comprise a series of steps which consist mainly of seeking initial views from individuals followed by voting rounds until the researcher is satisfied with the final results.

To ensure that everyone in the group participates, the researcher usually asks them to write the answers to a specific question. Lengthy answers (as may be the case in focus group interviews) are not encouraged. Responses are listed on a board or flip chart. To facilitate the process the researcher imposes a structure on the questions. For example, she may ask participants to write down five factors which contribute to their job satisfaction rather than asking them broadly what contributes to job satisfaction. In the early part of the NGT process, responses are listed but not discussed. Once a 'workable' list is drawn, discussion can begin in order to inform the voting, until finally (often after several rounds) a consensus is reached.

The advantage of the NGT is that it is a cheaper and quicker way to collect views than individual interviews. All participants have to contribute responses to the discussion since the researcher asks questions to each one of them. Although this may give the impression that the views of each participant have equal weightings, one must take into account the group dynamics and the 'status' of participants in the sample. Anonymity and confidentially are also not guaranteed with the NGT since the process involves face-to-face interaction. As with other designs and methods, the NGT can be used not as a substitute for others, but for achieving the desired ends of researchers.

Examples of the use of the NGT include studies by:

- Gibson and Soanes (2000) on the development of 'clinical competences for use on a paediatric oncology nursing course'.

- Elliott and Shewchuk (2002) on the identification of the 'problems experienced by persons living with severe physical disabilities'.

- Dewar et al. (2003) on the assessment of 'chronic pain, patients' perceived challenges and needs in a community health region'.

For an example of the NGT in a study see Research Example 42.

Ethical implications of interviewing

Interviewing shares with experiments and postal questionnaires some of the ethical concerns discussed in previous chapters. Unlike the self-administered questionnaire, however, the researcher knows who she is talking to and the respondent cannot therefore remain anonymous. The researcher has a moral obligation to keep the respondent anonymous from others, and the data collected must remain confidential. Anonymity and confidentiality are only two of the many ethical issues that researchers and others must consider if the rights of individuals are not to be compromised. The behaviour of the interviewer before, during and after the interview has the potential of harming respondents.

RESEARCH EXAMPLE 42

The development of clinical competencies for use on a paediatric oncology nursing course using a nominal group technique
Gibson and Soanes (2002)

A study using the nominal group technique

In this study Gibson and Soanes (2000) used the nominal group technique (NGT) in the initial phase of the development of clinical competencies. The NGT was used to gather data about their detailed practice. Data were collected from two groups: 'one with senior staff/ward sisters on a haematology/oncology unit', and one with course members of a Paediatric Oncology Nursing Course.

Comments:

1 The reasons given for the choice of the NGT over other methods (such as the questionnaire, expert panels and the Delphi survey) were that the NGT could give 'quick results', was not 'too time-consuming', was 'cheap' and could resolve all their 'practical issues while also achieving consultation and consensus with a professional group'.

2 Gibson and Soanes (2000) follow the NGT steps proposed by Butterfield (1988). These were:

   (a) Introduce nominal group process to the group
   (b) Silent generation of ideas in writing
   (c) Round-robin listing ideas
   (d) Discussion of ideas on a flip chart
   (e) Rank ordering ideas
   (f) Total rankings
   (g) Discussion
   (h) Conclusion

3 Participants in each group were asked to identify the knowledge, decision-making skills, and clinical attributes essential for successful performance as a paediatric oncology nurse.

   One group generated 46 ideas and the other 66. Each group was subsequently asked to rank their top eight items. This process was useful in the development of competency statements and performance criteria.

Before the interview

The issue of consent, especially in relation to patients as a captive population, has been discussed in earlier chapters. Even when people are interviewed in their own homes, they can still feel obliged to help health
professionals, either because they are grateful for the services they have
received or because they may require them later on. Interviewing as a method
of data collection puts particular pressure on respondents to take part. The
physical presence of researchers or the sound of their voice over the telephone
has more 'weight' than a questionnaire through the letter box. Interviews are
sometimes preferred precisely because they yield higher response rates than
questionnaires.

To obtain consent, researchers must give as much information as possible to
respondents to enable them to make up their minds. Among these may be
people who are bereaved, depressed, recovering from a suicide attempt, an
abortion or miscarriage, or have just been diagnosed as having a terminal
illness. They constitute a vulnerable population who may not be in a position
to fully comprehend and digest all the information given to them and may not
be able to give proper informed consent. Even when they are not experiencing,
or recovering from, an illness or a tragic event, the respondents' living conditions may make them vulnerable and open to exploitation. Many people who
live alone crave someone to talk to. Many researchers have been surprised to
find that they cannot take their leave because respondents want to carry on
talking.

During the interview

The interview process itself is potentially harmful. Individuals have a right to
privacy, which can be easily invaded once they have given consent. According to
Waltz et al. (1991), 'a generally accepted ethical position is that subjects should
be free to participate or withdraw from participation without recrimination or
prejudice'. It is unlikely that this right is frequently exercised. On the other
hand, a 'skilful' interviewer can make the respondent reveal intimate details
before the latter notices what is happening. Researchers must not use under-
hand tactics to achieve their ends. Smith (1992) suggests:

> researchers, who interview people and perhaps particularly women, need an
> awareness and a sensitivity to the fact that, although a subject may have
> agreed to take part in a study, it cannot be known for certain what that inter-
> view will uncover or give rise to. It could be argued that to be allowed a
> private view of another person's past or opinions or pain is a privilege.

Qualitative interviews depend on in-depth probing and, as such, have the
potential to violate the right to privacy. Fontana and Frey (1994) state:

> A growing number of scholars . . . feel that most of traditional in-depth inter-
> viewing is unethical, whether wittingly or unwittingly, and we agree whole-
> heartedly. The techniques and tactics of interviewing are really ways of
> manipulating respondents while treating them as objects or numbers rather
> than individual human beings.

Qualitative interviews, although individual-centred, operate on the basis that
respondents will reveal their inner thoughts if the researcher is skilful enough
and if a trust is built up with the respondent. However, in some cultures it is
offensive to probe into people's lives. Qualitative interviewers must pay particular attention to cultural norms in order to avoid violating the moral and ethical conduct of particular groups.

Interviews have the potential to reveal views, beliefs, attitudes and behaviours
that can be damaging to respondents. In the course of the study, the researcher's
view of the respondent may be confirmed or altered. This may not be very
important if the respondent never comes into contact with the researcher again,
but it has implications if, for example, the respondent is a student on a course
in which the researcher is involved. It is not unusual for research to be carried
out in order to make services more cost-effective, and this may eventually lead
to a cut in services.

Interviews, especially qualitative ones, can arouse emotions and lead to
catharsis. The subject matter of such interviews can be highly sensitive and
emotionally charged. In Smith's (1992) study of 'the help-seeking behaviours of
alcohol dependent and problem drinking women', 'the content of the discussions ranged over many areas and included references to events which could
only be described as highly personal, emotionally charged and, in some cases,
unresolved: for example, the giving up of children for adoption; rape; violence
to themselves as well as being violent towards others'.

Smith (1992) believes that the researcher has 'an ethical responsibility to
handle such material with sensitivity and judgement'; she 'can listen and
acknowledge the event but she must not probe in such a way as to produce and
encourage emotional pain'. The author also contends that 'to interview and then
leave someone in emotional distress without adequate support or safeguards is
morally wrong' (Smith, 1992).

In one-to-one interviews, the researcher is in a position to observe overt or
subtle changes in the verbal and non-verbal behaviours of the respondent and
may therefore respond to them. In focus group interviews, it is difficult for her
to observe and respond to the distress of some individuals. Smith (1995)
believes that 'when discussing sensitive topics, it is important to have a coleader
with clinical experience to adequately monitor the group's comfort level'. In
structured interviews, researchers may use questionnaires or other tools that can
also arouse emotions and cause distress.

The interview can have the effect of raising expectations and changing
respondents' perceptions. In asking them about the services they do or do not

use, the interviewer may create expectations that they should avail themselves of these. Similarly, interviews may make respondents aware of their plight and leave them to consider their sad state of affairs. Buckeldee (1994) found this in her study of 'carers in the community'. She writes:

> not only did most carers willingly talk with me but many also freely talked about themselves, including personal and intimate matters. At times this process also resulted in participants exploring new feelings and ideas they had not previously considered or acknowledged. This commonly occurred when we explored their feelings and perceptions of their caring role.

As part of a course, a student carried out a case study during which she interviewed a technician and her boss. The student soon became aware that issues (such as the appraisal of the technician's work) had not been considered by the boss prior to the interview and, because she raised them, it was likely thereafter to have implications for the technician. In doing the student a favour by granting her the interview, she (the technician) created the conditions that could potentially alter her working practice.

The interview process gives rise to a number of dilemmas that researchers have to face and which may cause themselves stress as well. Buckeldee (1994) gives an idea of her own feelings when exploring the feelings of her respondents. She describes the 'depth of sorrow and sadness', which she felt at times was 'overwhelming'. Respondents may tell researchers in confidence things which can become difficult to ignore and overlook. For example, a respondent may tell the interviewer of her intention of committing suicide or may describe the abuse of patients that she has recently witnessed. The researcher faces the dilemma of doing nothing about it or breaking the confidentiality. Nurse researchers often have to deal with the conflict between their roles as nurses and as researchers. There are numerous examples in the nursing literature (see Smith, 1992; Wilde, 1992; Buckeldee, 1994) of the implications of this conflicting role and of how researchers have dealt with it. Wilde (1992) reports that 'most authors advocate that the researcher resists the temptation to make interventions during the interview, and that they postpone answering questions or making comments until the end of the interview'.

After the interview

What happens after the interview also has ethical implications. Should researchers care about their respondents when the interview is over? What responsibilities do researchers have towards respondents after the interview? Buckeldee (1994), referring to her study, expresses this dilemma:

> Having 'got my data' I did not know whether I should leave the carers in the hope that they would solve or deal with their problems in their own way or

whether, having caused them to realise feelings not previously acknowl-edged, I had a responsibility to help them in some way. If the latter was the case I needed to know what the nature of that responsibility was.

What happens to the data after they are collected is also important. There is the possibility that the views of respondents may be misrepresented. According to Smith (1992), 'it is clear that the interpretation of interview data is never wholly objective and dispassionate despite any effort made to be so' and that 'data interpretation is influenced by life experience and intellectual ability'. This is why some researchers go back to respondents for them to validate their (the researcher's) interpretation of what was said. Since, usually, not all respondents are consulted in this exercise, could it be that interviewers go back to those who are more receptive and hospitable and avoid those who are controversial?

It has also been suggested that debriefing sessions are necessary to deal with some of the stresses that respondents face. Researchers also need such help to relieve some of their stresses as well. In focus group interviews, individuals may be distressed and frustrated if they feel that they have not been able, for what-ever reason, to express their views. Researchers can help to allay some of these frustrations by talking to them individually afterwards.

The safety of group members must also be of concern to the researcher. Some of the participants may be open to victimisation for the views they have offered. Researchers must be sensitive to these issues. Buckeldee (1994) gives an exam-ple from her study of a case where the husband insisted that his wife (his carer) be interviewed in his presence. Buckeldee explains how this 'inhibited her responses', that 'with hindsight she should have anticipated that this could happen' and that she could have arranged the interview when the client was out. While this may have solved a methodological problem, it could, unwittingly, have caused a conflict between the couple had the husband become aware that his wife was asked questions related to his care behind his back.

How interview data are reported can also have ethical implications. Alderson (2001) points to the possibility of qualitative reports causing distress to people 'who took part in the research by identifying them more readily than numerical quantitative reports are likely to do'.

Much of the potential harm to participants can be prevented by interviewers who are thoughtful, sensitive and alert to their discomfort, especially when this is not overtly manifested. Corbin and Morse (2003) emphasise the importance of the interviewer's skill in not provoking distress, in recognising signs of distress and in taking measures to diffuse it if necessary.

These are some of the main ethical issues in interviewing. In some cases, the worst possible scenarios have been described and, of course, they do not neces-sarily apply to all types of interview. They are discussed here for researchers and others to be alert and sensitive to the ethical implications of what could be seen as harmless activities, for which some researchers think (often wrongly) that no approval from an ethical committee is required.

Critiquing interviews

Critiquing or evaluating interviews is problematic, mainly because very often little information is provided on what takes place between the interviewer and the interviewee. No two interviews are the same. Researchers must therefore describe the interview process in some detail. For example, in structured interviews, although the list of questions is predetermined, structured and standardised, readers need to know whether the input of the interviewer (or interviewers) was the same across all the interviews and, if not, how this affects the data. In qualitative interviews, one can ask whether the researcher was more or less directive, whether she used disclosures to encourage respondents to talk, whether the same questions were asked of all of them or whether the researcher built upon issues raised in the previous interview. Answers to these questions can help to determine how much the topics discussed reflect the interviewer's or the respondents' perspective. For semi-structured interviews, one can question the extent to which the prepared list of questions provided a loose or a rigid structure. For example, were respondents simply asked to provide answers to open-ended questions or did the researcher follow up issues raised in these answers? This is to determine whether there was limited or ample scope for respondents to talk freely. In focus group interviews, the rationale for adopting this approach as opposed to personal interviews, as well as information about the size and relevant profile of the group and how the participants were recruited, must be provided. Readers can decide whether the group seemed too large for the interviewer to handle and, depending on the purpose of the group interview, whether the recruitment method was biased or not.

The duration of the interview is often an indication of whether or not it was rushed. While it is not possible to say with certainty that in a two-hour interview respondents were able to talk freely, it is difficult to comprehend how a qualitative interview can last less than 30 minutes, especially when only one interview is carried out per respondent. It takes that length of time for the interviewer and interviewee to exchange 'civilities' and begin to engage in a conversation, let alone talk 'in depth' about anything.

As with other methods of data collection, researchers are better able than readers to reflect on whether their data can be taken at face value. Only they can tell whether their dress, appearance, accent, gender, race and other characteristics, or other events, had any bearings on the data collected.

Researchers must also explain how informed consent was obtained, access to respondents negotiated and respondents' privacy respected. They also have to report on where the interview took place and who else was present.

Measures taken for ensuring the validity and reliability of data must be fully explained. These should give an indication of the length to which the researchers have gone in order to ensure the credibility of their data. Finally, researchers should reflect on the limitations of their studies and indicate whether their findings can apply to other settings or whether they should be treated with caution.

SUMMARY

Summary and conclusion

The interview is one of the main methods of data collection and takes different forms. In structured interviews, the questions are predetermined, standardised and highly structured, with only limited scope for clarification and elaboration.

Qualitative interviews are characterised by flexibility and versatility, the researcher moulding the interaction in order to obtain in-depth information about phenomena. Semi-structured interviews combine elements of both of these types: they give respondents some freedom to express themselves while answering a set number of questions. Finally, focus group interviews make use of group dynamics to obtain a variety of perspectives cheaply and quickly on the same phenomenon.

Each of these interviews has its value and limitations. We have discussed the strategies that researchers adopt to ensure that the data they collect are credible. They should describe the interview process in relevant detail to enable readers to evaluate these data.

Finally, interviews, whatever the type, have ethical implications that researchers must seriously consider. Respondents' human rights must always take precedence over any research consideration.

References

Alderson P (2001) *On Doing Qualitative Research Linked to Ethical Healthcare*, vol. I (London: Wellcome Trust).

Barriball K L and While A (1994) Collecting data using a semi-structured interview: a discussion paper. *Journal of Advanced Nursing*, **19**:328–35.

Bennett L (1991) Adolescent girls' experience of witnessing marital violence: a phenomenological study. *Journal of Advanced Nursing*, **16**:431–8.

Bloor M, Frankland J, Thomas M and Robson K (2001) *Focus Groups in Social Research* (London: Sage).

Brown S and Williams A (1995) Women's experiences of rheumatoid arthritis. *Journal of Advanced Nursing*, **21**:695–701.

Buckeldee J (1994) Interviewing carers in their own homes. In: J Buckeldee and R McMahon (eds), *The Research Experience in Nursing* (London: Chapman & Hall).

Butterfield P G (1988) Nominal group process as an instructional method with novice community health nursing students. *Public Health Nursing*, **5**:12–15.

Carter H, MacLeod R, Brander P and McPherson K (2004) Living with a terminal illness: patients' priorities. *Journal of Advanced Nursing*, **45**, 6:611–20.

Cartwright A (1986) *Health Surveys in Practice and Potential*, 2nd edn (London: King Edward's Hospital Fund for London).

Chenitz W C (1986) The informed interview. In: W C Chenitz and J M Swanson (eds), *From Practice to Grounded Theory: Qualitative Research in Nursing* (Maidenhead: Addison-Wesley).

Corbin J and Morse J (2003) The unstructured interactive interview: issues of reciprocity and risks when dealing with sensitive topics. *Qualitative Inquiry*, **9**, 3:335–54.

Davis A J (1980) Research as an inactional situation: objectivity in the interview. *International Journal of Nursing Studies*, **17**:215–20.

Deutscher I (1966) Words and deeds: social science and social policy. *Social Problems*, **13**:233–54.

Dewar A, White M P, Posade S T and Dillon W (2003) Using nominal group technique to assess chronic pain, patients' perceived challenges and needs in a community health region. *Health Expectations*, **6**, 1:44–52.

Elliott T R and Shewchuk R M (2002) Using the Nominal Group Technique to identify the problems experienced by persons living with severe physical disabilities. *Journal of Clinical Psychology in Medical Settings*, **9**, 2:65–76.

Fitzgerald M, Pearson A, Walsh K, Long L and Heinrich N (2003) Patterns of nursing: a review of nursing in a large metropolitan hospital. *Journal of Clinical Nursing*, **12**:326–32.

Fontana A and Frey J H (1994) Interviewing: the art of science. In: N K Denzin and Y S Lincoln (eds), *Handbook of Qualitative Research* (Newbury Park, CA: Sage).

Friedman D B and Hoffman-Goetz L (2003) Sources of cancer information for seniors: a focus group pilot study report. *Journal of Cancer Education*, **18**, 4:215–22.

Garbett R and McCormack B (2001) The experience of practice development: an exploratory telephone interview study. *Journal of Clinical Nursing*, **10**, 1:94–102.

Gibson F and Soanes L (2000) The development of clinical competencies for use on a paediatric oncology nursing course using a nominal group technique. *Journal of Clinical Nursing*, **9**:459–69.

Gözüm S and Ünsal A (2004) Use of herbal therapies by older, community-dwelling women. *Journal of Advanced Nursing*, **46**, 2:171–8.

Gray M (1994) Personal experience of conducting unstructured interviews. *Nurse Researcher*, **1**, 3:65–71.

Green A J and Holloway D G (1997) Using a phenomenological research technique to examine student nurses' understandings of experiential teaching and learning: a critical review of methodological issues. *Journal of Advanced Nursing*, **26**, 5:1013–19.

Hanson E J (1994) An exploration of the taken-for-granted world of the cancer nurse in relation to stress and the person with cancer. *Journal of Advanced Nursing*, **19**:12–20.

Hogston R (1995) Quality nursing care: a qualitative enquiry. *Journal of Advanced Nursing*, **21**:116–24.

Holbrook A L, Green M C and Krosnick J A (2003) Telephone versus face-to-face interviewing of national probability samples with long questionnaires. *Public Opinion Quarterly*, **67**, 1:79–81.

Holloway I and Fulbrook P (2001) Revisiting qualitative inquiry: interviewing in nursing and midwifery research . . . including commentary by C Bailey. *Nursing Times Research*, **6**, 1:539–51.

Hume D (1969) *A Treatise of Human Nature: Being an Attempt to Introduce the Experimental Method of Reasoning* (London: Pelican Books).

Hyman H H (1954) *Interviewing in Social Research* (Chicago: University of Chicago Press).

Jones S (1985) Depth interviewing. In: R Walker (ed.), *Applied Qualitative Research* (Aldershot: Gower).

Kitzinger J (1994) The methodology of focus groups: the importance of interaction between research participants. *Sociology of Health and Illness*, **16**:103–21.

Kitzinger J (1995) Introducing focus groups. *British Medical Journal*, **311**:299–302.

Kitzinger J and Barbour R E (1999) Introduction: the challenge and promise of focus groups. In: R S Barbour and J Kitzinger (eds), *Developing Focus Group Research: Politics, Theory and Practice* (London: Sage).

Klapowitz M D (2000) Statistical analysis of sensitive topics in group and individual interviews. *Quality and Quantity*, **34**:419–31.

Kuremyr D, Kihlgren M, Norberg A, Astrom S and Karlsson I (1994) Emotional experiences, empathy and burnout among staff caring for demented patients at a collective living unit and a nursing home. *Journal of Advanced Nursing*, 19:670–9.

Kyngäs H (2003) Patient education: perspective of adolescents with a chronic disease. *Journal of Clinical Nursing*, 12:744–51.

Larsson M, Hedelin B and Athlin E (2003) Lived experiences of eating problems for patients with head and neck cancer during radiotherapy. *Journal of Clinical Nursing*, 12:562–70.

McLafferty I (2004) Focus group interviews as a data collection strategy. *Journal of Advanced Nursing*, 48, 2:187–94.

Neadley A W, Kendrick D C and Brown R (1995) Health and memory in people over 50: a survey of a single-GP practice in England. *Journal of Advanced Nursing*, 21:646–51.

Nolan M, Owens R G and Nolan J (1995) Continuing professional education: identifying the characteristics of an effective system. *Journal of Advanced Nursing*, 21:551–60.

O'Connor H and Madge C (2003) Focus groups in cyberspace: using the internet for qualitative research. *Qualitative Market Research*, 6, 2:133–43.

Perry C, Thurston M and Green K (2004) Involvement and detachment in researching sexuality: reflections on the process of semistructured interviewing. *Qualitative Health Research*, 14, 1:135–48.

Reid D, Angus J, McKeever P and Miller K (2003) Home is where their wheels are: experiences of women wheelchair users. *American Journal of Occupational Therapy*, 57, 2:186–95.

Schaefer K M (1995) Struggling to maintain balance: a study of women living with fibromyalgia. *Journal of Advanced Nursing*, 21:95–102.

Scholl N, Mulders S and Drent R (2002) On-line qualitative market research: interviewing the world at a finger tip. *Qualitative Market Research*, 5, 3:210–23.

Sechrist K and Pravikoff D (2002) *Cinahl Information Systems* (Glendale, CA).

Sim J (1998) Collecting and analyzing qualitative data: issues raised by the focus group. *Journal of Advanced Nursing*, 28, 2:345–52.

Smith L (1992) Ethical issues in interviewing. *Journal of Advanced Nursing*, 17:98–103.

Smith M W (1995) Ethics in focus groups: a few concerns. *Qualitative Health Research*, 5, 4:478–86.

Sudman S and Bradburn N (1974) *Response Effects in Surveys* (Chicago, IL: Aldine).

Tsiboukli A and Wolff K (2003) Using focus groups interviews to understand staff perceptions from training in the therapeutic community model. *Journal of Drug Education*, 33, 2:143–57.

Van de Ven A H and Delbecq A L (1972) The nominal group as a research instrument for exploratory health studies. *American Journal of Public Health*, 69:337–42.

Vandendorpe F (2000) Funderals in Belgium: the hidden complexity of contemporary practices. *Mortality*, 5, 1:18–33.

Walker J M, Hall S and Thomas M (1995) The experience of labour: a perspective from those receiving care in a midwife-led unit. *Midwifery*, 11:120–9.

Waltz C F, Strickland C L and Lenz E R (1991) *Measurement in Nursing Research*, 2nd edn (Philadelphia, PA: F A Davis).

Webb C and Kevern J (2001) Focus groups as a research method: a critique of some aspects of their use in nursing research. *Journal of Advanced Nursing*, 33, 6:798–805.

Wengraf, T (2001) *Qualitative Research Interviewing* (Thousand Oaks, CA: Sage Publications).

Wilde V (1992) Controversial hypotheses on the relationship between researcher and informant in qualitative research. *Journal of Advanced Nursing*, 17:234–42.

Wilhelmsson S and Foldevi M (2003) Exploring views on Swedish district nurses' prescribing – a focus group study in primary health care. *Journal of Clinical Nursing*, 12:643–50.

Wright D (1994) Boys' thoughts and talk about sex in a working-class locality of Glasgow. *Sociological Review*, 42:702–37.

Observations 15

OPENING THOUGHT ▶ Where observation is concerned, chance favours only the prepared mind.

Louis Pasteur

Introduction

In a practice-based profession such as nursing or midwifery, observation is perhaps the most important method of collecting information. As a research tool for the study of human behaviour, it is invaluable on its own or when used in conjunction with other methods. In this chapter, we will explore briefly the use, value and limitations of observation in nursing practice and nursing research. The main two types of observations, structured and unstructured, will be described and discussed. We will examine the ethical implications of using observation to collect data on people in general, and patients and nurses in particular. Finally, some suggestions will be made to facilitate those who undertake a critical reading of observational studies.

Observation and nursing practice

Researchers did not invent observation. Adler and Adler (1994) remind us that, 'for as long as people have been interested in studying the social and natural world around them, observation has served as the bedrock source of human knowledge'.

Although observation is part of daily life, some professionals, in particular nurses, need to be skilled at it. Without observation effective nursing care is not possible. The process of nursing care, from assessment to evaluation, depends a great deal on precise and accurate observation. The ability to observe, although naturally possessed by some, can be developed with training. While observation is usually associated with sight, the other four senses (hearing, touch, smell and taste) are also involved. These senses vary as to the extent to which they are used in nursing practice. Sight and hearing are understandably the most frequently used, although touch and smell provide valuable information as well.

Humans have also devised aids to increase their ability to observe. The most common ones include telescopes, microscopes and sound amplifiers. In nursing practice, thermometers, sphygmomanometers and stethoscopes are but some of a whole array of devices and equipment designed to make observations of body functions and changes as precise and accurate as possible, and to venture where normal human senses cannot reach.

To assess and monitor clients, practitioners have to observe verbal and non-verbal signs. Many of the clients whom nurses treat, however, are either not able or unwilling to speak. The ability to assess their conditions and attend to their needs depends greatly on the observational skills of nurses. According to Rose-Grippa (1979), 'non-verbal communication, or the transmission of messages without the use of words, is the most basic form of communication' and 'it is estimated that in everyday communication between people, only one third of the message are transmitted verbally, while two thirds are transmitted nonverbally'.

'Doing the obs' is a well-known expression in nursing which normally means recording the temperature, pulse, respiration and blood pressure of the patient. Many of the observations carried out by nurses involve the use of more than one sense simultaneously. In 'taking' blood pressure, the nurse may use touch to find a vein, listen for the 'beats' and watch the movement of the 'needle' or 'mercury'. Apart from occasions when nurses are asked to 'observe' or 'special' a patient or to carry out specific observations, they are, according to Peplau (1988), participant observers in most relationships in nursing. As she explains:

> This requires that she use herself as an instrument and as an object of observation at the same time that she is participating in the interaction between herself and a patient or a group. The more precise the nurse can become in the use of herself as an instrument for observation, the more she will be able to observe in relation to performances in the nursing process.

Nurses also use a large number of tools or instruments to record nursing activities, assess and monitor patients' condition.

Observation in nursing research

The purpose of observations in nursing practice differs from that in nursing research. Nurses use observations to collect information to attend to the needs of clients while researchers conduct observations for the purpose of answering research questions. Many nursing observations, such as the monitoring of temperature, pulse and respiration or blood pressure require utmost rigour and precision. However, many other observations are casual, accidental or haphazard. They are made, as Peplau (1988) described above, during everyday interactions between nurses and patients. Therefore observations are made as part of the process of care and are not necessarily the focus of interactions. On the other hand, researchers' main purpose is not to deliver care but to observe. Therefore interactions are a means to an end, which is to collect research data. Adler and Adler (1994) explain how lay observations differ from research observations:

> What differentiates the observations of social scientists from those of everyday life actors is the former's systematic and purposive nature. Social science researchers study their surrounding regularly and repeatedly, with a curiosity spurred by theoretical questions about the nature of human action, interaction, and society.

As the nature of nurses' work requires them to observe all the time, a knowledge of how and why researchers carry out observations can enhance nurses' understanding of the complexity and implications of this method of collecting information. Some of the issues which will be raised in this chapter should, hopefully, help you to reflect on your own knowledge of, and skill in, observation. Like interviews, observations can be carried out in surveys, experiments and case studies. They are used in inductive, deductive, qualitative and quantitative research. They are more suited to some phenomena than others and can be used in conjunction with other methods such as questionnaires and interviews. The need to choose the most appropriate method, however, cannot be overemphasised. Observations are particularly suited to the study of psychomotor activities and other non-verbal activities, while knowledge, attitudes and beliefs are better studied by questionnaires and interviews. Observations are most suited for studying the behaviour of patients and health professionals, in particular interactions, communication and performance. Not all observations need to be of people. Gould and Ream (1994), in a study of infection control, used a 'ward facilities checklist' to document the availability of resources. Observation of behaviour in its natural setting provides an insight into the context in which it occurs. Researchers have the opportunity to sample the physical, cultural, psychological and social environment in which the behaviour takes place.

Although observations on their own can tell us a lot about human behaviour, they can increase our understanding when used in combination with other methods such as interviews or document analysis. This is because, with observation, researchers can see and interpret behaviour but cannot have access to the meaning which participants give to their own behaviour. Researchers and practitioners interested in the link between knowledge, attitude and practice often find that there are discrepancies between these. Salmon (1993) points out that 'in nursing care as in other aspects of behaviour, attitudes have been found to be a poor guide to behaviour'. He carried out observations of 27 nurses and administered a questionnaire to all them in his study of the 'interactions of nurses with elderly patients' to find out if there was a link between their attitudes and the way they interacted with patients. Another reason for using multiple methods is because different methods often reveal different realities. For example, Lowe (1992) carried out semi-structured interviews and participant observation 'in order to investigate the interventions used by psychiatric nurses when faced with challenging behaviour'. In the interviews he paid particular attention 'to situations in which the observations of different witnesses to the same event were conflicting' (Lowe, 1992).

On the other hand, interviews on their own are limited in studying behaviour. There are a number of problems with asking people about their behaviour. These include, among others, perception bias, memory gaps, ulterior motives or that respondents may not be aware of how they behave.

Some phenomena which have been studied by means of observation include: 'the work behaviour of head nurses' (Drach-Zahavy and Dagan, 2002), 'nurse–patient interactions associated with pain assessment' (Manias et al., 2002), 'patient teaching' (Barber-Parker, 2002), 'washing and dressing of stroke patients' (Booth et al., 2001), 'patient care in intensive care setting' (Turnock and Gibson, 2001) and 'interaction between individuals with dementia and aggressive behaviour and caregivers' (Skovdahl et al., 2003).

Limitations of observations

Observation, as with other methods, has its own limitations and ethical implications (discussed in a later section). One of the main problems is the effect of the observer on the 'observed'. The awareness of being observed is likely to lead people to be self-conscious and may influence them to behave in ways that they would not normally behave. In a classic study by Roethlisberger and Dickson (1939), in which they set out to find the effect of illumination levels on productivity at the Hawthorne plant of Western Electric in Chicago, they experimented with different levels of lighting over a period of two and a half years and found that no matter what the levels were, productivity continued to increase. Roethlisberger and Dickson (1939) concluded that the workers produced more, mainly because they were being observed rather than as a result of different lighting. This type of observer effect is now known popularly as the 'Hawthorne effect'.

In an observation study of 'patient care in intensive care units', Turnock and Gibson (2001) queried whether the impact of their presence upon staff behaviour would have been different if they had been 'either true researchers or practitioners'. They described one incident which confirmed their suspicion that the observer's presence may have led to fewer nursing interventions than expected. To test this 'hypothesis',

> After one 1 hour of observation, the observer changed position. The same patient was observed for a second hour but from a position much further away from the bed area. Once the new position was taken up, several activities/interventions began to take place.

They explained that 'this may have been a coincidence, but was more likely due to the influence of the observer's presence on staff behaviour' (Turnock and Gibson, 2001).

While the effect of the observer's presence cannot be fully eliminated, researchers found that it is not always possible for people to change their normal behaviour and sustain it for long periods. They noticed that after a while, the observer can become 'part of the furniture'. In Cormack's (1976) study, in which he observed the work of the charge nurse in an acute psychiatric setting, he reported clues which led him to believe that his presence as an observer did not entirely affect the behaviour of those he studied. These clues included 'tea drinking staff groups, which left the entire ward without nursing supervision or observation', staff playing cards among themselves, derogatory remarks made about patients, and patients discussing issues in his presence which they insisted were 'highly confidential to be shared with the doctor only'.

Mulhall (2003) believes that while the Hawthorne effect is an obvious drawback, its effect in participant observation can be over-emphasised. Based on her experience, she explains that 'most professionals are too busy to maintain behaviour that is radically different from normal'.

Some of the strategies to reduce this effect will be discussed later. Researchers are also best placed to know if they are aware that their presence influenced the data they collected and must reflect on it. There is no perfect method and some trade-off is often necessary for the collection of valid and reliable data. To some extent the video can be used to reduce observer's effect (this is discussed further on).

Another problem with observations is that they can be costly and impractical over long periods of time. For example, watching and waiting for aggressive behaviour to happen can be time-consuming. The researcher's ability to observe with precision can wane over time, as fatigue sets in. The difficulties of observing different aspects of the same phenomenon, which occur at the same time, and the ways in which researchers cope with these and other problems are discussed further in the next section.

Structured observation

A *structured* observation is one in which aspects of the phenomenon to be observed are decided in advanced (i.e. predetermined). For example, if nursing activities are to be observed, the researcher can break down 'activities' into a number of *units* or *categories*.

In their observation of 'medication-related activities of nursing staff' in a neonatal unit, Ridge and While (1995) used the following categories to observe:

- Key responsibilities
- Drug selection
- Charting
- Clerical

- Preparation
- Clarification – medication
- Checking
- Administration

- Relative counselling
- Related communication
- Other

Each of these categories was described further in order to help the observer to distinguish between categories. The following explanation was provided for the category 'Checking':

Checking

(i) Observing another nurse in the process of preparation of a drug prior to administration of a medication to a specific neonate.

(ii) Checking that a medication is to be administered to the correct neonate.

(iii) Checking the treatment care for due medications, etc.

The reason for specifying aspects of the phenomenon in advance is mainly to find out if they are present and, if so, to what extent. The same type of data is required from each observation, thereby introducing standardisation in the process.

To carry out structured observation a 'checklist' or 'schedule' is devised. It is similar to a questionnaire and can be highly or loosely structured. For example, in a study of touch in nurse–patient interaction, the observer could be asked to indicate the 'site' of touch without providing her with any categories of site. She has to decide which term she wants to use to describe where the touch was applied. Alternatively, as Oliver and Redfern (1991) did, 'site of touch' was further divided into: 'head, face, shoulder, axilla, arm, hand, chest, abdomen, back, leg, foot, bottom and genitals'. The observer had simply to select the appropriate category. This avoids the problem which arises when different observers use different terms to describe the same site. A highly structured observation schedule leaves little for the observer to interpret other than to 'tick' the appropriate columns or boxes.

Observation units or categories have been described as 'molar' and 'molecular' (Lobo, 1992). *Molar* units are broad and sometimes abstract, making the task of the observer more difficult since the category is not defined in enough detail for it to be instantly recognised. An example of molar categories comes from a study by Salmon (1993) of 'interactions of nurses with elderly patients', in which 'interactions with patients were subdivided into: positive (informing, questioning, general conversation) negative (ordering, rebuking) and neutral'. 'Informing' itself is a broad term which can be subdivided into further categories. The observer in this case has to decide first what constitutes informing, before deciding whether the behaviour is positive. *Molecular* units, on the other hand, are more detailed and precise, and therefore allow for more accurate recording. In a study by Fuller and Conner (1995) of 'the effect of pain on infant behaviors', 'cries' were described as follows:

> Cry duration. A single phonation with more than 3 seconds of silence preceding and following another phonation was defined as a cry. Phonations with less than 3 seconds separating each other were labelled subcries. A cry bout is a series of subcries separated by more than 3 seconds from a cry or second cry bout. The duration in seconds was measured for all cries, subcries, and cry bouts contained on each videotape.

The more molecular categories there are, the more structured the checklist is. Some phenomena lend themselves more to molecular subdivisions than others.

To facilitate recording and analysis, categories are given codes. The following example of the use of codes is taken from Turnock and Gibson (2001) in their observation of patient exposure:

Code	Area exposed
1	Chest
2	Front genitalia
3	Buttocks
4	Legs
5	None
6	Other (state)
7	More than one

While codes are helpful in making it easier and quicker to record a category, especially in observations where behaviours are happening simultaneously, they nevertheless have to be memorised. This can be a difficult and challenging task for observers in studies where a large number of codes are used.

In structured observation, the phenomenon to be studied must be operationally defined. The categories or units depend on the particular definition which the researcher chooses. An existing definition can be used or researchers may formulate their own after reviewing the literature. Felce et al. (1980), in their study 'measuring activity of old people in residential care', formulated their definition of 'engagement in purposeful activity' by 'using the literature on behavioral observation, available manuals on measuring engagement in various settings, and the authors' informal observations of residents' behavior in the homes for the elderly'. Whatever the definition it must represent adequately the phenomenon and it must be operationally feasible (see Chapter 9). This means that it must describe behaviours which *can* be observed. Booth et al. (2001) offer the following operational definition of 'doing for' in their observational study of 'washing and dressing of stroke patients':

Doing for: All actions which are 'done to' or 'on' the patient by a member of staff. The patient is passive and makes no active contribution.

Structured observations and structured interviews are similar in that both use predetermined, structured and standardised tools. The observer and interviewer also adopt a non-participative or non-interventionist stance. As with the administration of questionnaires, the observer stands 'outside' what is being observed and tries not to influence events or behaviours in any way. Fitzpatrick et al. (1996) found that avoiding interaction during non-participant observation was a real challenge. They pointed out that 'by choosing not to respond may result in observer alienation from the field setting'. Turnock and Gibson (2001) explained how they 'experienced problems in maintaining a detached, researcher role' as non-participant observers. They were 'asked to keep an eye on the patient for a minute'. Turnock and Gibson (2001) also found it 'morally impossible to ignore the requests of patients not involved in the study'. Although researchers may not be able to keep a completely non-participant, detached stance when doing observations, they should be sensitive to the possible effects of such interactions on the data collected.

In structured observations, researchers seek to quantify specific aspects of the phenomena being observed. Usually they want to find the presence or absence of a particular behaviour or characteristic, and the frequency or intensity with which they may happen. For example, in Salmon's study of nurses' interactions with elderly patients, he set out to find, among others, the number of nurses' interactions which involved patients and the proportion of these interactions which 'were concerned with physical care (medication, meals and dressing)' or 'informal reality orientation periods' (Salmon, 1993). Structured observations adopt mostly a deductive approach since the behaviour or activity is observed against units of observation which are specified in advance. The underlying assumption in the use of structured observations is that researchers know what constitutes the behaviour or activity and only seek to discover to what extent they are present in the population under study.

Sampling in structured observation

It is not always feasible or possible to observe every behaviour or activity on a continuous basis. Prolonged observation of patients and nurses can cause unnecessary stress to them. Therefore researchers resort to time sampling, where appropriate. Nurses are familiar with the concept of time sampling. Patients are monitored at set intervals as in the case of four-hourly recording of temperature, pulse and respiration. In the same way if patient activities are being observed, the researcher may decide to carry out observations during the first 15 minutes of each hour for the duration of the shift. This can be done if it is believed that these periods of 15 minutes are able to give an accurate and representative picture of activities over the whole shift. In their study of what elderly people do in hospital, Birchall and Waters (1996) carried out observations for periods of 2.5 hours each on different days of the week until a record of their activities for the period between 8.00 am and 9.30 pm was completed. They explained that although this information did not reflect a continuous day's behaviour, it provided 'an example of the activities that were occurring at any particular time of day'. In their study of medication-related activities of nursing staff, Ridge and While (1995) found that medication administration happened four times more frequently 'between 08.00 and 09.59 hours' than between '02.00 and 03.59 hours'. Therefore the 'former 2 hr period was observed four times more frequently' (Ridge and While, 1995). The selection periods of observation must be justified as it is likely that some behaviour or activities may happen at certain times only.

Intermittent observation, as in the case in time sampling, may not be appropriate in cases where the behaviour or activity happens rarely or unpredictably. For example, if a researcher wants to observe aggressive behaviour among psychiatric patients, then continuous observation would be advisable. This can be achieved either by observing whole shifts or by dividing the day into, for example, four-hourly sessions from 8.00 am to midnight. The researcher then carries out the 8.00 am to 12.00 midday observation on day one and the 12.00 midday to 4.00 pm session on day two. This is continued until all four sessions are covered. In this way data for the whole period between 8.00 am to midnight are obtained, although not in one day. Patients and nurses do not have to 'suffer' the presence of the researcher for one whole day.

Alternatively, the researcher may want to observe aggressive behaviours during specific 'events' such as meal times or in discussion groups. In this case these events become the focus of the study. However, not all meal times may be observed. The researcher may select a sample of meal times, as for example, lunch on Monday and Friday, dinner on Tuesday and Saturday and breakfast on Wednesday and Sunday. Thus a sample of mealtimes can be chosen to represent mealtimes in general in that particular ward. This is known as event sampling; the event becomes the sampling unit.

Limitations of structured observations

Behaviours and activities happen simultaneously and the observer may not be able to notice and record all of them. The position of the observer may be such that the behaviour may be outside her observation range or she may be obstructed, as in the case where a nurse is in the observer's line of vision and the patient cannot be observed. Some movements or change may be so subtle or rapid that the researcher is unable to capture it. For example, eye contacts can be fleeting or a facial expression can last a fraction of a second. As Lobo (1992) explains:

If the behavior occurs very infrequently, it may be missed altogether because the length of the observation is not sufficient to capture the behavior. Or if the event is fleeting and the observation is over a long period of time, a fatigued observer may miss the event.

In a busy environment, it is possible for the observer to be distracted, especially if she is concerned about what happens to other people. In continuous observation, fatigue may set in, leading to lack of concentration. According to Porter et al. (1986), 'circadian variation may affect the accuracy of the observer at different times of day'.

One of the major problems with structured observations is the difficulty of deciding which category or unit the observed behaviour or activity belongs to. Some categories are not adequately defined. In Porter et al.'s (1986) study, the observers found difficulty in recording the 'patient response to touch' because, as the authors admitted, 'response-type' 'was not sufficiently well operationally well defined'. Some categories require the observer to make more subjective judgements than others. For example, in the above study, there was more agreement between observers on such categories as 'duration of touch' or 'type of touch' than on 'response type' or 'intensity of touch'. This was because the observers had to subjectively decide what constituted 'response-type' or 'intensity of touch'. On the other hand, 'duration of touch' can be measured by a stopwatch and 'type of touch' was sufficiently well defined for the observers not to rely too much on their subjective judgement. In a recent study by Fader et al. (2003), in which the frequency and intensity of erythema (reddening of the skin) were observed, there were disagreements between observers relating to grade 0 ('no erythema') and grade 1 ('barely perceptible erythema'). It was acknowledged that 'these discrepancies could be real (i.e. the skin colour changed slightly during the lapsed time period) or as a result of error (because the degree of difference between the two grades was very slight and therefore difficult to accurately grade' (Fader et al., 2003).

Researchers can overcome some of above problems by providing adequate operational definitions, by piloting their observation schedule, by training observers and by making use of audio- and videotaping where possible, appropriate and ethical.

Mason and Redeker (1993) suggest videotaping as an answer to observer fatigue. Video recording has the advantage of providing continuous data over long periods of time. It can record more details than a human observer can. It has 'frame by frame', 'close-up' (useful for subtle movements) and 'play-back' facilities. Videotapes can be made available for other researchers to analyse the data. Latvala et al. (2000) list two main limitations of video recordings: mechanical faults and the influence that the camera may have on people's behaviour. In their study of 'nursing report sessions and interdisciplinary team meetings' in a psychiatric unit they use videotaping as a method of data collection. They found that some nurses 'changed their habits and presented their ideal selves' when being taped (Latvala et al., 2000). Videotaping in the natural environment can be difficult if those being filmed are on the move rather than static.

A number of ethical issues should be considered when video recording is used in research studies. Participants must not feel under pressure to take part and must be free to withdraw after viewing the tapes. Researchers have the responsibility to keep the tapes in a safe place and destroy them when data have been analysed. For examples of studies using video recordings see Latvala et al. (2000) and Skovdahl et al. (2003).

Validity and reliability of structured observation

When structured observations are carried out 'the reliability and validity of observations depend upon the reliability and validity inherent in the observational aids and in the ability of the observer to identify and record the specified behaviors or events' (Waltz et al., 1991). For structured observations to have validity the observer must observe what she is supposed to observe. Observation schedules can be assessed for content validity in the same way as for questionnaires (see Chapter 13). The operational definition of the phenomenon must be clear and precise and the categories or units must represent the phenomenon. To ensure content validity, the observation schedule can be given to a panel of experts for review.

The observer's presence can also affect the validity of the data. As mentioned earlier, the observer's effect can be reduced when those observed 'get used' to the presence of the observer. Sometimes the observer spends little time in the setting prior to the observation and therefore has little or no opportunity for 'settling in'. The personal attributes – such as gender, sex, race, dress or manner – of the observer may influence how people behave when they are observed. Researchers must be sensitive to this possibility and make allowance for this when they analyse and interpret data.

When a number of people witness an accident, it is unlikely that their individual accounts of the event would be entirely consistent, even if it happened five minutes earlier. Police officers are familiar with instances when witnesses give different descriptions of the same burglary or assault. Research observers are not immune to such inconsistencies. The observation schedule, the instructions to observers and the opportunity to record behaviours as they happen, facilitate the observation process. However, observers are human and can be influenced by a number of factors that can distort their perception or they may simply make mistakes.

Reliability in structured observations refers to the consistency with which the observer matches a behaviour or activity with the same unit or category on the observation schedule and records it in the same way each time it happens. *Intra-observer* reliability is the consistency with which one observer records the same behaviours in the same way on different occasions. Often observations in the same study are carried out by two or more observers. It is important that they observe, interpret and record the same behaviour or activity in the same way. *Inter-observer* or *inter-rater reliability* can be monitored by asking two or more observers to record the same behaviours and their findings are then computed. A '1.00' indicates total agreement and thereby excellent reliability while a score of below 0.60 (an agreement in six instances out of ten) is of doubtful reliability. However, each study may set its own acceptable levels of reliability depending on the type of phenomenon. The more difficult they are to observe the less likely it is to achieve a score close to 1.00. There is normally a consensus in the research literature on what constitutes an acceptable reliability level depending on the complexity of the observational task.

A high level of agreement between two or more observers usually means that they consistently recognised and recorded the same behaviour in the same way. However, they could also be consistently wrong. In their study of 'interpersonal communication between nurses and elderly patients', Oliver and Redfern (1991) reported that two observers 'recorded that no non-verbal response' to touch had occurred during their observations. Oliver and Redfern (1991) explained that:

> This is unlikely to be true; it is much more likely that the non-verbal responses that did occur were not observed because the observers were busy recording other components. Non-verbal responses contain such a range of behaviours that they require a more focused and 'close-up' observation technique than was used in this study. Videorecording would be an appropriate technique for this.

Different types of errors may affect the reliability of observation data. The most common error is when the same researcher faced with the same behaviour or activity interprets it differently or when different observers use different categories to classify the same phenomenon. Another error is when, due to the lack of concentration or because the behaviour happens too quickly, observers use the wrong codes (especially when there are a large number of them).

The observers' interpretation of behaviour can be influenced by their experience and prejudices. Our professional backgrounds often make us see things differently from others. Assertiveness can be interpreted as aggressiveness by different people. Lobo (1992) gives this example of how prejudices can influence observation:

> if mother–baby interaction is observed and the data collector knows that all of the mothers have had histories of drug use, the observer may score all of the mothers lower, or if the data collector knows the mothers are all upper middle class and highly educated, the scores may be higher.

The training of observers is crucial if a high level of reliability is to be achieved. In their study of nurse performance, in which they carried out 297 observation sessions lasting 742.5 hours, Fitzpatrick et al. (1996) concluded that observer training emerged as one of the most important strategies for addressing the challenges posed by this method.

When observations do not match, observers must discuss their perception of the particular behaviours or activities in dispute and arrive at an agreed interpretation of it. The validity and reliability of structured observations depend mainly on how the observation schedule is constructed and used. Clear operational definitions, although not the answer to all the problems associated with structured observations, can help to ensure the validity and reliability of the tools. For a useful study on the inter-rater reliability of a structured tool (the adapted Waterlow scale) see Cook et al. (1999). For an example of the use of structured observations see Research Example 43.

Unstructured observation

Maupassant, a French novelist, in a preface to *Pierre and Jean* in 1887, wrote:

> In everything there is an unexplored element because we are prone by habit to use our eyes only in combination with the memory of what others before us have thought about the thing we are looking at. The most significant thing contains some little unknown element. We must find it.

According to Kirk and Miller (1986),

> In science, as in life, dramatic new discoveries must almost by definition be accidental ('serendipitous'). Indeed, they occur only in consequence of some kind of mistake.

They relate how radioactivity was discovered when Henri Becquerel 'tossed the uranium salts into a drawer with his photographic materials and knocked off work'. Alexander Fleming also found that 'some kind of mold got into his staphylococcus culture and ruined the bacteria' and accidentally discovered penicillin (Kirk and Miller 1986).

Although the ability to understand what happens is based on prior knowledge, these examples also show the need to study phenomena with fresh eyes and an open mind. By adopting a deductive approach, researchers collect data to test what is already known. The categories to be observed are formulated in advance, based on previous knowledge. Alternatively researchers can observe phenomena without any predetermined categories and allow these to emerge from the data collected.

When we observe people's behaviour in buses we do not have categories to 'tick'. Instead we record and analyse mentally what we watch. We may notice that some people sit by themselves rather than join others, younger people sit at

RESEARCH EXAMPLE 43

Observing washing and dressing of stroke patients: nursing intervention compared with occupational therapist. What is the difference?
Booth et al. (2001)

A structured observation

In this study, non-participant structured observation was used to compare the intervention of qualified nurses with that of occupational therapists during morning care with a group of stroke patients.

An existing tool adapted for use in this study consisted of 46 items covering the following areas: position, movement, washing/grooming, dressing, elimination and physiotherapy. The observer had to differentiate between these seven categories of physical interaction: 'no contacts', 'supervision', 'prompting/ instructing', 'providing articles', 'facilitation', 'giving physical assistance' and 'doing for'.

Comments:

1   A structured observation tool or schedule was used to observe only pre-determined aspects of morning care and categories of interactions (see Booth et al., 2001, p.105). The researcher was required to 'tick' the relevant boxes or columns as they occurred.

2   Structured observation schedules should be designed with as much precision as possible to facilitate observation and recordings. Therefore the operational definition of terms used in the observation schedule is of vital importance. For example, in this study the category 'giving physical assistance' was defined as: '. . . actually helping the patient to carry out an activity. The actions of the helper must be rehabilitative in nature e.g. helping somebody stand up and providing physical support while the patients pull up their trousers'.

3   'Event sampling' was used because the researchers knew exactly what they wanted to focus on. The event selected was 'morning care activities (personal hygiene, grooming and dressing, in particular)'. Dates and times were agreed with the participants (including the patients involved), after consent was obtained.

4   To avoid 'professional' bias and reduce 'problems of inter-rater reliability', one researcher who was neither a nurse nor an occupational therapist carried out the observational sessions.

5   To remain detached (and objective) the following strategy was used: if patients or staff spoke to the observer whilst he was observing, 'he would respond verbally but indicate that he was not able to engage in conversation at that time'.

the back, some sit comfortably while others sit at the edge of their seat or some people read while others meditate or talk to others. We would have, in fact, carried out 'unstructured' observations. In the latter the researcher does not start with any predetermined categories, but instead constructs them while she observes or after all the observations have been made. Unstructured observations therefore adopt an inductive approach and are described as qualitative observations.

Unstructured observations are appropriate in cases where little is known about the phenomenon. The knowledge gained can be used afterwards to construct categories for structured observations. In the above example, a researcher can thereafter try to see whether people in buses in fact behave as described above. To do so she has to construct an observation schedule containing the various behaviours mentioned above and record their presence or absence and their frequency.

Unstructured observations are also undertaken when researchers believe that existing knowledge of phenomena is either lacking or not valid. For example, Samarel (1989), in her study of how hospice nurses meet the needs of terminally ill and acutely ill patients, in which she used unstructured observations, found that the 'observed interactions of the participant nurses differed from that suggested by the literature regarding ways nurses interact with dying patients'. In this case unstructured observations provided data to challenge existing knowledge.

In structured observations the boundaries of what is to be observed are set prior to data collection. Observers are only expected to collect information required in the schedule or checklist. Each observation session lasts about the same amount of time and the researcher also carries out the same observation for each and every session. Unstructured observations are less standardised and more flexible. Each observation session is treated as a unique event and no two sessions are considered the same. What is learnt in the first session can be built upon in the later sessions, as is the case with qualitative interviews. In everyday life, we learn by accumulating 'facts' which are confirmed or rejected as we come across the same event time and again. This 'cumulative' process of confirmation and validation is adopted by researchers as they move from one observation to the next. Barber-Parker (2002), in her study of patient teaching, used the data from the initial observations to generate questions which were explored in later observations. The purpose of an unstructured observation is to arrive at as complete an understanding of the phenomenon as possible. For this to happen, researchers must be flexible enough to make the most of the observation situation and should not feel constrained to observe only the categories decided in advance.

Unlike the case in structured observations, no specific research questions, objectives or hypotheses are set at the beginning of unstructured observations. Researchers decide during the observation what to focus on. Usually the initial observations are 'unfocussed and general in scope', and later when observers become more familiar in the settings their attention may be more focused (Adler and Adler, 1994). According to Mulhall (2003) researchers 'may have some ideas as to what to observe', but these 'may change over time as they gather data and gain experience in the particular setting'.

Unstructured observations are also flexible in the duration of the sessions. They do not all necessarily have to be carried out over the same period of time. In a study by Hewison (1995) of 'nurses' power in interactions with patients', the unstructured observation sessions 'ranged from 2½ to 4 hours in duration'.

In structured observations, researchers make recordings on the schedule or enter the data directly into a portable computer. These 'tools' are essential; without them no observation can take place, in the same way that one cannot conduct a survey without a questionnaire or a checklist. In unstructured observations researchers take notes in a variety of ways. As explained before, in a qualitative study the researcher is herself a tool of data collection and analysis during the process of data collection. This is sometimes supplemented by note taking in one form or other. These can range from scribbles to extensive descriptions and tape recordings. Usually notes are taken as inconspicuously as possible so as not to disturb the normal flow of events. In a study of care in a secure forensic unit, Clarke (1996) went 'to the unit lavatory inconspicuously, either to make notes or speak in a miniature dictaphone'. Barber-Parker (2002) describes how, in her study, only brief notes were taken in the presence of others, but 'planned time alone to create detailed notes, including quotes, context and personal thoughts'. Whatever the practice adopted for taking notes, it should not interfere with the flow of the observation, inhibit participants in behaving in their normal ways or raise suspicions about the actions and motives of the observer.

Analysis of data collected by unstructured observations is similar to that for qualitative interviews. There are many examples in the literature of the analysis of unstructured observation data (see e.g. Barber-Parker, 2002 and Skovdahl et al., 2003). Barber-Parker (2002) gave a summary account of the process of data analysis in her study of patient teaching.

> Through repeated reading of the notes, the investigator identified the who, what, where, when, why and how of teaching activities. Incentives and barriers for patient teaching were searched for in the data and a third category emerged, that of facilitators for patient teaching. The critical attributes (items that appeared repetitively) of teaching activities were identified and the investigator created a precise operational definition of patient teaching for this setting. The entire analysis remained concrete and well grounded in the data.

Other researchers have used the phenomenological method (Hallberg et al., 1995) and grounded theory method (Hewison, 1995) in their analysis of data from observations.

One of the main problems with unstructured observations is that one can be selective in what to focus on, and this may reflect the personal interest of the researcher. Observational data are not more 'factual' than other types of data (from interviews, questionnaires, documents or records). They are interpretations of researchers, and as such must be treated with the same caution as other data.

Hewison (1995), commenting on the limitations of his study of 'nurses' power in interactions with patients', points out:

> While every effort was made to overcome the selective inattention (Spradley 1980) which can result in obvious everyday activity being overlooked, what was actually observed also constitutes a limitation. The selection of interactions to be recorded was mediated by what was felt to be pertinent to the research problem.

Analysis of data can also be a problem. By not deciding in advance which aspects to observe it is likely that a large mass of data will be collected. This can make data analysis particularly difficult, laborious and time-consuming, as is the case with qualitative interview data as well.

The problem of observer's effect is also real in unstructured as it is in structured observation. To offset this limitation researchers have to use strategies to 'blend in' with the environment and reflect on the effect of their presence.

Validity and reliability of unstructured observations

By not seeing behaviours and activities through the lens of predetermined categories, it is possible to some extent to observe a phenomenon 'as it is'. The purpose of unstructured observations is to seek as many different ways in which the phenomenon manifests itself. As explained earlier, each observation builds on the previous one by providing data which contribute towards an in-depth understanding of the phenomenon.

The flexibility of unstructured observations allows the researcher to search for the 'truth' whenever she can find it. This means that she can observe for longer or shorter periods in some sessions if the data are considered valuable. Thus the validity of unstructured observations is increased. The selectivity bias present in this type of observation is one of the main limitations. As explained earlier, there is little doubt that different researchers are likely to collect different data while observing the same phenomenon.

It is not possible for others to replicate unstructured observational studies. However, their data can be compared with those collected by different methods and in similar settings. The validity and reliability of unstructured observations will be further discussed in the next section.

So far observation methods have been presented in the form of two ideal types: structured and unstructured. While this may be helpful for the purpose of teaching and learning, they do not adequately describe what happens in practice. Mulhall (2003), for example, emphasises that 'the label "unstructured" is misleading'. As with unstructured interviews, unstructured observations are not totally without structure or focus. The process of unstructured observation, in any particular study, rarely remains the same. It is likely that observers, as they become interested in some ideas, events or issues, impose more structure on the observations than they do at the start of a study. Examples were given earlier of how researchers doing 'structured' observations could not remain totally detached and are instead drawn into interaction by participants. Observations can also vary in terms of the degree of structure imposed by the researcher. This has led some researchers to label their observations as semi-structured (see e.g. Sarantakos, 1998 and Drach-Zahavy and Dagan, 2002) in the same way that this label is applied to interviews. It is more helpful, as Turnock and Gibson (2001) suggest, 'to describe the role of the observer rather than struggle to identify the "correct" theoretical label'. According to them, readers can make their own judgement about the validity and reliability of the study if they are able 'to follow the decision making trail'. For an example of a study using unstructured observation see Research Example 44.

Participation in observation

Observers can adopt a detached role or can participate fully in the activities which they observe. In between these two stances, there are a number of positions which observers can occupy. Gold (1958) suggested the following four roles: 'the complete participant, the participant-as-observer, the observer-as-participant and the complete observer'. Adler and Adler (1994) describe the complete observer role as:

> researchers who are fundamentally removed from their settings. Their observations may occur from the outside, with observers being neither seen nor noticed. Contemporary varieties of this role might include the videotaping, audiotaping, or photographing noninteractive observer. This role most closely approximates the traditional ideal of the 'objective' observer.

The complete participant role is described as one in which the researcher is one of the participants in the activities or events which are observed without, however, revealing that in fact she is also carrying out research observations while being part of the group. This covert role has serious ethical implications which will be discussed later. The rationale on which this covert, total participative role is based is that observers can never fully avoid the effect of their presence. They believe that, by revealing their role as researchers, they are not observing what would have normally happened if they were not present, and thereby do not collect valid data.

The other two roles, participant-as-observer and observer-as-participant, are similar. The former reflects a more participative role while the latter, a more

Observation of pain assessment and management – the complexities of clinical practice

Manias et al. (2002)

Unstructured observations

This observational study investigated 'nurse–patient interactions associated with pain assessment, and management' in a surgical unit. Twelve field observations were carried out by one non-participant observer. A portable audio-recorder was used to record all observations 'and to allow for rapid descriptions of actions'. Nurses were also asked to clarify decisions and the context in which they were made. Four major themes were identified after data were transcribed and analysed.

Comments:

1 Observation was selected as a method because of the authors' perceived limitations of self-reports (in interviews) as the latter may 'differ from what occurs in actual clinical practice'. They explained that 'observational studies may provide a more effective means of describing some of the complex issues that influence pain assessment and management'.

2 According to Manias et al. (2002), previous observation studies of pain in clinical settings 'focused on issues that were preconceived prior to data collection'. This study, using unstructured observations, allowed the themes to emerge out of the data. The observer did not use a predetermined and structured observational schedule to record what was happening.

3 Each observation period lasted two hours and various observation times were selected to 'cover' the whole spectrum of activities which occur over a 24-hour period.

4 All nurses in the unit and each patient involved in the observation 'were invited to consent to participate in the data collection process and to allow their medical records to be accessed for relevant demographic information'.

5 The authors concluded that the observational method was 'invaluable for exploring work demands in clinical areas, levels of accountability surrounding pain assessment and management, and the complexity of competing demands between nurses, doctors and patients'.

research role. Gold's classifications (which are four points on a continuum with complete participant at one end and complete observer on the other) are ideal types; in practice these four roles may be more problematic than one might think. For example, although researchers may be overt about their role, how much they reveal can affect the data. Some observers ask permission to observe but do not reveal the exact nature of their study. Nurse researchers may also conceal the fact (or do not volunteer the information) that they are trained nurses. Making others aware that one is a researcher is not enough to remove the charge of 'covert' research.

The nature of participation differs from observer to observer even when they adopt a participant-as-observer role. For example, a trained nurse's participation in this role will differ from that of a non-nurse. Her participation in nursing care and access to information would be different from that of, for example, Millman, a sociologist (in a study of 'life in the backrooms of American medicine'), who could only 'follow' surgeons around in operating theatres and attend ward rounds and various staff meetings (Millman, 1976). Had she been a surgeon she would have participated in their conversations in a way which a sociologist could not, and although she may not have carried out operations, the 'surgeon researcher' would have taken part in other activities as well. In being allowed or able to do some tasks, the surgeon researcher would have some experiential understanding of what she observes in a way that Millman could not.

Finally, in the same study, it is not always possible or desirable to maintain the same degree of participation in the pursuit of valid data. Samarel (1989) describes how her participation varied as her study of 'caring for the living and the dying' progressed:

> The primary mode of data collection was participant observation with the role of the researcher ranging from observer-as-participant to participant-as observer . . . During the early phase of data collection the researcher was present in the hallways, lounges, offices, nurses' station and at staff meetings . . . After two months of observation in this manner, the investigator's presence began to be accepted by the staff as natural. The investigator then began to take a more active role (observer-as-participant).

Samarel (1989) went on to explain that, thereafter, she had minimal participation 'in informal patient care conferences in which patients' needs were discussed and nursing care planned'. She also 'assisted the participant nurses with such aspects of patient care as moving, bathing or bed making'. Randers and Mattiasson (2004) explain how participating in the care of patients at meal times and assisting in bedmaking helped to 'offset the impression as just an observer'. On the other hand, not integrating in the setting and not being 'accepted' by participants can affect the 'quality and quantity of data gathered through participant observation' (Drury and Stott, 2001).

Participant observation and ethnography

The term 'unstructured observation' is often used interchangeably with that of participant observation. They should not be confused, as it is possible to observe a phenomenon inductively (without predetermined categories) and yet refrain from taking part in the action.

Participant observation is the choice method in ethnographic studies. Layder (1993) describes the benefits sociologists derive from such an approach:

> The method of 'participant observation' allows the closest approximation to a state of affairs wherein the sociologist enters into the everyday world of those being studied so that he or she may describe and analyse this world as accurately as possible. Participant observation represents the ideal form of research strategy because this method requires that the sociologist for all intents and purposes 'becomes' a member of the group being studied.

Davies (1995) explains that 'ethnographic research uses observational skills that people use in their everyday lives' and that 'we constantly make sense of speech, body movement and facial expressions in different social settings'.

To get a glimpse of people's feelings and behaviour, ethnographers not only have to be present where the action is but also, as much as possible, be part of their environment and become an insider. The purpose of participating is to try to see things from the subjects' point of view and to understand how (and why) they behave in their social and cultural groups. The participant observer aims to perceive and feel things in the same way as the participants do.

The ethnographer can never fully participate in the action in the same way as those she studies. The sociologist cannot do what the doctor does, but can be close enough to get an understanding of the world of doctors. In her study of 'life in the backrooms of medicine', Millman (1976) describes how this became possible:

> By spending so much time with individuals and by accompanying them through their entire days for weeks or months at a time I was able to get a feeling for the texture and quality of staff life in the hospital. I was able to observe how the various groups of doctors viewed and gave meaning to the situations which arose, and how they chose to pay attention to some things and not to others.

One of the strengths of the ethnographic approach is that observations and interviews go hand in hand. This allows for a more complete understanding of what is being studied. Thus the ethnographer can ask why people behave the way they do and clarify inconsistencies which arise between what people say and do. Ethnographic interviews take the form of normal conversations, as is the case when a student spends a day 'shadowing' or accompanying a community nurse on her visits. However, formal interviews can also be carried out. An important feature of the ethnographic approach is that participants can ask questions of the researcher. According to Frankenberg (1982), it often happens to the field worker that the questions he is asked are more important than the questions he asks.

One of the problems with ethnography is overidentification of the researcher with the participants in the study. This is what Frankenberg (1982) describes as 'going native'. The danger, as Alderson (2001), explains, is 'becoming too much of an accustomed insider instead of a questioning stranger'.

Ethical implications of observation

Privacy, confidentiality and anonymity

Research observation, whether overt or covert, is an intrusion into other peoples' privacy. When informed consent is given the observer has the duty to keep the confidentiality of the information obtained. Johnson (1992) makes clear the distinction between privacy and confidentiality:

> Privacy would allow the individual nurse, for example, to carry out work without the scrutiny of a researcher, just because people ought to be able to avoid the inconvenience of observation if they so choose. Confidentiality would mean that a person having agreed to be observed, those observations would not be disclosed to others in any identifiable way.

With all the best intention and goodwill it is not always possible to maintain confidentiality. Mander (1995), drawing from her own research experience, concludes that 'in the course of research, confidentiality carries many benefits for all parties, but may present the researcher with some practical difficulties'. She added:

> Data, including personal experience seeking access, collected during my recent studies indicate that the implementation of confidentiality is difficult, inconsistent and occasionally falls short of the recommended standard. It is necessary to conclude that in research, the practice of confidentiality does not always equate with that which is preached.

Obtaining informed consent to enter the private world of others does not give the right to researchers to treat the data as they like.

Reporting observation data carries some threats to anonymity and confidentiality. Since observation studies are usually carried out in one or two settings, it is sometimes possible for readers to identify the setting and some of the personalities in them. Researchers must continue to respect participants' rights and ensure that there is no breach of confidence even well after the data are collected.

Intervention by observers

Compared with other methods of data collection, observational studies may create more dilemmas for researchers regarding whether they should intervene or not when patient safety is compromised. As a rule participants' well-being and safety should take precedence over research objectives. However, deciding what constitutes 'threats' to their well-being and safety is not always as straightforward as it seems. In their study of nurse performance, Fitzpatrick et al. (1996) decided that preventing 'a patient from falling out of bed' and informing staff of 'completed intravenous infusion' necessitated intervention by the observer, while 'lack of attention regarding infection control policies' did not. Fitzpatrick et al. (1996) found that it was important for the research team to reflect on these experiences in order 'to achieve equilibrium between one's role as a researcher and one's role as a nurse'.

There is also the question of whether to report malpractices and unsafe practices. This can lead to the investigation and suspension of the very people who granted access in the first place. Mason and Redeker (1993) point out that 'videotaping may also raise ethical and legal issues in health care delivery settings, where the videotaping or observation may record errors in health care practices'.

Covert observation

Covert observation brings with it particular ethical implications. Three main, not mutually exclusive, reasons are given to support this type of observation. Firstly, some researchers believe that the only way to obtain valid data is not to let participants know they are being observed. In this way it is possible to observe things 'as they are' normally, unaffected by the observer's presence. Secondly, access to research sites may be denied by gatekeepers for various reasons. For example, the owners of a private nursing home may not want a researcher to 'pry' around. Thirdly, there are those who believe that research is a political act and the results benefit some people at the expense of others, especially the more deprived groups such as the mentally ill, those with a learning difficulty and the elderly in institutions. Those who carry out covert research may believe that although the rights of some participants are infringed, the findings will benefit a larger number of people in similar situation as theirs. To some extent, according to this argument, the rights of the few can be sacrificed for the benefit of the many. Johnson (1992), discussing some of the ethical implications of a study by Field (1989), in which a research student worked as a nursing auxiliary to collect data on dying patients, concludes that 'it is impossible to say whether Field's approach is absolutely right or wrong'.

Covert observations are often discussed in terms of 'either/or'. However, even when participants are made fully aware that they are being observed, it is impossible to give everyone concerned all the details of a project. Sometimes what researchers focus on in the later part of a project was not foreseen at the beginning of the project. There are also cases where a semi-covert approach is used. In a study by Turnock and Gibson (2001) on patient care in an intensive care setting, the authors 'employed a degree of cover by not informing staff about which particular aspects of their activity were being observed'. Therefore it is possible to be 'open' by informing participants about the 'broad' focus and 'covert' by not revealing the 'specific' focus. Participants would have to be debriefed afterwards and given the right to withdraw. Researchers must balance 'harm' and 'benefits' when taking a decision to use a degree of concealment. Research ethics committees will consider the arguments and advise accordingly.

Political issues with observations

Another problem relates to the selection of some and not all the patients in the same ward or clinical area. While many would not be affected, others may feel that they are being 'neglected' and that those who are observed are getting all the attention. For example if in one study ten out of 21 patients in a ward are observed and no explanation is given to those who are not observed, this may cause some concern to them or their visiting relatives.

Obtaining informed consent from everyone in the setting where the study is carried out can be problematic. Visitors and other professionals can drop in and out. It is not practical to inform each and every one of the purpose of the study and to seek informed consent from them. Another issue is the right of participants to withdraw from the study. This may cause considerable inconvenience if participants, after seeing the tape recording, decide they do not want the data to be used. The right of patients to withdraw should be respected even if it means that the study is not completed.

The political implications of observations are many. Johnson (1992) points to the potential 'political and managerial gain from use or misuse of information' from observations. The image of particular institutions can be tarnished if observational data show deficiencies in services. It is likely that managers and others may want to take some actions to remedy the situation and this may affect some of the individuals who took part in the study. Although researchers should not identify by name the setting where observations are carried out, it is not possible to keep anonymity when a study is carried out in full view of others.

Research data can be used to inform decision making. Data from observations may therefore be used to alter the very situation which the researcher was granted access to observe. By providing the researcher with information, the working conditions and even the livelihood of those observed could be seriously at risk. Davies (1995), referring to her ethnographic study of 'initial encounters in a midwifery school', relates how some of her informants 'responded with amusement and others with initial consternation to the discovery that their friend and student researcher was "the person who had the power to close us down".' Davies was an officer of the Welsh National Board.

Many people are reluctant to have their working practices observed. Some would associate this type of research activity with the infamous 'time and motion' studies which are carried out to find ways of increasing production and reducing the workforce. Understandably, people may be suspicious of the motives of researchers, many of whom do not show any concern for those they observe once the data are collected, and would, probably, not allow others to observe their (researchers') own practices.

Critiquing observation

To evaluate data from structured observations, readers need to know exactly what phenomenon was observed and how it was defined. Researchers must also provide adequate information on how the observations were carried out. This includes information relating to how the research tool was constructed and comments on its content validity. If an observation checklist is provided, you can attempt to assess its face validity. Researchers must also explain how intra- and inter-reliability were achieved, and what other steps were taken to ensure the validity and reliability of the instrument.

The context in which the observations are conducted and the strategies designed to reduce the observer effect need to be explained; the sampling of periods to be observed must be justified. For example, is one hour's observation every four hours appropriate for a study of ward teaching? If the observations take place at 9.00 am, 1.00 pm, 5.00 pm and 9.00 pm, it is likely that the last three sessions may not be appropriate as they could be the times that staff are at lunch, on coffee breaks and handing over to the next shift, respectively.

The observer is also in a position to explain whether or not difficulties were experienced when observing certain behaviour or events. If this was the case she must discuss how this may have affected the collection of valid and reliable data. In Day et al.'s (1993) study of handwashing, the researchers acknowledged the difficulty of observing certain behaviours and recommended the use of video cameras. They were also concerned that because 'after washing, the children received a stamp on the back of their hands from a common stamp and stamp pad', this may have affected the results as 'organisms from the stamp and pad were transmitted to each child'. As one of the objectives of this study was 'to compare the incidence of infectious illness', the use of a common stamp and pad would have been a serious limitation of the study.

For unstructured observations, researchers must provide information on the type of observation and their degree of involvement with the participants. The thought processes and the actions of the observer during the observation must be conveyed for readers to have an idea of what happened. Information on how the participants were recruited, the reasons for their selection as well as a description of the setting must also be provided. Finally, the measures taken to ensure rigour and respect for peoples' rights (this applies to structured observations as well) should be described in detail.

SUMMARY

Summary and conclusion

Observations provide useful information for clinical and research purposes. They are particularly suited to the study of verbal and non-verbal behaviour. They are used in qualitative and quantitative studies and in both experimental and non-experimental designs. As a quantitative tool, observation can be structured, predetermined and standardised. Researchers know in advance the data required and use a schedule or checklist, constructed prior to the collection of data. Qualitative researchers prefer not to be influenced by prior knowledge and instead allow phenomena to unfold before their eyes. From the data collected, they aim to formulate themes, conceptual models, hypotheses and theories. The degree of researcher participation with the people, and in the setting where the observations take place, varies according to the aims of the study. Each type of observation has its value, limitations and ethical implications. As with other research methods, the challenge to researchers is to find ways to collect useful data without infringing people's rights.

References

Adler P A and Adler P (1994) Observational techniques. In: N K Denzin and Y S Lincoln (eds), *Handbook of Qualitative Research* (Newbury Park, CA: Sage Publications).

Alderson P (2001) *On Doing Qualitative Research Linked to Ethical Healthcare*, vol.1 (London: Wellcome Trust).

Barber-Parker E D (2002) Integrating patient teaching into bedside patient care: a participant-observation study of hospital nurses. *Patient Education and Counselling*, 48:107–13.

Birchall R and Waters K R (1996) What do elderly people do in hospital? *Journal of Clinical Nursing*, 5, 3:171–6.

Booth J, Davidson I, Winstanley J and Waker K (2001) Observing washing and dressing of stroke patients: nursing intervention compared with occupational therapist. What is the difference? *Journal of Advanced Nursing*, 33, 1:98–105.

Clarke L (1996) Covert participant observation in a secure forensic unit. *Nursing Times*, 92, 48:37–40.

Cook M, Hale C and Watson B (1999) Interrated reliability and the assessment of pressure-sore risk using an adapted Waterlow Scale. *Clinical Effectiveness in Nursing*, 3:66–74.

Cormack D (1976) *Psychiatric Nursing Observed* (London: Royal College of Nursing).

Davies R M (1995) Introduction to ethnographic research in midwifery. *British Journal of Midwifery*, **3**, 4:223–7.

Day R A, St Arnaud S and Monsma M (1993) Effectiveness of a handwashing program. *Clinical Nursing Research*, **2**, 1:24–40.

Drach-Zahavy A and Dagan E (2002) From caring to managing and beyond: an examination of the head nurse's role. *Journal of Advanced Nursing*, **38**, 1:19–28.

Drury J and Stott C (2001) Bias as a research strategy in participant observation: the case of intergroup conflict. *Field Methods*, **13**, 1:47–67.

Fader M, Clarke-O'Neill S, Cook D, Dean G, Brooks R, Cottenden A and Malone-Lee J (2003) Management of night-time urinary incontinence in residential settings for older people: an investigation into the effects of different pad changing regimes on skin health. *Journal of Clinical Nursing*, 12:374–86.

Felce D, Powell L, Lunt B, Jenkins J and Mansell J (1980) Measuring activity of old people in residential care. *Evaluation Review*, **4**, 3:371–87.

Field D (1989) *Nursing the Dying* (Tavistock: Routledge).

Fitzpatrick J M, While A E and Roberts J D (1996) Operationalisation of an observation instrument to explore nurse performance. *International Journal of Nursing Studies*, **33**, 4:349–60.

Frankenberg R (1982) Participant observers. In: R G Burgess (ed.), *Field Research: A Sourcebook and Field Manual* (London: Allen & Unwin).

Fuller B F and Conner D A (1995) The effect of pain on infant behaviors. *Clinical Nursing Research*, **4**, 3:253–73.

Gold R L (1958) Roles in sociological field observations. *Social Forces*, **36**:217–23.

Gould D and Ream E (1994) Nurses' views of infection control: an interview study. *Journal of Advanced Nursing*, **19**:1121–31.

Hallberg I R, Holst G, Nordmark A and Edberg A (1995) Cooperation during morning care between nurses and severely demented institutionalized patients. *Clinical Nursing Research*, **4**, 1:78–104.

Hewison A (1995) Nurses' power in interactions with patients. *Journal of Advanced Nursing*, **21**:75–82.

Johnson M (1992) A silent conspiracy? Some ethical issues of participant observation in nursing research. *International Journal of Nursing Studies*, **29**, 2:213–23.

Kirk J and Miller M L (1986) *Reliability and Validity in Qualitative Research* (Newbury Park, CA: Sage Publications).

Latvala E, Vuokila-Oikkonen P and Janhonen S (2000) Videotaped recording as a method of participant observation in psychiatric nursing research. *Journal of Advanced Nursing*, **31**, 5:1252–7.

Layder D (1993) *New Strategies in Social Research* (Cambridge: Polity Press).

Lobo M L (1992) Observation: A valuable data collection strategy for research with children. *Journal of Paediatric Nursing*, 7, 5:320–8.

Lowe T (1992) Characteristics of effective nursing interventions in the management of challenging behaviour. *Journal of Advanced Nursing*, **17**:1226–32.

Mander R (1995) Practising and preaching: confidentiality, anonymity and the researcher. *British Journal of Midwifery*, **3**, 5:289–95.

Manias E, Botti M and Bucknall T (2002) Observation of pain assessment and management – the complexities of clinical practice. *Journal of Clinical Nursing*, **11**:724–33.

Mason D J and Redeker N (1993) Measurement of activity. *Nursing Research*, **42**, 2:87–92.

Millman M (1976) *The Unkindest Cut – Life in the Backrooms of Medicine* (New York: Morrow Quill).

Mulhall A (2003) In the field: notes on observation in qualitative research. *Journal of Advanced Nursing*, **41**, 3:306–13.

Oliver S and Redfern S J (1991) Interpersonal communication between nurses and elderly patients: refinement of an observation schedule. *Journal of Advanced Nursing*, **16**:30–8.

Peplau H E (1988) *Interpersonal Relations in Nursing*, 2nd edn (London: Macmillan Education).

Porter L, Redfern S, Wilson-Barnett J and Lemay A (1986) The development of an observation schedule for measuring nurse–patient touch, using an ergonomic approach. *International Journal of Nursing Studies*, **23**, 1:11–20.

Randers I and Mattiasson A (2004) Autonomy and integrity: upholding older adult patients' dignity. *Journal of Advanced Nursing*, **45**, 1:63–71.

Ridge H E and While A E (1995) Neonatal nursing staff time involved with medication-related activities. *Journal of Advanced Nursing*, **22**:623–7.

Roethlisberger F J and Dickson W J (1939) *Management and the Worker* (Cambridge, MA: Harvard University Press).

Rose-Grippa K (1979) Nurse communicator. In: F L Bower and E O Bevis (eds), *Fundamentals of Nursing Practice: Concepts, Roles and Functions* (St Louis, MO: C V Mosby).

Salmon P (1993) Interactions of nurses with elderly patients: relationship to nurses' attitudes and to formal activity periods. *Journal of Advanced Nursing*, **18**:14–19.

Samarel N (1989) Caring for the living and dying: a study of role transition. *International Journal of Nursing Studies,* **26**, 4:313–26.

Sarantakos S (1998) *Social Research*, 2nd edn (Basingstoke: Macmillan).

Skovdahl K, Kihlgren A L and Kihlgren M (2003) Dementia and aggressiveness: video recording morning care from different care units. *Journal of Clinical Nursing*, **12**:888–98.

Spradley J (1980) *Participant Observation* (New York: Holt, Rinehart & Winston).

Turnock G and Gibson V (2001) Validity in action research: a discussion on theoretical and practice issues encountered whilst using observation to collect data. *Journal of Advanced Nursing*, **36**, 3:471–7.

Waltz C F, Strickland O L and Lenz E R (1991) *Measurement in Nursing Research*, 2nd edn (Philadelphia, PA: F A Davis).

Making Sense of Data

Introduction

Collecting data is a crucial part of the research process, but data in themselves do not answer research questions or support or reject hypotheses. Researchers have to make sense of them before presenting them to readers in ways that they, in turn, can understand. In this chapter, some of the common methods of data analysis and presentation in quantitative and qualitative studies are examined. A brief outline of some of the descriptive and inferential statistics in quantitative analysis is given. Finally, some of the ways in which researchers make sense of, and report, qualitative data are described.

What does making sense of data mean?

In Chapter 2, it was explained that data means all the information collected during the process of research for the purpose of answering questions, testing hypotheses or exploring a phenomenon. In the course of a study, a large mass of data are collected. All the individual bits of information from questionnaires, interviews or observations are known as 'raw' or 'crude' data. In themselves, crude data do not immediately make sense. The answers to research questions do not 'jump out' of the pile of questionnaires; they have to be 'teased out' or analysed, a process called data analysis.

The analysis of data in quantitative studies tends to take place after all the data have been collected. However, it is not an afterthought but an integrated part of the research design. The level of research (descriptive, correlational or experimental), the research questions, objectives or hypotheses and the type of data collected determine which type of analysis is required. Those who have left decisions about data analysis to the end phase of a research project have learnt that this can be a serious mistake.

In qualitative research, data analysis begins during the data collection phase. The researcher processes the information, looks for patterns during the interview or observation and selects themes to pursue. Data analysis continues between interviews and after all the data are collected. In the first part of this chapter, we will focus mainly on data analysis in quantitative studies.

Quantitative data analysis

In Chapter 3, it was explained that the purpose of quantitative research is to measure phenomena. Some of these can be measured more accurately and easily than others. For example, we can measure respondents' weight with more precision than we can measure their satisfaction with nursing care. For measurement to take place, there must be numbers. Some measures are already in the form of numbers. For example, weight is expressed in grams and height in centimetres. Others have to be converted into numbers if they are to be analysed quantitatively. For example, if health visitors are asked to rate the degree of importance of research to their practice according to whether it was 'high', 'moderate' or 'low', these categories would be allocated numbers to reflect their order of importance.

Quantitative analysis can only be carried out with numbers, but numbers in some cases have no intrinsic worth: they have to be given meaning by those using them. For example, number 1 can mean 'first' or 'most important' or it can be the lowest value on a scale of 1 to 10. To make sense of numbers, they are given a value, usually according to a scale. For example, when respondents are asked to rate, in order of importance, their sources of health information on a scale of 1 to 10, the researcher must specify whether 1 is the most important or the least important.

Levels of measurement

To measure one needs a scale. As explained earlier, not all phenomena are readily amenable to measurement, nor can they all be measured with the same degree of precision. The scales devised to measure them also differ in their degree of precision. Mathematicians have classified scales into a hierarchy of four levels. The lowest is nominal, followed by the ordinal, interval and ratio.

Nominal scale

Some of the variables with which quantitative researchers deal cannot in themselves be measured, although some aspects of them can. For example, being male cannot be measured against being female, although their weight, height and attitudes can be measured and compared. In the same way, when a researcher asks respondents to state their professional qualifications, she cannot measure and compare adult nursing with mental health nursing; for example, it would be arbitrary and controversial to assign more value to one qualification than to the other. However, these variables (gender or qualifications) are given a number for the purpose of quantitative analysis. When researchers code their questionnaires for manual or computer analysis, they may assign numbers as follows:

Adult nursing	1
Mental health nursing	2
Care of people with learning disability	3
Children's nursing	4

While the scale is 1 to 4, the numbers in this case have no value: 4 does not mean twice as good or as many as 2. It is simply a way of labelling or coding the variable 'qualification'. This type of scale is known as 'nominal'. The *Oxford Dictionary* describes 'nominal' as 'existing in name only, not real or actual'. The numbers on a nominal scale are therefore in name only and do not have any real worth or value: they serve only to distinguish one category from another.

Ordinal scale

Sometimes respondents are asked to state whether or not they are satisfied with the care or treatment they receive, using a scale similar to the one below:

Very satisfied
Satisfied
Neither satisfied nor dissatisfied
Dissatisfied
Very dissatisfied

The ranking of these categories from 'very satisfied' to 'very dissatisfied' implies a hierarchy or ordering of satisfaction. In coding responses from this type of question, the researcher may allocate numbers as follows:

Very satisfied	5
Satisfied	4
Neither satisfied nor dissatisfied	3
Dissatisfied	2
Very dissatisfied	1

While those allocated number 5 have a higher satisfaction than those with a 4, there is no equal distance implied between the numbers. Those who are satisfied (4) are not twice as satisfied as those who are dissatisfied (2), only more satisfied. The ordinal scale is different from a nominal scale in that the numbers signify the order or hierarchy of these variables. The higher numbers indicate that the respondents have more of the property (in this case, satisfaction) than do the lower numbers, but the scale cannot specify by how much.

Interval scale

An interval scale is a more precise ordinal scale. In it, the distances between the numbers on the scale are known. A thermometer is an example of an interval scale; the degrees are numbered in such a way that the distance between 5 degrees and 10 degrees is the same as between 75 degrees and 80 degrees. In this example, the centigrade or Fahrenheit thermometers have no absolute zero, since there are degrees below zero. Zero degrees centigrade does not mean 'nil' temperature. Twenty degrees is warmer than 10 degrees, but it does not mean that it is twice as warm: it means that it is 10 degrees warmer.

Ratio scale

A ratio scale is an interval scale with an absolute zero. For example, rulers and weighing scales have an absolute zero. A zero on a ruler means no length and 20 centimetres is twice as long as 10 centimetres. Therefore, the numbers on a ratio scale tell us not only the amount by which they differ (i.e. by 10 degrees) but also by how many times (twice as long or four times as heavy).

The distinction between these four levels is usually made because there is a view that 'the level of measurement specifies the type of statistical operations that can be properly used' (Waltz et al., 1991). The choice of statistical techniques should also relate to the research question asked. We will pursue this theme later in this chapter.

To sum up, the purpose of quantitative research is to measure, and measurements are carried out by scales consisting of numbers. There are different levels of measurement and different levels of scale. The meaning of the numbers differs from scale to scale: numbers can be used as labels, as indicating order or rank, or can have values.

Statistical levels

How data are analysed and presented depends on the type of question which researchers ask. In Chapter 10, three levels of quantitative research were identified – descriptive, correlational and experimental. The types of question that can be asked depend on these levels.

There are two types of descriptive question that are usually asked. The first refers to the sample, especially its demographic characteristics (for example: how many respondents are there in the sample?, what is their age and gender distribution?). The second type refers to their responses (for example: how many respondents indicated a preference for primary nursing rather than team nursing?, what were the scores of respondents on the 'assessment of pain scale'?).

At the correlational level, researchers are mainly interested in finding answers to two types of question: whether there is a relationship between variables (for example between educational background and compliance with treatment) and whether there are differences between groups (for example, is there a difference between male and female nurses' attitudes to nursing research?).

At the experimental level, the main question asked is whether changes in one or more independent variables actually cause changes in one or more dependent variables (for example, does an educational programme cause an increase in patients' knowledge of diabetes?).

Descriptive statistical analysis is carried out to answer descriptive questions, while correlational and causal relationships are explored by the use of inferential statistics.

Descriptive statistics

Statistics has a language and logic of its own. If you were asked to describe a car to someone who has not seen it, you can convey a picture of it by referring to its colour, size, make, engine capacity, age and number of doors. These main features are essential to adequately describe the car. Similarly, when researchers describe data, they normally report the main features, which can give an idea of what the data consist of without the need to see the crude data.

To describe quantitative data, researchers use terminologies for which there are agreed meanings. Some layman's terms, such as 'average' or 'majority', are vague and may not have the same meaning for everyone. Statisticians have not only devised terms that describe the essential features of data, but also have explained precisely what they mean. The three main features that researchers use to describe and summarise data are:

- frequency
- central tendency
- dispersion.

Frequency

The most basic analysis of quantitative data involves counting the number of times a value appears in the data. Samples are described in terms of frequency – as, for example, in a study of 'nurses' attitudes towards lesbians and gay men' by Röndahl et al. (2004), in which they reported:

A total of 212 participants responded to the question about the causes of homosexuality. A majority (58%, $n = 124$) believed homosexuality to be congenital, 35% believed it to be acquired and 7% chose the 'other' responses.

This extract shows that frequency can be reported both in terms of percentages and absolute numbers (represented by n).

It is sometimes difficult to compare absolute numbers. If 20 out of 60 male students and 12 out of 48 female students prefer lectures to seminars, the difference between these numbers is not immediately obvious since the sizes of the groups are not similar. When converted to proportions or percentages, they can make more sense. Fink (1995) defines a proportion as 'the number of observations or responses with a given characteristic divided by the total number of observations'. In the above example, the proportion of male students who prefer lectures is:

$$\frac{20 \ \text{(number who prefer lectures to seminars)}}{60 \ \text{(total number of observations)}} = \frac{1}{3}$$

and for female students

$$\frac{12}{48} = \frac{1}{4}$$

Thus by converting these numbers into proportions, it is possible to see that proportionately more male than female students prefer lectures.

Percentages also facilitate comparisons. A percentage is a proportion multiplied by 100. In the above example, the percentage of male students is:

$$\frac{1}{3} \times 100 = 33.3\%$$

Frequencies are commonly reported in the form of tables, bar charts and pie charts. An example of data reported in tabular form (Table 16.1) comes from a study by Karlsson and Nordström (2001), entitled 'Nutritional status, symptoms experienced and general state of health in HIV-infected patients'. In this table, the authors give a frequency distribution of responses in absolute numbers and in percentages.

Tables facilitate the presentation of large amounts of data in a concise way. To report the data from the above table in the text would require many sentences, which would have to be read a number of times to be fully comprehensible and digestible. A quick glance at the table (below) not only gives the frequency of the different responses, but also enables instant comparisons between items in the health index.

Table 16.1 Description of a general state of health (reproduced by kind permission of the *Journal of Clinical Nursing*)

Health index	Very/rather good n	(%)	Very/rather poor n	(%)
1 Energy	9	(36)	16	(64)
2 Temper	14	(56)	11	(44)
3 Fatigue	5	(20)	20	(80)
4 Loneliness	18	(72)	7	(28)
5 Sleep	19	(76)	6	(24)
6 Vertigo	16	(64)	9	(36)
7 Bowel function	10	(40)	15	(60)
8 Pain	14	(56)	11	(44)
9 Mobility	20	(80)	5	(20)
10 Health	8	(32)	17	(68)

Diagrammatic presentation of data is designed to attract readers' attention and give a sense of proportion; this is important if the purpose is to compare data. A bar chart is one type of diagram used for this purpose. An example of a bar chart (Figure 16.1) comes from a study by Röndahl et al. (2004) on nurses' attitudes towards lesbians and gay men. The bar chart shows the number of nurses who held negative, neutral or positive attitudes. At a glance it is possible to clearly see that most nurses in this study held positive attitudes towards lesbians and gay men. The sense of proportion is conveyed graphically by the relative height of the bars. Some bar charts can have multiple bars and can be presented sideways as well.

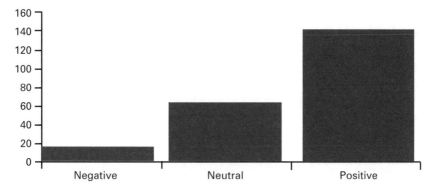

Figure 16.1 Categorisation of scores on Attitudes towards Homosexuality scale (reproduced by kind permission of the *Journal of Clinical Nursing*)

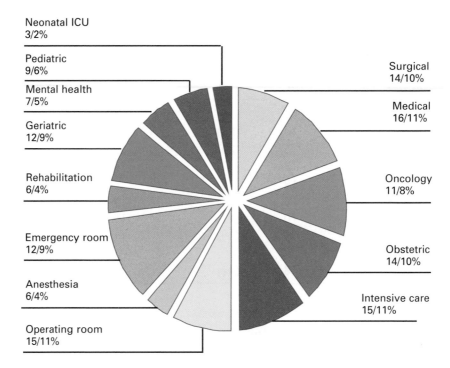

Figure 16.2 Number and proportion of respondents by nursing specialty ($n = 140$) (reproduced by kind permission of the *Journal of Advanced Nursing*)

Pie charts, although less popular and less versatile than bar charts, are also used to convey the sense of proportion in data. Unlike bar charts, the numbers must be converted into proportions or percentages before the pie chart is constructed, although absolute numbers can additionally be included. An example of a pie chart (Figure 16.2) is taken from a study by Gudmundsdottir et al. (2004). The segments show the number and proportion of respondents in each nursing specialty.

Bar charts and pie charts have an advantage over textual reporting in that they can present large amounts of data in a concise and visual form. They must, however, be clearly labelled and, where appropriate, properly shaded, as shading often fades in the process of photocopying. Tables, bar charts and pie charts must not be overloaded with data and should require little effort on the part of readers to understand them.

Central tendency

To make sense of information, we use such concepts as 'average', 'typical' or 'common'. We may ask, 'How many people, on average, are admitted to the casualty department of the local hospital on a Saturday night', or 'What is the "typical" injury or illness with which they attend the casualty department?'. In effect, in statistical terms, we are looking for the central tendency rather than for extreme cases. The statistical measures of central tendency are the mode, median and mean. To explain these terms, we will use Example A. Suppose ten patients on a medical ward were administered a 'satisfaction with nursing care scale' and the scores (from 0 to a possible 100) for each patient (represented here by the letters A to J) were as follows:

Example A

A	B	C	D	E	F	G	H	I	J
50	40	60	50	70	40	20	50	90	60

The *mode* is the most frequent value. It can be used on any scale of measurement and is unaffected by extreme values. In the above example, the value '50' occurs three times and no other value occurs as many times. Therefore the mode is 50. However, knowing that the mode is 50 does not tell us anything about the other scores (if we did not have access to them, as is normally the case). The mode is therefore of little value, especially if we do not know what percentage of respondents had this typical score.

The *median* is the midpoint value when the scores are arranged in ascending order, as shown below. It can be used on interval or ordinal level data and, like the mode, is unaffected by extreme values.

20	40	40	50	50	50	60	60	70	90

Since there are ten scores, there is no one single midpoint. Therefore the average of the two middle values is the median, which in this case is 50 (this is calculated by adding the two middle values and dividing the total by 2). Fifty per cent of the values fall below and 50 per cent above the midpoint. By knowing that the median is 50, we also know that half of the respondents scored below and half above 50.

The *mean* is the arithmetic average of a set of values and can be used on interval or ratio level data. It is calculated by adding all the scores and dividing by the number of responses. The total score in the above example is 530 and the number of responses is ten. Therefore the mean is:

$$\frac{530}{10} = 53$$

Unlike the mode and the median, the mean is actually determined by a calculation that takes into account all the other scores and thus can be distorted by a single extreme score in one direction. If one score is greatly increased or reduced, it may not affect the mode or median but it will change the mean. For example, if the score of patient 'J' were 90 instead of 60, the mode and the median would remain 50 while the mean would increase to 56.

The limitations of the mode, median and mean can be demonstrated by Example B, showing the satisfaction scores of the same ten patients:

Example B

A	B	C	D	E	F	G	H	I	J
20	30	20	30	40	70	90	90	90	90

The mode is 90
The median is (40 + 70)/2 = 55
The mean is 570/10 = 57

The mode in this case gives the impression that patients scored very high, yet only 40 per cent did. The median indicates that five patients scored less than 55, but it fails to show that some patients scored very low and others very high. The mean of 57 is deceptive as it suggests that the level of satisfaction of these ten patients is medium (57), yet as the crude scores show, none of them had medium-level satisfaction. What these measures of central tendency do not tell us is how the scores vary. In Example A, the scores bunched around 50 (with only two extreme scores – 20 and 90) and the mean was 53. In Example B, there were four very low and four very high scores, and the mean was 57. We may conclude that the patients in Example B were more satisfied with the care they received (mean 57) than the patients in Example A (mean 53), yet only one patient scored below 40 in Example A, while four patients in Example B did.

Dispersion

Central tendency measures are, therefore, not enough to make sense of the data. We need to know the variance of the scores (i.e. how they vary). The three measures which can describe variance are:

● range

● interquartile range

● standard deviation.

The *range* is the easiest way to measure the variation in a set of data. This is simply the difference between the highest and lowest values in a data set. In Example B, the range would be:

90 – 20 = 70

The problem with using the range is that it uses only two values in the data set and ignores all other scores in the distribution. Thus it can be easily affected by extreme scores and is considered to be an unreliable measure of variability.

The *interquartile range* gives a better description of variation in the data. If you recall, the median is the score that divides a distribution exactly in half. Using the same technique, scores in a distribution can be divided into four equal parts using quartiles. The first or lower quartile (Q1) is the midpoint between the lowest value and the median (second quartile, Q2), and the upper quartile (third quartile, Q3) is the midpoint between the highest value and the median. We can refer to Example A to show the lower and upper quartiles. The scores (arranged in ascending order) of the ten patients were as follows.

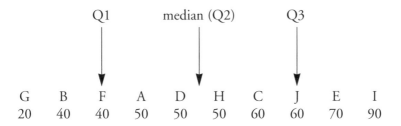

The median is 50. This was obtained by arranging the scores in ascending order and selecting the midpoint score. As the number of values is even (ten), there are two midpoint scores: 50 and 50. The median lies between them, as shown above.

The lower quartile (Q1) is calculated by finding the midpoint of the scores below the median. There are five scores and the midpoint is 40. Similarly, the upper quartile (Q3) is the midpoint of the five scores above the median, in this case 60.

The interquartile range is the distance between the first quartile and the third quartile. In the above example the interquartile range is 20.

Q3 – Q1 = 60 – 40 = 20

The semi-interquartile range is half the difference between the upper and lower quartiles. It provides a descriptive measure of the 'typical' distance of scores from the median.

$$\text{Semi-interquartile range} = \frac{Q3 - Q1}{2} = \frac{60 - 40}{2} = 10$$

The measure most widely used for describing the spread of a distribution is the *standard deviation* (SD). The SD is a 'kind of average deviation of the observations from the mean' (Moore, 1985) and takes into account all values in the distribution. The SD is always reported in conjunction with the mean.

If the scores are homogenous, there is little or no deviation from the mean and therefore the SD is zero or close to zero. The larger the SD, the more the scores deviate from the mean. This deviation from the mean can be positive or negative. If the mean of ten scores is 65 and the SD is 1.75, this means that the scores are closely bunched around 65. If, on the other hand, the mean is 65 and the SD 30.5, many of the individual scores are far from the mean. In general, almost 70 per cent of all scores in a distribution fall within 1 SD of the mean. Below is an example of how SD is reported, from a study by Williams (1989) on empathy and burn-out in male and female helping professionals:

> The subjects ranged in age from 23 to 80 (M = 37.4, SD = 10.6) and had practised from 1 to 44 years (M = 12, SD = 9).

Frequency, central tendency and dispersion are the main measures of descriptive statistics. Together, they can convey the main features of data, although the most commonly reported ones are frequency, mean and standard deviation.

Finally, the term 'normal distribution', needs to be explained. In normal distribution, most of the scores cluster around the mean, and the extreme scores are few and are more or less equally distributed above and below the mean. This is illustrated in Figure 16.3 and is referred to as a 'bell-shape' distribution.

A normal distribution has the following characteristics: 34 per cent of all scores fall between the mean and 1 SD on either side of the mean; similarly, 28 per cent of all scores fall between 1 SD and 2 SD from the mean, as in Figure 16.3.

The 'normal distribution' is crucial in statistics because many statistical techniques were developed on the assumption that scores were bell-shaped or normal. As explained later on, some statistical tests can only be performed if the distribution is normal, although techniques may generally be applied to data that are only roughly bell-shaped without losing too much accuracy.

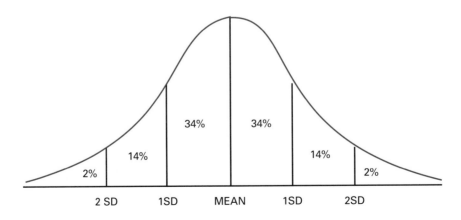

Figure 16.3 A normal distribution curve

Inferential statistics

Researchers using quantitative approaches such as surveys and experiments seek to find relationships between variables and, where possible, to establish the exact nature of these relationships, with the aim of making predictions. They also seek to generalise the findings from their samples to equivalent populations. To do so, they resort to inferential statistics.

To find out whether there are relationships between variables, researchers formulate hypotheses. A null hypothesis (H_0) states that there is no actual relationship between variables whereas a research (or alternative) hypothesis (H_1) predicts some relationship between the variables. Data are collected to accept or reject the null/alternative hypothesis.

Errors are sometimes made in the testing of hypotheses and two possibilities are presented here. A type I error happens when a statistically significant relationship is found, in the study sample, between two variables (for example educational attainment and the practice of breast self-examination) when, in fact, no such relationship exists in the population. A type I error can result in the researchers making a false report of a treatment effect. A type II error occurs when no such relationship is found in the sample when, in fact, it exists in the population. In this case the researcher could conclude that a treatment had no effect when in fact it did (see Figure 16.4).

To establish statistical significance, researchers can select from a number of tests, some of which will be described later. The results from these tests will signify whether or not there are relationships between variables. However, there is always a probability that the results were obtained by chance. You have perhaps seen the following:

$p > 0.05$

The symbol > denotes 'greater than' and the letter p is used to denote the probability of a chance occurrence. The figures and decimal points (e.g. 0.05) are the levels set by researchers above which they will accept the null hypothesis and conclude that there is no relationship between the variables. Researchers can use several levels of probability, but 0.05 is a standard level, above which no researcher should claim significance for the result.

	Actual situation	
	No effect H_0 true	Effect exists H_0 false
Researcher's Reject H_0	Type I error	Decision correct
decision Retain H_0	Decision correct	Type II error

Figure 16.4   Testing of hypotheses

Selecting a test

The choice of statistical tests depends, among others, on sample size and sampling method (i.e. random or not), on the level of measurement (nominal, ordinal, etc.) and on whether the variables to be measured in the sample are normally distributed in the population. For parametric tests, the variable has to be normally distributed, while for non-parametric tests no such assumption is made. Munro et al. (1986) explain:

> The main difference between these two classes of techniques is the assumptions about the population data that must be made before the parametric tests can be applied. For t-tests and analysis of variance (ANOVA), for example, it is assumed that the variable under study is normally distributed in the population and that the variance is the same at different levels of the variable. The nonparametric techniques have relatively few assumptions that must be met before they can be used.

In this section, we will take a brief look at some of the commonly used tests in nursing research, namely Pearson product moment correlation coefficient, *t*-test and chi-square test.

The Pearson product moment correlation coefficient

The Pearson product moment correlation coefficient is the 'most usual method by which the relationship between two variables is quantified' (Munro et al., 1986) and it relates to parametric data. Correlation coefficients (represented by the letter *r*) can be positive or negative. They vary between +1 (a perfect positive relationship) and −1 (a perfect negative or inverse relationship). Published statistical tables can be used to interpret the significance of the correlation coefficient but Fink (1995) suggests the following interpretation:

0 to +.25 (or −.25) = little or no relationship
+.26 to +.50 (or −.26 to −.50) = fair degree of relationship
+.51 to +.75 (or −.51 to −.75) = moderate to good relationship
over +.75 (or −.75) = very good to excellent relationship

Chan and Yu (2004) used a Pearson product moment correlation to examine relationships between items in the Quality of Life (QoL) Scale and the Brief Psychiatric Rating Scale (BPRS). All of the correlations reported were negative and less than 0.5. They concluded:

> that total BPRS score was significantly and negatively correlated to overall score for perceived QoL. Participants with poorer mental health had lower scores for many aspects of perceived QoL. However, the correlations were not strong.

The *t*-test

The *t*-test is a parametric test to compare the means of two samples, for example the mean knowledge scores of one group of patients who were given verbal information about their illness and of another group who were given written information.

According to DePoy and Gitlin (1994), the '*t*-test must be calculated with interval level data and should be selected only if the researcher believes that the assumptions for the use of parametric statistics have not been violated'. As they explain:

> The *t*-test yields a *t* value that is reported as $t = x$, $p = 0.05$ where x is the calculated *t* value and *p* is the level of significance set by the researcher. There are several variations of the t-test.

To find whether a *t* value is statistically significant, it has to be compared to the critical value of *t* reported in statistical tables. This critical value is the level the *t* value must equal or exceed to be deemed statistically significant. Tables of critical values are readily available, but we assume that most researchers will now be using appropriate computer software to calculate statistical values and tell you if they are statistically significant. The level of the critical value is determined by the significance level set by the researcher and the degrees of freedom (df). Both of these values need to be known and are always reported alongside the *t* value. It is beyond the scope of this book to explain what degrees of freedom are. What is important to know is how they are calculated and how to use them. The df in a *t*-test for independent groups is calculated by summating the number of subjects in each group together and subtracting two.

An example of the use of a *t*-test is from a study by McCleary and Brown (2003) that investigated barriers to paediatric nurses' research utilisation. They reported:

> Rating of the organization as a barrier to research was higher among nurses who had completed a course about reading or using research than those who had not taken a course (mean 2.73 vs. 2.52; $t = 1.98$, d.f. 163, $p = 0.05$).

The chi-square test for independence

The chi-square test for independence (χ^2) can be used to test whether or not there is a relationship between two variables and is normally used with non-parametric data. For example, 100 smokers attend anti-smoking sessions and only 60 stopped smoking after a month, while in another group of 80 smokers, who received no sessions, 20 stopped smoking (Table 16.2). The χ^2 statistic is used to test if the differences are statistically significant (i.e. did attendance at an anti-smoking session enable more people to stop smoking?). The χ^2 statistic for the example in Table 16.2 is calculated (by computer software) to be 20.52.

Table 16.2   Effect of anti-smoking sessions

	Stopped smoking	Did not stop	Total
Number attending a session	60	40	100
Number not attending a session	20	60	80
Total	80	100	180

The df are calculated by subtracting 1 from the number of rows and multiplying this by the number of columns minus 1. This can be expressed as:

$$(R - 1) \times (C - 1)$$

where R = rows and C = columns.

In the example in Table 16.2, there are two columns and two rows. Therefore df is $(2 - 1) \times (2 - 1) = 1$. Once the df value and the p value (a level set by the researcher) are known, it is possible to compare the calculated χ^2 value with the critical value of χ^2 from the appropriate statistical table. The calculated χ^2 value must equal or exceed the critical value to be deemed statistically significant.

McCleary and Brown (2003) used the χ^2 test in their study investigating barriers to paediatric nurses' utilization. They reported:

> while just under half of the paediatric nurses reported that their feeling incapable of evaluating the quality of the research was a barrier (47.8%), they were less likely to report this barrier than nurses in the US sample (69.9%, $\chi^2 = 21.9$, d.f. 1, $p < 0.001$) or the UK sample (59.3%, $\chi^2 = 7.4$, d.f. 1, $p. < 0.01$).

For the above example, McCleary and Brown (2003) reported their results to be statistically significant because the value of their χ^2 statistics were greater than the critical values of χ^2 using the appropriate df and probability level.

It is beyond the scope of this book to explain how these tests are carried out or to discuss other tests. If you are in doubt about statistical data, you should consult a statistics text or a statistician. Three useful references are Hicks, *Research and Statistics: A Practical Introduction for Nurses* (1990), Reid, *Health Care Research by Degrees* (1993) and Scott and Mazhindu, *Statistics for Health Care Professionals: An Introduction* (2005).

Qualitative data analysis

Quantitative research is described as objective partly because it is believed that the research process, including data analysis, can be replicated. If the crude data are made available to other researchers, it is possible for them to carry out the same statistical tests and obtain the same results. It is also possible to carry out other tests or challenge the original tests. Qualitative data analysis is to some extent subjective, although researchers have developed strategies to allow others to follow and validate their actions.

In quantitative research, data analysis starts once all the data are collected. In qualitative research, data analysis takes place during data collection and thereafter. The researcher processes the data as they are received and makes judgements relating to aspects of the phenomenon to pursue. For example, as she carries out more and more interviews, she has to remember some of what was said in previous interviews. She analyses and synthesises the information while talking to respondents. However, once all the data are collected, she will systematically analyse the data in order to make sense of what participants said or what she observed. Therefore one of the main features of qualitative data analysis is that data collection and analysis are carried out both concurrently and after data collection is completed.

Textual data analysis

Qualitative researchers record their data in a number of ways. The term 'field notes' is frequently used to refer to data kept by researchers prior to, during and after their interaction with their participants. Audio-tape recordings are commonly used to record the interviews 'verbatim' (word by word). These are normally transcribed and analysed thereafter. Other methods of data recording include memos and diaries in which researchers (and sometimes participants) keep notes of their thoughts, ideas, chronology of events, patterns or trends. Field notes, transcripts, memos, diaries, letters, leaflets, and case notes all constitute the 'texts' which qualitative researchers analyse.

Types of data analysis

There are different types of data analysis in qualitative research depending on how structured the questions are. Different approaches are used for the analysis of data from open-ended questions (in questionnaires), semi-structured interviews, documents and unstructured interviews or observations.

Open-ended questions can be specific or broad. An example of a specific, open-ended item from a questionnaire is: 'Please list the sources of information which you access regarding sexual health'. A researcher analysing the data will list as many sources as provided by respondents and their frequency of access. This is not different from quantitative analysis. In fact it is likely that researchers will seek to find correlations between 'sources of information' and other demographic variables such as education or gender. A broad open-ended item could be: 'Briefly explain how you felt when you were told of the diagnosis'. The responses are likely to be in the form of a description of the respondent's feelings, experiences and whatever they think they should tell the researcher. In this case researchers will have to sort, decipher and interpret the responses. Therefore the broader the question, the more complex the data analysis is. The same applies to the analysis of data from semi-structured interviews. The questions guide the search for answers.

Any text can be subjected to quantitative or qualitative analysis or a mixture of both. An example of quantitative analysis of qualitative data comes from Klapowitz (2000). He carried out a study to test the null hypothesis that participants in focus groups raise sensitive issues as frequently as those in individual interviews. Klapowitz (2000) compared data from 12 focus groups and 19 individual interviews. The study investigated participants' use, understanding and perceptions of their 'shared mangrove ecosystem'. 'Sensitive issues' were defined as 'mention' of relevant 'conflicts' or 'complaints'. He then counted the number of times conflicts and complaints were mentioned. Using a chi-square test, he concluded that individual interviews were 'more likely to raise socially sensitive discussion topics than focus groups'. This study demonstrates the use of numbers and frequencies in qualitative research. The quantitative treatment of qualitative data and vice versa demonstrate the value of going beyond the quantitative–qualitative divide in pursuit of answers to our research questions.

Qualitative analysis of data from unstructured interviews and observations is a process which is rarely described in detail. It is a lonely journey which many researchers undertake and for which, often, they receive little training. There are a number of textbooks (see e.g. Miles and Huberman, 1994; Gibbs, 2002) which have taken up the challenge of preparing researchers for this task. Although each textbook or guideline has its own number of steps or procedures which researchers can follow, the purpose of analysing qualitative data is the same. Researchers have to 'unravel' and make sense of phenomena they are investigating.

The process of qualitative data analysis

Strauss and Corbin (1998) explain their three levels of coding in the analysis of grounded theory data:

> Open coding: The analytic process through which concepts are identified and their properties and dimensions are discovered in data.

> Axial coding: The process of relating categories and their sub-categories, termed 'axial' because coding occurs around the axis of a category, linking categories at the level of properties and dimensions.

> Selective coding: The process of integrating and refining theory.

A second example of different levels of theme extraction comes from Attride-Stirling (2001). These are:

Basic theme: This is the most basic or lowest order theme that is derived from the textual data . . . Basic Themes are simple premises characteristic of the data, and, on their own they say very little about the text or group of texts as a whole. In order for a Basic Theme to make sense beyond its immediate meaning it needs to be read within the context of other Basic Themes. Together, they represent an Organizing Theme.

Organizing Theme: This is a middle-order theme that organizes the Basic Themes into clusters of similar issues . . . they are more abstract and more revealing of what is going on in the texts.

Global Theme: They are sets of Organizing Themes . . . they tell us what the texts as a whole are about within the context of a given analysis.

Drawing from these and other frameworks one can summarise the process of analysis of data from unstructured interviews and observations in the following three stages. To start the process of data analysis researchers have to 'open up' or break the data into as many parts or categories as they can identify. This is followed by grouping together some of these parts into manageable themes based on their similarities. The final part of the process is to put the themes together in order to describe the 'whole'. Thus one can say that there are three levels of analysis: basic, intermediate and higher. These levels are neither distinct nor linear. They facilitate a process which began during data collection. Researchers continually move forward and backward between these levels or stages, until a comprehensive understanding of the phenomenon as a 'whole' is ready to be reported.

Below is a hypothetical example to illustrate these three levels of analysis. Suppose a researcher carries out in-depth interviews about nurses' perceptions of obstacles to, and facilitators of, research utilisation in their practice. Once the transcripts are available, she reads them and begins to 'open-up' the data by noting all the parts she comes across. These may include:

- Skills to appraise research
- Manager's support
- Resources
- Time to read and update
- Support to attend courses
- Autonomy to make change
- IT skills
- Understanding of research
- Time to make changes to practice
- Permission to introduce change
- Funding to go to conferences
- Good leadership
- An organisation which recognises and rewards initiative

This list is likely to be much longer. Already, by comparing these individual parts she can begin to group them. For example 'support to attend courses' can be put together with 'funding to go to conferences'. She may decide to have a category called 'support', which has sub-categories such as support for courses, support for conferences, support to undertake a research project and so on. This exercise is repeated with other categories such as 'time', 'training', 'education' or 'attitudes to research'.

At the next level all the categories can be further grouped into themes. For example, the researcher may find that a number of categories, such as education, training and attitudes, have something in common in that they are related to characteristics of nurses. She could label them 'personal' factors. In the same way she may group the others into themes such as 'research', 'organisation' and 'settings'. At this level researchers engage in intellectual activities such as identifying, defining, delineating, differentiating and comparing categories or concepts which emerge. By this process categories and sub-categories are formed before they are grouped into a number of themes.

At the third level of analysis, the researcher begins to explain how the themes are interrelated. For example, is one of these themes more important than the others? How does the 'organisation', create a 'setting' which encourages 'personal development'? How does leadership influence research utilisation? The researcher has to constantly read the scripts and look for relationships, links, patterns, transitions, stages, phases, preconditions or outcomes in the data. This is when a number of techniques, such as mapping, constructing networks (of relationships between concepts) or using diagrams, are useful in helping researchers to keep control of the large number of categories and themes in order to make sense of the data. In presenting and discussing the findings researchers often make selective use of direct quotes from respondents.

Codes, themes and categories

The terms 'codes', 'categories' and 'themes' are sometimes used interchangeably in the literature. Coloured highlighter pens are used to differentiate between categories, and the purpose of different colours is only to group categories which have similar meanings. Numbers, colours and verbal descriptions are commonly used for coding purposes. Because a word is used as a code it becomes a variable rather than a representation of a variable. For example, if 'support' is used as a code, it has meaning of its own, similar to a category.

Weber (1983) describes a category as a 'group of words which have similar meanings and/or connotations'. Perhaps one should add 'group of statements' or 'phrases' as well. He describes 'theme' as a cluster of words with different meanings or connotations that taken together refer to some theme or issue.

Using specific frameworks to analyse qualitative data

A number of authors have proposed frameworks for the analysis of grounded theory data (e.g. Glaser and Strauss, 1967; Stern, 1980; Strauss and Corbin, 1998) and data from phenomenological studies (e.g. VanKaam, 1966; Colaizzi, 1978; Giorgi, 1985; Ricoeur, 1991). Strauss and Corbin (1998) describe in detail the techniques and procedures for developing grounded theory. The types of coding they propose, such as open coding, axial coding and selective coding, were described earlier in this chapter. An example of the use of this technique to analyse data comes from Jacobsson et al.'s (2004) grounded theory study of 'emotions, the meaning of food and heart failure'. They describe below how they analysed their data:

> Analysis was carried out in three stages: open, axial and selective coding, which in practice were more or less interwoven. The purpose of open coding was to capture the substance of the data, and to break it up into smaller segments through identifying and joining together substantive codes or concepts to form abstract categories. Substantive codes were made up of statements such as 'I force myself to eat, otherwise I'm done for', 'Even though it tastes good, I can't eat', 'I eat less food' and 'I am quickly sated'. A search was made to find ideas or codes that summarised the material. In this way, connections, courses of events and hidden messages were identified. The next stage, axial coding, involved sorting the information and searching for patterns. At this stage, data were combined into a larger whole, by means of associations between categories and their subcategories.
>
> Connections or patterns describing cause and effect emerged from the empirical data. Examples of axial coding were: 'I eat [strategy] because I have to [circumstance], not because it tastes good . . . or because I am hungry [phenomenon] . . . but because otherwise I would die [consequence]'. The final stage, selective coding, resulted in two core categories: 'emotions' and 'the meaning of food', which emphasized the main problems of the phenomena.

Jacobsson et al. (2004), in their article, went on to illustrate graphically how axial coding was carried out.

Researchers who use a phenomenological approach draw from a variety of philosophical sources such as Husserl (1970), Merleau-Ponty (1964), van Manen (1997) and Gadamer (1994). Others such as Colaizzi (1978), Giorgi (1985) and van Kaam (1966) have developed detailed procedures which can be used to analyse phenomenological data. One of the more common frameworks used in nursing research is that of Colaizzi (1978). In a study of 'staff perceptions of the behaviour of older nursing home residents and how these perceptions govern their decision making on restraint use', Hantikainen (2001) describes how Colaizzi's procedures were followed:

> Analysis was based on a phenomenological method adapted from Colaizzi (1978) and involved the following stages:
>
> 1   All transcripts were read in order to gain an overall view and feeling for them;

2 Significant statements were extracted from each protocol;
3 Formulated meanings were extracted from each significant statement;
4 Formulated meanings were clustered into themes;
5 The results of everything so far were integrated into an exhaustive description of the investigated phenomenon;
6 Findings were validated by returning them to the participants.

As well as proceeding through these steps, the analysis in this study included the stage of extracting from the clusters the main themes that helped to provide a clearer overall view of the results.

Hantikainen (2001) went on to give examples of how two main themes were extracted from the data. For a comparison of the methods proposed by Colaizzi (1978), Giorgi (1985) and van Kaam (1966), see Beck (1994). Whatever the method used for the analysis of qualitative data, the scripts have to be read and reread. They have to be 'opened up' to reveal the various parts. These 'parts' are analysed in the context of the 'whole'. Thereafter, a process of synthesis takes place whereby the parts are reconstituted in order to present a new understanding of the phenomenon.

Computer-assisted qualitative data analysis

Computer packages for the analysis of quantitative data are an established feature. In contrast, researchers have been slow in using qualitative data analysis software, despite their availability for almost a decade. Recently there has been a noticeable increase in their use, perhaps partly because they offer more features and because there are more opportunities for acquiring the skills to use them.

A wide range of software programs has been developed over the years. These include: Ethnograph, HyperQual, HyperResearch, Hypersoft, Qualpro, Atlas-ti, NUD*IST and N-Vivo. They differ in the functions they offer, and new versions of these programs come on to the market quite regularly. The earlier packages operated more as an indexing system, while the later ones, responding to the needs of qualitative researchers, are designed to facilitate theory building. Some are more appropriate for particular qualitative approaches. For example, NUD*IST has been used for the analysis of data in grounded theory studies (see e.g. Morison and Moir, 1998).

The main advantage of using computer-assisted qualitative data software (CAQDAS) is that it helps researchers to manage large amounts of data which can be indexed, coded, stored and retrieved. Manual data analysis can be overwhelming and time-consuming. The more recent software versions facilitate conceptual mapping and networking. In a study of 'families' experiences of living with a young person who wets beds', Morison and Moir (1998) found the NUD*IST package they used was 'helpful for data storage, searching and retrieval and certain aspects of concept organisation and theory testing'. But they pointed out, among other things, that the use of computer packages may lead to a 'rigid and unreflexive' approach to data analysis. One can use the analogy of completing a questionnaire to explain this concern. In answering the questionnaire, there is a tendency to fit the answers in the specific formats in which the questions are structured.

Webb (1999), who reviewed the background to, and advantages and disadvantages of, computerised approaches, suggests that

> The technique offered by CAQDAS should be used as mechanical tools and not seen as monsters which take over the analysis. The thinking and creative part belongs to the researcher and provided the software is used appropriately CAQDAS is within the control of her/him.

This, however, requires that the researcher is perceptive and experienced in the analysis of qualitative data. This is why Webb (1999) concluded that 'beginning researchers conducting small-scale studies would be best recommended to use a manual approach in order to gain insight into the intuition aspects of analysis'.

In the UK, the Economic and Social Research Council (ESRC) has funded the CAQDAS Networking Project (http://caqdas.soc.surrey.ac.uk/) which provides 'practical support, training and information in the use of a range of software programs which have been designed to assist qualitative data analysis'.

Ensuring rigour in data analysis

Researchers report a number of strategies which they use to ensure rigour in the analysis of qualitative data. One of their first tasks is to make sure that the transcription of audiotapes is an accurate version of what was said during the interviews. Transcribing is an arduous task and is often carried out by secretaries with little experience of research. Accents, the 'pace' of speech and other speech mannerisms can all affect this process. Some transcripts contain paralanguage as well (e.g. 'uums', 'aahs', pauses, half-words or silences). When transcribing and translating (in cases where the interview is in a different language than the one being used in transcription) happens at the same time, more than one translator is often required to ensure inter-translator reliability.

Expert validation is the process whereby one or more 'experts' (in the methodology and/or the subject matter) are called upon to 'verify' the findings. This is usually done by giving all the scripts to experts and letting them analyse the data. Findings can thereafter be compared. More often the researcher will make a sample of scripts and the themes extracted available to the expert for confirmation (or discussion thereafter in cases of different interpretations). Expert validation has been the subject of much discussion (see e.g. Sandelowski, 1998; Cutcliffe and McKenna, 1999, 2004). The problems with expert validation relate to a number of issues including the definition of 'expert' and the different analytical processes which more experienced researchers (than less experienced ones) use. Also, researchers' decisions during data analysis are not easy to articulate as they are often made at a subconscious level (Cutcliffe and McKenna, 2004). Sandelowski (1998) questions if experts, 'no matter how impressive their credentials', are 'in any position to certify as valid the findings in studies in which they played no part'. One of the main differences in quantitative and qualitative data analysis is that in the latter, the process of analysis starts with the very first opportunity of data collection. This process is even more difficult to articulate and convey to others. Sandelowski (1998) concludes that 'no outsider-expert can confer the validity stamp of approval on a project, but they can provide expert criticism of a project'.

Some researchers (see for example Hantikainen, 2001) ask some of their participants 'to verify the interpretations made of their descriptions for validation of the findings'. This is known as 'participant validation'. There are also a number of contentious issues with this practice including the difficulties in, and cost of, going back to all participants or deciding who to sample, in case this is not possible. Disagreements between participants may not be easy to resolve. Sandelowski (1998) points out that 'participants may not understand an interpretation intended for an audience of researchers'.

Issues of rigour in qualitative research will be discussed further in the next chapter.

SUMMARY

Summary and conclusion

In this chapter, the purpose and process of quantitative and qualitative data analysis were described. In quantitative studies, descriptive and inferential statistics help researchers and readers to make sense of the data. The main measures in descriptive statistics are frequency, central tendency and dispersion. Inferential statistics help researchers to determine whether relationships exist between variables and whether there are differences between groups.

In qualitative research, the process of data analysis is laborious and on-going. It starts during data collection and continues after the field notes and/or tapes have been transcribed. Grounded theory and phenomenology provide frameworks that researchers can use to analyse qualitative data. Researchers have also developed ways of allowing others to understand their thinking processes and actions. The purpose of qualitative analysis is ultimately to gain insights into phenomena. The themes, patterns and categories generated can lead to the development of hypotheses and theories.

References

Attride-Stirling J (2001) Thematic networks: an analytic tool for qualitative research. *Qualitative Research,* **1**, 3:385–405.

Beck C T (1994) Reliability and validity issues in phenomenological research. *Western Journal of Nursing Research,* **16**, 3:254–67.

Chan S and Yu I W (2004) Quality of life of clients with schizophrenia. *Journal of Advanced Nursing,* **45**, 1:72–83.

Colaizzi P (1978) Psychological research as the phenomenologist views it. In: R Valle and M Kings M (eds), *Existential Phenomenological Alternative for Psychology* (New York: Oxford University Press).

Cutcliffe J R and McKenna H P (1999) Establishing the credibility of qualitative research findings: the plot thickens. *Journal of Advanced Nursing,* **30**:374–80.

Cutcliffe J R and McKenna H P (2004) Expert qualitative researchers and the use of audit trawls. *Journal of Advanced Nursing,* **45**, 2:126–33.

Dawkins R (1988) *The Blind Watchmaker* (London: Penguin).

DePoy E and Gitlin L N (1994) *Introduction to Research* (St Louis, MO: C V Mosby).

Fink A (1995) *How to Analyse Survey Data* (Thousand Oaks, CA: Sage).

Gadamer H-G (1994) *Truth and Method,* 2nd rev. edn (New York: Continuum Publishing).

Gibbs R G (2002) *Qualitative Data Analysis: Explorations with Nvivo* (Philadelphia, PA: Open University Press).

Giorgi A (1985) *Phenomenology and Psychological Research* (Pittsburg, PA: Duquesne University Press).

Glaser B G and Strauss A L (1967) *The Discovery of Grounded Theory: Strategies for Qualitative Research* (Chicago: Aldine).

Gudmundsdottir E, Delaney C, Thoroddsen A and Karlsson T (2004) Translation and validation of the nursing outcomes classification labels and definitions for acute care nursing in Iceland. *Journal of Advanced Nursing,* **46**, 3:292–302.

Hantikainen V (2001) Nursing staff perceptions of the behaviour of older nursing home residents and decision making on restraint use: a qualitative interpretative study. *Journal of Clinical Nursing,* **10**:246–56.

Hicks C M (1990) *Research and Statistics: A Practical Introduction for Nurses* (London: Prentice Hall).

Higgins L W (1999) Nurses' perceptions of collaborative nurse–physician transfer decision making as a predictor of patient outcomes in a medical intensive care unit. *Journal of Advanced Nursing,* **29**, 6:1434–43.

Husserl E (1970) *Logical Investigation* (New York: Humanities Press).

Jacobsson A, Pihl E, Martensson J and Fridlund B (2004) Emotions, the meaning of food and heart failure: a grounded theory study. *Journal of Advanced Nursng,* **46**, 5:514–22.

Karlsson A and Nordström G (2001) Nutritional status, symptoms experienced and general state of health in HIV-infected patients. *Journal of Clinical Nursing,* **10**, 5:609–17.

Klapowitz M D (2000) Statistical analysis of sensitive topics in group and individual interviews. *Quality and Quantity,* **34**:419–31.

Marshall K, Thompson K A, Walsh D M and Baxter G D (1998) Incidence of urinary incontinence and constipation during pregnancy and postpartum: survey of current findings at the Rotunda lying-in hospital. *British Journal of Obstetrics and Gynaecology,* 105:400–2.

McCleary L and Brown G T (2003) Barriers to paediatric nurses' research utilization. *Journal of Advanced Nursing,* **42**, 4:364–72.

Merleau-Ponty M (1964) *The Primacy of Perception and Other Essays* (Evanston, IL: Northwestern University Press).

Miles M B and Huberman A M (1994) *Qualitative Data Analysis: An Expanded Sourcebook*, 2nd edn (London: Sage).

Moore D S (1985) *Statistics: Concepts and Controversies*, 2nd edn (New York: W H Freedman).

Morison M and Moir J (1998) The role of computer software in the analysis of qualitative data: efficient clerk, research assistant or Trojan horse? *Journal of Advanced Nursing*, **28**, 1:106–16.

Munro B H, Visintainer M A and Page E B (1986) *Statistical Methods for Health Care Research* (Philadelphia, PA: J B Lippincott).

Reid N (1993) *Health Care Research by Degrees* (London: Blackwell Scientific).

Ricoeur P (1991) *From Text to Action: Essays in Hermeneutics*, vol. II, trans. K Glamey and J Thomson (Evanston, IL: Northwestern University Press).

Röndahl G, Innala S and Carlsson M (2004) Nurses' attitudes towards lesbians and gay men. *Journal of Advanced Nursing*, **47**, 4:386–92.

Sandelowski M (1998) The call to experts in qualitative research. *Research in Nursing and Health*, **21**:467–71.

Scott I and Mazhindu D (2005) *Statistics for Health Care Professionals: An Introduction* (London: Sage).

Stern P N (1980) Grounded theory methodology: its uses and processes. *Image*, **12**, 1:20–33.

Strauss A and Corbin J (1998) *Basics of Qualitative Research: Grounded Theory Procedures and Techniques*, 2nd edn (Thousand Oaks, CA: Sage).

van Manen M (1997) *Researching Lived Experience: Human Science for an Action Sensitive Pedagogy* (London: Althouse Press).

van Kaam A (1966) *Existential Foundations of Psychology* (Pittsburg, PA: Duquesne University Press).

Waltz C F, Strickland O L and Lenz E R (1991) *Measurement in Nursing Research*, 2nd edn (Philadelphia, PA: F A Davis).

Webb C (1999) Analysing qualitative data: computerized and other approaches. *Journal of Advanced Nursing*, **29**, 2:323–30.

Weber R P (1983) Measurement models for content analysis. *Quality and Quantity*, **17**:127–49.

Williams C A (1989) Empathy and burnout in male and female helping professions. *Research in Nursing and Health*, **12**:169–78.

Evaluating Research Studies

Introduction

The previous chapters have described, explained and discussed the basic concepts and the research process in qualitative and quantitative research. Issues relating to the validity and reliability of methods and findings have been extensively covered. Where appropriate, suggestions have been made on how to critique particular aspects of research studies.

This chapter provides a structure for the evaluation of research studies and a summary of the relevant questions to ask. Sources of bias and some of the common practices in the reporting of research are identified. In addition, the role of researchers in facilitating evaluation will be raised.

Critiquing skills

The terms 'critique', 'appraise' and 'evaluate' will be used interchangeably here to mean making a value judgement on what is reported. By now, readers should have the necessary knowledge and comprehension to begin to read research studies critically. In particular, they should be able to describe the aim of the research, its methodology and findings. However, description is only the first step towards evaluation. The latter requires a judgement on the part of the reader of the actions and interpretations of the researcher. This can be done mainly by weighing what was done against accepted practice by researchers, although new and unconventional approaches should be considered on their own merit. For example, there is consensus among researchers that if, in quantitative studies, samples are not randomly selected, the findings cannot be generalised to the target population. Therefore, if a researcher states that her findings can be generalised when the sample is one of convenience, the reader can question the validity of this claim. Although individual readers may critique a study differently, the criteria they use during their evaluation must be objective. One cannot state that a literature review is inappropriate or inadequate without giving reasons to explain why. The task of critiquing is a challenging one and can only be acquired through practice.

Although nurses are expected to implement research findings in their practice, it is unsafe to base their decision on one single study, however good it is.

Reviewing studies with a view to using them in practice must also be done by experienced practitioners and researchers. The Cochrane Collaboration and the NHS Centre for Review and Dissemination are two of the organisations who carry out reviews to facilitate health practitioners in using research findings.

One may question if all nurses should possess the skills to critically appraise research studies, particularly since this requires an in-depth knowledge of a wide range of research methodologies. The answer to this question lies in the purpose of the exercise. Nurses need to have a questioning attitude and the skills to critically read relevant literature including research studies. Although they may not be expert in research, they should be able to know, appraise, and keep up to date with what is written in their particular field of work. They should be able to distinguish between opinionated, one-sided arguments and poor research, and well-balanced articles or good research. Guidelines for policy and practice based on evidence should be developed by experienced researchers and practitioners after a systematic review and appraisal of the literature. They may sometimes require the help of more experienced colleagues to understand or interpret what researchers report. The benefits of research awareness and research-mindedness have been fully discussed in Chapter 1.

A structure for evaluating quantitative studies

Individuals may approach the evaluation of a study in different ways. Beginners sometimes prefer to be guided through the process. A step-by-step guide is provided here for this purpose. Only a summary of the main questions to ask is included, as relevant chapters already have a section on critiquing; readers are strongly advised to consult these for more details. The following headings (based on the format in which quantitative studies are most often reported) provide a structure for the evaluation of research articles:

- Title of article
- Abstract
- Literature review
- Methodology
- Results
- Discussion and interpretation
- Recommendations

Title of article

The title should draw readers' attention to the precise area of study and make reference to the population from whom data are collected. For example, the title 'comparison of the experiences of having a sick baby in a neonatal intensive care unit among mothers with or without the right of abode in Hong Kong' (Yam and Kan, 2004) makes clear the phenomenon being investigated (experiences of mothers having a sick baby in a neonatal unit) and the population (mothers with or without right of abode). This title also suggests that the purpose of the study is to 'compare' experiences.

Too much information in the title can make it long and inelegant. For example, 'Nurses' creativity, tedium and burnout during one year of clinical supervision and implementation of individually planned nursing care: comparisons between a ward for severely demented patients and a similar control ward' (Berg et al., 1994) is very informative, but some of the details could perhaps be confined to the abstract. Titles can be misleading or confusing.

Abstract

An abstract is a short summary of a study (the number of words is normally stipulated by the journal). The purpose of an abstract is to give readers enough information for them to decide whether or not the article is of interest to them. The abstract should state briefly the background and aim of the study, the design, including the method(s), sample(s) and sampling, and the main findings. This information is essential as it describes what the study is about, how it was carried out and what was found. The importance of succint and brief summaries has increased since the advent of on-line databases. The information contained in abstracts helps readers to decide whether they should access the whole article or not. Readers should not ask too much from an abstract as details are provided in the rest of the article.

Literature review

Readers may want to know why the current study is important, what research, if any, has been carried out previously and what the study will contribute. The four functions of a literature review described in Chapter 7 can be used as a framework for evaluation. In particular, the following questions may be asked:

- Is a rationale provided? If so, what is it? How convincing are the reasons? Does the author support it with evidence such as research findings, statistical data and, to a lesser extent, expert opinion?
- Does the author provide a critical overview of similar research carried out?
- Are the relevant concepts and issues dealt with adequately?
- Is there a conceptual framework? How does the author propose to use it?
- Is there reliance on primary or secondary sources? Are the references dated?

- Is it likely there may be more recent material? Has the author been selective in her review of the literature?

Remember that the author is restricted by word limits, but if the lack of information affects your understanding of the study, it is a good indication that the information should have been provided.

The title, abstract and literature review have little bearing on the reliability and validity of the findings. Readers are advised not to spend too much time critiquing them. The methodology of the study determines the quality of the research and, as such, deserves the most attention.

Methodology

The philosophical assumptions, methods of data collection and techniques of data analysis can be used to find out whether the study is qualitative, quantitative or a mixture of the two.

Questions to ask of the methodology include:

- Are the research questions, objectives or hypotheses clearly stated?

- Are the operational definitions adequate? The criteria of clarity, precision, validity, reliability and consensus (see Chapter 9), can be used for this purpose.

- Is the design the most appropriate for the phenomenon under study? If, for example, the researcher uses a cross-sectional design to study the difficulties that mothers face breastfeeding in the first six months, is a longitudinal design more appropriate? What are the limitations of a cross-sectional design for this study (see Chapter 10)?

- What are the methods of data collection? Are there any instruments (questionnaires, interviews or observation schedules) used in this study? Are they constructed for the purpose of the current study? Do they have face, content or other forms of validity? How was this achieved? Where do the items in the instruments come from?

- Is the instrument reliable? Was a test–retest or a split-half test, if appropriate, carried out (see Chapter 13)?

- Was the instrument borrowed? What is its established validity and reliability? How extensively has it been used in other similar studies?

- If the borrowed instrument is modified for the purpose of the current study, what are the changes made? How do they affect the validity and reliability of the original instrument? What are the measures taken to ensure the validity and reliability of the modified instrument?

One important aspect of methodology on which researchers sometimes omit to provide information is the sampling method. It is not unusual to find that a random sample is used without any explanation of how participants were selected and what the target population was. Although such terms as 'systematic', 'stratified' or 'random' have specific meanings, they are not self-explanatory in the context of individual studies. The questions to ask are:

● Who was selected? From what population were they selected? What was the precise method of selection? What implications does the sampling method have for generalisability of the findings?

● What was the response rate? What implications does the non-responses rate have for the findings?

In addition to the above aspects of methodology, researchers must describe the steps taken to ensure that the rights of individuals are respected and whether approval from an ethical committee, where appropriate, was obtained. They must also explain how access to the study population was obtained as this may have implications for the data.

Results

The method of data analysis must be described and justified. Researchers are often selective in their presentation of results. Readers should refer back to the questions or hypotheses set at the start of the study to find out whether they are addressed in the results section. Tables and figures must also make sense. The way in which some results are presented can be misleading. Stevens et al. (1993) give the following example:

> [W]hen an author writes that sixty per cent of respondents state that they drink alcohol because of stress, it must be explained that they were asked to choose from a list of reasons provided by the researcher. By not stating the format of the question, i.e. whether it was an open or a multiple-choice one, it is difficult for the reader to put the responses in context.

Beginners may find it difficult to understand statistical tests and jargon. A good journal referee should query mistakes or inconsistencies in the analysis. If you are in doubt about some of the calculations, you should, if possible, consult someone who knows about statistics. What is more important is for the author to explain what the results mean.

Discussion and interpretation

Results can be presented on their own or with discussion and interpretation. Whatever the choice of presentation, it is important that results are explained, discussed and interpreted. One of the first tasks of a critical reader is to find out if the research questions, objectives or hypotheses set at the start of the study have been addressed, and, if not, reasons should be provided. Sometimes researchers only discuss results in which they are interested and/or support their particular views. As far as possible all results, positive or negative, should be discussed. To contribute to the pool of knowledge, results should be compared with findings from other studies and when these are different, possible explanations should be offered.

It is not enough to report that the results are statistically significant; researchers must also explain the clinical significance of the results or identify why the results are not (perhaps on their own) clinically significant. It may be that the results of the study show that, with the new treatment, people are cured of their illness more quickly. However, their degree of discomfort with the new treatment may be greater than with the usual one.

The discussion and interpretation of data often reflect the subjective opinion of researchers. To evaluate this aspect of a study, Stevens et al. (1993) suggest the following questions:

- Can you follow the steps leading to the conclusions?

- Are there any gaps in the development of the arguments?

- How consistent are the arguments?

- Is the author contradicting himself?

- Do the arguments make sense according to your experience?

- Does your experience lead you to see different meanings in the data?

- Overall, do you agree with the data and/or the interpretation of the author?

Recommendations

Readers must first ask whether the recommendations are based on the research findings of the present study. Researchers are often in favour of certain policies or practices and they peddle them in the form of recommendations even when the findings of their studies are not conclusive. The recommendations must also be practical, feasible and well thought out. In fact, researchers should be expected to discuss the limitations of their recommendations rather than simply state them.

Validity and reliability in quantitative studies

In quantitative studies, 'validity' and 'reliability' are two of the most important concepts used by researchers to evaluate the rigour with which they are carried out. These concepts have been described in previous chapters. Therefore, in evaluating these studies, readers must look for measures taken to produce valid and reliable results. These include strategies to avoid bias and to enhance objectivity.

Biases represent the greatest threat to the reliability and validity of data. To ensure rigour, researchers must avoid bias or, if this is not possible, account for it. The main sources of bias are:

● respondents

● researchers

● methods of data collection

● the environment

● the phenomenon.

Respondents' motivation, perception, social class affiliation, personal and collective agendas or even communication skills (or their lack of), among others, can bias the results. Similarly, researchers' own prejudices, values, beliefs or lack of research skills, and other factors, can affect the collection, analysis and presentation of data. Questionnaires may contain leading or ambiguous questions, and interview and observation schedules may not be valid or reliable. The environment can also influence the findings. Captive populations (such as patients in hospitals) may yield different data than if they were studied in their own homes. In experimental studies, data contamination can occur when subjects in the control group share information with those in the experimental group, especially when both are on the same ward. Finally, the phenomenon may not reveal itself in its usual form on days when it is studied. For example, if the researcher sets out to observe aggression among patients, it may not necessarily occur in the way it normally does while the researcher is present. These and other sources of bias are extensively discussed in this book. The few examples given are only a reminder to readers.

In quantitative studies the quality of the tools determines the validity and reliability of the findings, provided sources of bias are controlled. Quantitative researchers are also expected to remain detached (objective) from the respondents and the environment in which data are collected. Therefore so long as the tools are valid and reliable, that they are administered in an objective way and that the data/analysis techniques are appropriate the quality of the findings is assured. The main task of critical readers is to make a judgement on the extent to which this is achieved. The second task is to find out how 'generalisable' the findings are. This is assessed by examining the sampling technique, and the size and characteristics of the sample.

Evaluating qualitative studies

We can use the same headings, as above, for evaluating qualitative studies since they are commonly reported in the same way as quantitative ones. The questions to be asked about the abstract and title are also the same.

Purpose, aim or research questions

Qualitative researchers seek to 'explore' phenomena from the perspectives of participants. They may not know the precise questions to ask in advance of data collection. They must, however, make clear what the area of enquiry is, and what they are focusing on. Readers can, thereafter, assess whether the aim is achieved.

Literature review

There are different views about whether the literature should be reviewed before a qualitative study is carried out. This was dealt with in Chapter 7. When a qualitative study is reported in a journal, readers need to be introduced to the rationale and background to the study, in particular to the gaps which it seeks to fill. Therefore this section should demonstrate the particular contribution the study makes in terms of adding to current knowledge in that field. When a different methodology (than in previous studies) is proposed, the rationale for its use should be stated. The author should also explain how the aim of the study evolved.

Methodology

The research process must be detailed as much as possible for readers to understand the decisions for the actions taken and the rationale on which they are based. Articles are limited in length, depending on the type of journal in which they are published. This should not be an excuse for omitting vital information, which often takes only a few words to describe.

One aspect of the methodology which is often not well described is the sampling strategy and the profile of participants. In Webb's (2004) analysis of all papers published in the *Journal of Advanced Nursing* in 2002, she found that 'the type of sample was rarely stated'. When the sampling is described as 'purposive' and no other information provided it is assumed that the term is self-explanatory.

Purposive sampling means that the researcher carefully selects the participants on the basis of the varied experience they may bring to the study. Readers need to know why and how particular participants were selected, and how 'varied' they were. Samples are chosen from a target population, yet in many studies there is little or no information about it. Information on samples is vital for readers to assess whether the study is relevant to their 'clinical' population. Theoretical sampling is another term which requires description and explanation (see Chapter 12).

The methods of data collection (such as interviews of observations) should be described in such a way that readers have a 'feel' of what happened. Often researchers only report the broad question they ask and leave readers in the dark about the interactions and the context in which they took place. Readers need to know the degree of control over the interview agenda that the researcher or the participants had.

Readers should also look for the researcher's awareness of the ethical implications of the study and how these were dealt with.

Findings

This is often a difficult section to evaluate since qualitative researchers report their 'findings' in a variety of ways. Sandelowski and Barroso (2002), in a review of qualitative studies of women with HIV infection, found that it was difficult to find the findings. Often there were 'lengthy description and many quotes, but virtually no interpretation of data'. This is similar to a quantitative researcher presenting readers with their SPSS print-outs. Researchers in qualitative studies should go beyond the raw data and provide answers to the research questions. For readers to critically appraise the findings of a qualitative study, these must be presented clearly and succinctly. If themes are presented, readers must look for an explanation of how they were developed out of the data. Participants' experience of a phenomenon is not fragmented into themes. Therefore a good study should show the interconnections between these themes (Sandelowski and Barroso, 2002).

Discussion

The questions to ask when evaluating this section are the same as those detailed earlier for quantitative studies. This section should put the findings in the context of previous knowledge, in particular existing themes. It should explore the extent to which the findings are new.

Recommendations for policy and practice

Readers should look at the match between the findings and the recommendations. One way to do so is to examine each recommendation and look for the findings which support it. A good study should also make realistic and feasible recommendations. It is easy to say that a particular service or intervention should be made available to everyone. The resource and other implications should also be taken into consideration.

Increasingly there is pressure on researchers to take dissemination of findings more seriously. This is now a requirement of funding organisations. Researchers should, therefore, be expected to suggest ways in which their findings can be used.

Ensuring rigour in qualitative studies

Researchers are still grappling with what constitutes rigour in qualitative research. As explained earlier, 'validity' and 'reliability' in quantitative studies refer to the tools of data collection and analysis. Valid and reliable findings depend on the degree of objectivity with which the tools are administered and on the extent to which sources of bias can be controlled. However in qualitative studies, the tools of data collection are not predetermined, structured and standardised. There may not be a 'visible' tool to test for validity and reliability. There can be differences in the content and wordings from one interview or observation to another. The researcher is also an instrument of data collection and analysis.

The notion of objectivity is also redundant in qualitative studies since researchers interact with the participants, and together they co-create the data produced. Therefore, far from attempting to remain 'detached', qualitative researchers aim to 'enter' the world of participants by getting close to them. Instead of 'controlling' the factors in the environment which may affect the results, qualitative researchers aim to find out how the context in which people live can influence their perceptions, experience or behaviour. Rejecting validity, reliability, objectivity and bias as conceptualised in quantitative studies, qualitative researchers have offered 'parallel' terms such as 'credibility', 'auditability', 'transferability', 'fittingness' and 'confirmability'. Credibility refers to the 'truth, value or believability of the findings' (Dreher, 1994). Auditability relates to the detail provided in the report to allow others 'to follow the methods and conclusions of the original researcher' (Streubert and Carpenter, 1999). Transferability or fittingness is the extent to which the findings of a qualitative study can be of use to other populations or settings similar to those in the study. Confirmability depends on participants and other 'experts' 'agreeing' with the researcher's interpretation (this was discussed in the last chapter).

Despite the use of different terms, one can detect some notions of validity, reliability and generalisability as used in quantitative studies. To some extent this is inevitable since researchers want their findings to reflect 'truthfully' the phenomenon they study and to contribute to knowledge that is useful to others.

To ensure rigour, qualitative researchers have proposed a number of strategies such as audit trail, reflexivity and validation by experts and/or participants. Audit trail was first described by Lincoln and Guba (1985), based on the work of Halpern (1983). As explained by Cutcliffe and McKenna (2004), audit trail, in that sense, means 'that an auditor (second party) will audit the decisions, analytical processes, and methodological decisions of the primary researcher (first party), and that this will occur *expost facto*'. Cutcliffe and McKenna (2004), after discussing the difficulties and implications of providing an audit trail, suggest that 'the absence of audit trails does not necessarily challenge the credibility of qualitative findings'. Auditing all the actions and decisions of qualitative researchers is an impossible task. However, where possible, researchers should give details and rationale for some of the key decisions taken. According to Koch (2004), 'an audit trail can be a creative way to shape the text, if signposts are offered along the way, readers can decide whether a piece of work is credible or not'.

There is a lot written about 'reflexivity' in the literature (see e.g. Koch and Harrington, 1998; Cutcliffe, 2003; Carolan, 2004; Hand, 2004; and Pellatt, 2004). If one takes the view that the researcher's presence, characteristics (including values and beliefs) and interpretations have an effect on the participants and the environment and vice versa, then reflexivity is the process of making this transparent. Drawing upon other authors' work, Sandelowski and Barroso (2002) describe reflexivity as:

> the ability to reflect inward toward oneself as an inquirer; outward to the cultural, historical, linguistic, political, and other forces that shape everything about inquiry; and, in between researcher and participant to the social interaction they share.

According to Cutcliffe (2003), 'there appears to be a clear perception among methodological researchers that the purpose of reflexivity, at least in part, is to enhance the credibility of the findings by accounting for researcher values, beliefs, knowledge, and biases'.

Reflexivity is important as it gives researchers the opportunity to account for their influence on the research process. There are examples in the literature of researchers describing their background (such as the fact that they are nurses) or political beliefs (e.g. feminism), expecting readers to read 'between the lines'. They should give examples of how their background affects the way they view phenomena, how it helped or hindered their understanding of what was happening. Within the context of a journal article, researchers are constrained by word limit to provide meaningful reflexive accounts. Cutcliffe (2003) is sceptical about the ability of researchers to engage in reflexivity mainly because they are not always totally conscious of their cognitive processes and because they draw on 'tacit' knowledge and intuition in their interpretation of phenomena. These processes do not lend themselves to detailed descriptions.

Sandelowski and Barroso (2002) found that describing the process of reflexivity can be taken too far in some studies. They believe that researchers should tell us more about their findings than about what they learnt about themselves.

When reading a study, it is important to know the actions and decisions taken by the researchers and the rationale for them. It is helpful when they are self-critical and aware of the different influences on the data collected.

Discussing their interpretations with participants, experts or others may help them to interpret data in unexpected ways. Thus audit or decision trail, reflexivity and validation by others are indications that the study was thoughtfully carried out. They can help readers to understand the findings better than if these issues were not explained and discussed. Ultimately the real value of the findings of a qualitative study rests upon its contribution to knowledge and how this knowledge is used thereafter. Its credibility and usefulness should stand the test of time. No doubt, in time, the findings will be built upon, adapted or rejected.

Omission and exaggeration

There are two types of omission – deliberate and unintentional. Deliberate omission is an attempt to deceive. Most omissions, however, are not intentional. Some of the common omissions identified in the earlier chapters include sampling methods, the description of interventions in control groups and the precise method of randomisation in RCTs. In qualitative studies, researchers often omit descriptions of the process of data collection as well as the rationale for their method of sampling. Sometimes researchers are so familiar with their studies that they assume that readers also are. Jargon and specialist terminologies, when not frequently used in the literature, must be avoided or explained. The lack of information about a study may lead readers to make their own assumptions. Stevens et al. (1993) point out:

> It is a common mistake on the part of readers to assume what the author means when the meaning is obscure. It is better to keep an open mind than to assume what the meaning is. The assistance of colleagues, fellow students and lecturers may be helpful in clarifying ambiguities.

Researchers are also prone to exaggeration in their reporting. Often they put their own 'spin' on the significance of their findings. For example, it is not unusual for one researcher to report '45 per cent of the population' as 'almost half the population' and another as 'less than half the population'.

The role of researchers in facilitating evaluation

It is the researchers' responsibility to present data clearly and in sufficient detail for others to understand how the research was carried out. Equally important is the researcher's own reflection on and evaluation of the study and its findings. Unfortunately, some researchers treat their findings as sacred and fail to be critical of them. If researchers were expected to include a section in their papers in which they attempted to falsify their own findings, readers would be better informed. In any case, researchers, as mentioned before, should be required to offer other plausible explanations for their findings. After all, it is they who know the circumstances in which the data were collected and are, therefore, in a position to identify possible sources of bias and error. They are also in possession of the raw data.

While the research enterprise is about asking questions, we must realise we cannot always find answers to them. However, in the process of inquiry, we come to learn more about ourselves and others and about the means by which we study people. We are, therefore, the richer for it. Very often, researchers and readers learn more from the process of research than from the findings. But we must not forget that the aim of research is to provide answers to the research question.

Journal editors and referees, too, have an important part to play in making sure that articles are written and presented in a form that informs rather than confuses readers. There is perhaps a case for some referees to be given training in evaluating research; some of them are clinical experts but have little research experience.

Finally, there is a lot to learn when reading research studies. The task of evaluation should be approached with an open and inquiring mind. As Parahoo and Reid (1988) conclude:

> Critical reading of research helps to develop a research imagination. With practice, the individual's sense of enquiry will be heightened as his or her disposition to passive acceptance of the written and spoken word diminishes. Healthy scepticism rather than negative, cynical attitudes will transform a fault finding activity into a learning experience which can only lead to the development of research-mindedness.

Frameworks and checklists for evaluation

Sometimes beginners need some guidance on how to approach the huge task of critically appraising a study. Different authors have produced models, checklists or frameworks designed to help this process. For example, Evans and Shreve (2000) propose the ASK (Applicability, Science and Knowledge) model for practitioners 'to quickly review and grasp the potential clinical significance of a journal study'. Others have offered guidelines to assess particular types of studies. For example, Loney et al.'s (1998) guidelines aim to 'determine the validity and usefulness of studies' on 'the prevalence or incidence of a disease or health problem'. Jadad et al. (1996) provide a checklist for the appraisal of randomised controlled trials. A number of frameworks and checklists to evaluate qualitative research have been also developed (see e.g. Treloar et al., 2000; Horsburgh, 2003; Spencer et al., 2003). A quick search on the internet will reveal a number of useful resources designed to facilitate the assessment of the quality and usefulness of research findings. One useful web-site is that of the Critical Appraisal

Skills Programme (CASP) (http://www.phru.nhs.uk/casp/appraisa.htm). It contains appraisal tools for systematic reviews, randomised controlled trials, qualitative studies, cohort studies, case control studies, diagnostic test studies and economic evaluation studies.

These checklists, frameworks and assessment tools can guide readers in the task of critically appraising research studies. However, training and practice in appraisal are still required.

SUMMARY

Summary and conclusion

In this chapter, the purpose of critiquing or evaluating research studies is outlined. The main aspects of quantitative and qualitative studies to look for in a review have been discussed. Issues and strategies relating to rigour have been examined. The role of researchers in facilitating evaluation has also been emphasised. Finally references to checklists and frameworks for critical appraised have been provided.

This book, as a whole, provides the necessary knowledge and insight to enable nurses and others to read, understand and critique research studies. It is hoped that by putting research in perspective, readers will realise the value, potential and limitations of research in contributing to the advancement of knowledge.

References

Berg A, Hansson U W and Hallberg I R (1994) Nurses' creativity, tedium and burnout during 1 year of clinical supervision and implementation of individually planned nursing care: comparisons between a ward for severely demented patients and a similar control ward. *Journal of Advanced Nursing*, **20**, 4:742–9.

Carolan M (2004) Reflexivity: a personal journey during data collection. *Nurse Researcher*, **10**, 3:7–14.

Cutcliffe J R (2003) Re-considering reflexivity in the case for intellectual entrepreneurship. *Qualitative Health Research*, **13**:136–48.

Cutcliffe J R and McKenna H P (2004) Expert qualitative researchers and the use of audit trails. *Journal of Advanced Nursing*, **45**, 2:126–33.

Dreher M (1994) Qualitative research methods from the reviewer's perspective. In: J M Morse (ed), *Critical Issues in Qualitative Research Methods* (Thousand Oaks, CA: Sage).

Evans J C and Shreve W S (2000) The ASK Model: a bare bones approach to critique of nursing research for use in practice. *Journal of Trauma Nursing*, 7, 4:83–91.

Halpern E S (1983) Auditing naturalistic inquiries: the development and application of a model. Unpublished doctoral dissertation, Indiana University (USA).

Hand H (2004) The mentor's tale: a reflexive account of semi-structured interviews. *Nurse Researcher*, **10**, 3:15–27.

Horsburgh D (2003) Evaluation of qualitative research. *Journal of Clinical Nursing*, **12**:307–12.

Jadad A R, Moore R A, Carroll D, Jenkinson C, Reynolds D J, Gavaghan D J and McQuay H J (1996) Assessing the quality of reports of randomized controlled trials: is blinding necessary? *Controlled Clinical Trials*, **17**, 1:1–12.

Koch T (2004) Expert researchers and audit trails. *Journal of Advanced Nursing*, **45**, 2:134–5.

Koch T and Harrington A (1998) Reconceptualizing rigour: the case for reflexivity. *Journal of Advanced Nursing*, **28**, 4:882–90.

Lincoln Y S and Guba E G (1985) *Naturalistic Inquiry* (Newbury Park, CA: Sage).

Loney P L, Chambers L W, Bennett K J, Roberts J G and Stratford P W (1998) Critical appraisal of the health research literature: prevalence or incidence of a health problem. *Chronic Diseases in Canada*, **19**, 4:170–6.

Parahoo K and Reid N (1988) Critical reading of research. *Nursing Times*, **84**, 43:69–72.

Pellatt G (2004) Ethnography and reflexivity: emotions and feelings in fieldwork. *Nurse Researcher*, **10**, 3:28–37.

Sandelowski M and Barroso J (2002) Finding the findings in qualitative studies. *Journal of Nursing Scholarship*, **34**, 3:213–19.

Spencer L, Richie J, Lewis J and Dillon L (2003) *Quality in Qualitative Evaluation: A Framework for Assessing Research Evidence – A Quality Framework* (London: National Centre for Social Research).

Stevens P M J, Schade A L, Chalk B and Slevin O D'A (1993) *Understanding Research* (Edinburgh: Campion Press).

Streubert H J and Carpenter D R (1999) *Qualitative Research in Nursing: Advancing the Humanistic Imperative*, 2nd edn (Philadelphia, PA: Lippincott).

Treloar C, Champress S, Simpson P L and Higginbotham N (2000) Critical appraisal checklist for qualitative research studies. *Indian Journal of Pediatrics*, **67**, 3:347–51.

Webb C (2004) Editor's note: Analysis of papers in JAN in 2002. *Journal of Advanced Nursing*, **45**, 3:229–31.

Yam B M C and Kan S (2004) Comparison of the experiences of having a sick baby in a neonatal intensive care unit among mothers with or without the right of abode in Hong Kong. *Journal of Clinical Nursing*, **3**, 1:118–19.

18 Utilising Research in Clinical Practice

Introduction

Despite the proliferation of research and the increase in research training and education of nurses and midwives, research findings are being used only sporadically in practice. This chapter discusses the barriers to, and facilitators of, the implementation of research and some of the strategies that have been used to facilitate its use. Theories of change and models of research utilisation are also introduced.

The meaning of research utilisation

There are many definitions of research utilisation in clinical practice (Weiss, 1979; Stetler and DiMaggio, 1991; Estabrooks, 1998). They all involve the transfer of knowledge generated by research to clinical practice. This can be achieved directly, indirectly and in ways which practitioners may not even be aware of. Weiss (1979) distinguishes between conceptual (or cognitive) use and instrumental use. For example, a study on 'cancer symptom transition periods of children and families' (Woodgate and Degner, 2004) provides useful insights for professionals working with this group of children. The substantive theory developed in this study 'provides nurses with a new perspective for childhood cancer', and could 'assist in the development of symptom relief strategies that will help to contain symptoms and improve overall quality of life for children and families' (Woodgate and Degner, 2004). The findings of a study may add, confirm or reject what the reader may already know or they may be totally new. Either way the study can affect the ways in which practitioners think. Closs and Cheater (1994) explain that 'the nature of many research projects is such that direct changes to practice are inappropriate – rather they may extend the way that nurses think about what they do, how they relate to the people they care for, and generally stimulate more reflecting and questioning attitudes'.

It is often difficult to describe when and how conceptual use takes place, and it is therefore difficult to assess how widespread it is. Practitioners may not be conscious of how their current practice is influenced by the sum total of what they read or experience. Conceptual use can be inferred from data on how often nurses access and read the research literature, take part in journal clubs, conferences and other discussion groups. It is implied that these activities may influence their practice. However, empirical evidence on conceptual use is hard to come by. Stetler and DiMaggio (1991), in a study of clinical nurse specialists, found that '75 per cent of the sample reported their most frequent level of use as "conceptual"' and that they 'used it to improve their understanding or influence their way of thinking about issues'. More studies need to be carried out to shed some light on the conceptual use of research in practice.

'Instrumental' use is the direct application of research findings into one's practice. If research shows that a particular treatment is the most effective in treating a certain condition, then it is expected that nurses will implement this finding by using the recommended treatment. It is instrumental use which is more commonly referred to when the term 'utilisation of research' is used. It is also relatively easier to study than other forms of research utilisation since it can be done by observing what practitioners do.

Other ways in which research can be useful to clinical practice include learning from the process of research. This type of use involves 'borrowing' research tools such as questionnaires or scales developed by researchers, to diagnose and assess health problems. Interview skills acquired while undertaking a research module may also be of value to those who routinely interview patients or clients in clinical practice. Another use of research, which Estabrooks (1998) calls 'persuasive use', is when practitioners collect data to influence policy at local or national levels.

The research–practice gap

The research–practice gap can be simply described as the failure of knowledge generated by research to be implemented in clinical practice. A gap is assumed to exist when there is sufficient research knowledge about a particular practice which is not used by practitioners. This seems to be an on-going problem. Hodnett et al. (1996) reported that despite excellent summaries of the best research evidence concerning helpful and harmful intrapartum practices that were available to practitioners, three studies in Southern Ontario hospitals revealed that intrapartum care was often not based on research findings.

The research–practice gap or 'the gap between producers and users of knowledge' (Caplan, 1982) exists in other professions as well. Hunt (1987) pointed out that nurses writing on this subject show no awareness that these are problems also identified by other occupational groups 'with more appropriate educational and research dissemination processes than have been developed in nursing systems'. The evidence-based practice movement was founded on the basis that despite an accumulating body of knowledge about the effectiveness of many clinical interventions, there is a gap between what is known and what is practised (Thompson, 1998).

Some much-quoted historical examples of the research–practice gap include the delayed uptake of lemon juice to prevent scurvy. According to Haines and Jones (1994), 'in 1601 James Lancaster showed that lemon juice was effective, but it was not until 1795 that the British Navy adopted the practice (and not until 1865, in the case of the Merchant Navy)'.

There is a gap between the time that knowledge is produced and the time when it is used. According to Drucker (1985), 'the lead time for knowledge to become applicable technology and begin to be accepted on the market is between 25 and 30 years' and 'this has not changed much throughout recorded history'. Drucker (1985) puts the 'lead time' down to 'the nature of knowledge'. Caplan (1982), on the other hand, points to other factors that influence the non-use of research findings:

> Simply because information is timely, relevant, objective and given to the right people in usable form, its use has not been guaranteed. Thus, the 'intelligence' value of the information conveyed does not directly relate to its utilization . . . Bureaucratic, ethical, attitudinal, and social considerations take precedence over the value of information in its own right.

The problem of non-utilisation of research findings is not confined to the present time, to any one discipline nor to any particular country. It continues to be a concern for the international community (Titler, 2004). One can, therefore, ask why it is perceived as a contemporary problem. The main reason seems to be that the volume of research has increased and that, through vastly improved means of communication, we are more aware of it. There is an expectation, therefore, that research utilisation should have increased significantly as a consequence.

Barriers to research utilisation

The reasons why clinicians do not use research in their practice as often as they are expected to do has been the subject of a number of studies and discussion papers (Funk et al., 1991; Le May et al., 1998a; Estabrooks, 1999; Hundley et al., 2000; Retsas, 2000; Parahoo and McCaughan, 2001; Estabrooks et al., 2004). The factors that act as barriers to, and facilitators of, the use of research in practice can be broadly grouped according to the following three overlapping headings:

- personal factors
- contextual factors
- factors related to research and its presentation.

Personal factors

Among the personal factors influencing the use of research are attitudes, knowledge, skills, motivation, critical thinking ability and readiness to change practice.

These factors are intertwined, as they tend to influence one another. For example, a nurse who has positive attitudes towards research may want to know more about research, while, on the other hand, reading research articles can foster a positive attitude towards research. The importance of attitudes as a variable in research utilisation has been demonstrated in a number of studies. In a US study, Champion and Leach (1989) found that attitude had the greatest correlation with research utilisation, while Lacey (1994), in a UK study, reported that attitude alone was a powerful predictor of utilisation. These findings were supported in Hicks's (1995) study of 550 midwives of all grades in England, Scotland and Wales. Studies on the attitudes of nurses and allied health professionals (AHPs) towards research have consistently reported positive attitudes. In a study on research utilisation among nurses in Northern Ireland, Parahoo (2000) compared his findings with those of a previous study in Northern Ireland using the same attitude scale. The results showed significantly more positive attitudes in 1997 than in 1990. Retsas (2000), in an Australian study, found that staff had a high level of readiness and shared a strong sense of valuing the contribution that research can make to improving practice. Hundley et al.'s (2000) study of nurses and midwives in four clinical areas in Scotland reported that the majority of participants expressed positive attitudes towards research and colleagues who carry out research. A study of occupational therapists also reported positive attitudes (Humphris et al., 2000).

While positive attitudes are important, it is difficult without knowledge to make use of findings. Nurses need to know about (be aware of) research studies and their findings. They also need the knowledge to understand, and the skills to evaluate, research. These two types of knowledge are not mutually exclusive. Evaluating research, although a prerequisite for the implementation of findings, is a skill that cannot easily be acquired. It can, however, be developed over a period of time through practice, often with the help of more experienced colleagues. Hundley et al. (2000) pointed out that 'despite the introduction of research methods into modern nursing and midwifery curriculae, lack of knowledge and skills remains a major barrier to reading research'.

The skills to access research literature with the use of information technology is crucial if clinicians are to maximise the potential of this medium in disseminating information. There is as yet very little research on how skilled nurses are in using information technology and how often they use it to access research and other information. Hundley et al. (2000) reported that less than a third of their participants had used electronic resources. Internet use at work among a sample of nurses in Alberta, Canada was reported to be low compared with physicians and the general public despite adequate workplace access (Estabrooks et al., 2003). In a UK study Veeramah (2004) reported that a number of respondents wanted 'more help with searching the literature, implementing research findings in practice and developing their critical appraisal skills further'.

Motivation, readiness to change and an inquisitive disposition are character-istics which can contribute towards research utilisation. The frequency with which nurses access the literature is often an indication of their thirst for knowl-edge. Thompson et al. (2001), who explored the sources of information which nurses accessed for decision making found that 'text-based and electronic sources of research-based information yielded only small amounts of utility for practising clinicians'.

Attitudes, knowledge and skills are prerequisites for, but cannot guarantee, research utilisation. Sleep (1992), referring to the non-implementation of find-ings in midwifery practice, warns that 'no matter how much clinicians learn about research in the educational setting, there is a problem about transferring this knowledge into the real world of practice'. Hunt (1987), who experienced many obstacles when undertaking a project aimed at evaluating and imple-menting research findings, points out the limitations of focusing solely on research education. She explains that 'the hope that if individual nurses could be educated to read research they could change their practice accordingly', seems to be 'too simplistic'.

Education is, therefore, a necessary but not sufficient condition for integrat-ing research and practice. The context in which implementation takes place is of utmost importance. As DeMey (1982) succinctly puts it: 'a solution which seems theoretically very sound and elegant might change into an awkward and inefficient scheme because in the "context of application" new and unforeseen factors drastically alter the picture'.

Contextual factors

The most frequently identified barriers to, and facilitators of, research utilisa-tion relate to the setting and the organisation where research is to be imple-mented. Funk et al. (1991) developed a Barriers to Research Utilization Scale, which has been used in a number of studies (see e.g. Funk et al., 1991; Walsh, 1997a, 1997b; Closs and Lewin, 1998; Dunn et al., 1998; Nolan et al., 1998; Nilsson Kajermo et al., 2000; Parahoo, 2000). The scale consists of 29 items divided into four sub-scales: characteristics of 'the adopter', characteristics of 'the organisation', characteristics of the 'innovation' and characteristics of 'the communication of research'.

In Funk et al.'s (1991) US study, all eight items in their Barriers to Research Utilization Scale relating to the characteristics of the setting were rated among the top ten barriers to using research findings in clinical practice. Parahoo (2000), in a similar study, also found that seven out of the top ten barriers reported by nurses in Northern Ireland were related to 'setting'. The main contextual factors identified by nurses, midwives and AHPs, in studies on research utilisation, were: time, managers' support, autonomy, access to libraries, training opportunities, a culture of critical enquiry and a comprehen-sive and operational research and development strategy.

Time

Studies in a number of countries and on different health professions (nursing, dietetics, occupational therapy, physiotherapy, speech and language therapy and midwifery) have reported lack of time as one of the major factors that impede research utilisation (Funk et al., 1991; Dunn et al., 1998; Closs and Lewin, 1998; Humphris et al., 2000; Parahoo, 2000; Retsas, 2000). 'Insufficient time on the job to implement new ideas' was ranked first in Dunn et al. (1998), second in Funk et al. (1991) and third in Parahoo (2000). Retsas (2000) concluded from his study of registered nurses in Australia, that 'if the use of research evidence by nurses is to increase, the most important organisational change that needs to occur is increasing the time available for nurses to achieve this goal'.

One can argue that it does not necessarily take more time to change one's practice. For example, using one type of dressing instead of another may not take more time. In fact if the new dressing is more effective it could save time in the long run. What nurses and other health professionals mean is that there is insufficient time due to workload levels and other demands to 'stop and think', to access and read the relevant literature and to go on training courses. According to Hundley et al. (2000) the finding that time is the main barrier is to be expected given the number of competing demands on practitioners. Expecting nurses to use their off-duty time to read and evaluate research makes research an optional and separate activity from practice, thereby enlarging rather than closing the theory–practice gap.

Managers' support

Titler et al. (1994) believe that managers can support staff by recognising those 'who participate in making practice changes, assisting staff by trouble shooting problems and by rewarding those staff members who serve as advocates for change through positive performance evaluations'. More crucially, middle managers have a leadership role as well as access to, and control over, limited resources. They can encourage or limit the autonomy of practitioners. They can take decisions to provide time for staff to engage in research or research-related activities. Yet in studies that have used the Barriers Scale two items which have consistently been rated high by practitioners are: 'the nurse does not feel she/he has enough authority to change patient care procedures' and 'lack of manager's support', (see e.g. Funk et al., 1991; Parahoo, 2000). In Funk et al.'s (1991) study the item 'administration will not allow implementation' was ranked 5th by practitioners and 24th by managers. Le May et al. (1998b) pointed to research evidence, albeit limited, which suggests that there is a gulf between practitioners and middle managers when support for the implementation of research is considered. Their study found that there was a dissonance in the way practitioners and managers perceive research in clinical practice.

The role of managers is pivotal in supporting staff, in particular by ensuring that resources and staffing levels are adequate, and facilitating staff training through time release, funding and by supporting them when there is opposition to change. Equally important are managers who, through leadership and support, create an environment where change, if appropriate, is seen as desirable. Nurses also identified management style, the need to listen to staff and to recognise achievements as facilitators of research utilisation (Parahoo, 2000). According to Bray and Rees (1995), policy directives frequently constrain practices, and authority may play an important part in what nurses are 'allowed' to do.

All changes involve a degree of disruption and discomfort. There is little surprise that there is often resistance to altering one's practice. Resistance to change is cited by several authors as a major influence inhibiting the introduction of research into clinical care (Sleep, 1992). Resistance can come from other health professionals as well as nursing managers and one's own colleagues. The pressure to conform to existing practices has been well documented in the nursing literature (Kane and Parahoo, 1994; Luker, 1984; Melia, 1984).

Autonomy

In studies on research utilisation nurses have also identified 'lack of authority to make changes', 'lack of autonomy' and 'doctors will not co-operate with implementation' as significant barriers to research implementation. Lack of autonomy is particularly felt by hospital-based nurses and those in lower grades. Lacey (1994) found that doctors were cited as potentially obstructive in the implementation of nursing research.

There may also be links between management systems and the use of research in clinical practice. Ersser and Tutton (1991) reported that clinical areas characterised by devolved authority and responsibility for care was linked to more innovative practice. In a study of five district nursing practices in the UK, Kenrick and Luker (1996) found that in one health district (where the organisational structure was flat) district nurses reported a higher extent of research utilisation than in the other four health districts (which had a strict hierarchical structure). Closs and Lewin (1998) concluded from their study of four therapies (dietetics, occupational therapy, physiotherapy and speech and language therapy) that, 'in contrast with findings from nurses, the problem of authority to change practices was less prevalent among therapists'. This may be because they have more autonomy in their practice than most nurses.

Access to information technology

Access to research information in developed countries has continued to improve. Universities and other nurse educational institutions provide web access to their students to relevant databases. At practice level too there is evidence of accessibility of electronic resources (Hillan et al., 1998; Hundley et al., 2000). Information on the extent to which nurses and midwives actually access these sources of information, how they use them, and for what purposes, is only beginning to emerge (Hillan et al., 1998; Royle et al., 2000).

Factors related to research and its presentation

The research itself and the way in which it is presented and communicated can determine whether or not it is eventually used. No matter how skilful nurses are at evaluating research, how positive their attitudes are or how much support they get from their managers, if the research itself (the product) is not known to nurses, is of poor quality, is not relevant to their practice or is hardly comprehensible, it will not be used.

The failure to find studies relating to clinical practice has been reported to be a common impeding factor (Pettengill et al., 1994). The nurses in Funk et al.'s (1991) study also reported that accessibility of the research and the way it was presented was a problem. They suggested that research be reported in journals frequently read by clinicians and written so as to give more specific explanations of the clinical implications in a 'how to' format.

The best studies are of little value if they are incomprehensible to those who could benefit most from them – practitioners. The language and style of research reports often present difficulties for practitioners. Funk et al. (1991) made the following observations:

> Research reports are commonly full of research jargon intended for other researchers, not clinicians; they emphasise the reliability and validity of measurements rather than what was actually measured; they focus on the statistical tests performed rather than on the meaning of the findings; they rarely indicate what information may be applicable to practice, even when supporting research has been published.

Edwards-Beckett (1990) suggested that 'for results to be of interest to clinicians, researchers need to spell out the meaning of their results in their manuscripts, identify previous studies that contributed to the current findings and clearly state the limits of generalisability'.

One cannot expect nurses and other health professionals to implement findings if they do not exist. Estabrooks (1999) pointed out that there are insufficient synthesised research findings and 'sound integrative literature reviews that would provide clinicians with digestible and readily available material'. Even when findings are available one can question how readily they can be applied to clinical practice, given that some of the studies have small samples of population which may or may not be similar to the patients or clients which nurses work with in their clinical environments. Rolfe (1996) goes further when he remarked that 'few academics stop to consider that perhaps the theory–practice gap is a result not of the failure of nurses to put theory into practice, but of the inadequacy of the theory itself; that perhaps theoreticians are out of touch with the needs and realities of clinical practice and are generating theories and models which either have no relevance to practising nurses, or else which are impossible to translate into practice'.

Hunt (1996) points out that less attention is given to the responsibility for non-utilisation held by researchers, mainly that they:

- do not produce their findings in usable form;
- do not study the problems of practitioners;
- do not manage to persuade or convince others of their value;
- do not develop the necessary programmes for the acceptance and introduction of innovation;
- do not have the necessary authority/access.

Hughes and McNeish (2000) reviewed the process of integrating research in social care practice. They identified the following strategies which researchers need to address. Many of these issues are similar to those faced by nurses.

- Provide accessible summaries of research.
- Keep the research report brief and concise.
- Publish in journals or publications which are user friendly.
- Use language and styles of presentation which engage interest.
- Target the material to the needs of the audience.
- Extract the policy and practice implications of research: where possible, this should be done in partnership with practitioners and policy-makers.
- Tailor dissemination events to the target audience and evaluate them: use feedback to inform future dissemination events.
- Use the media.
- Use a combination of dissemination methods.
- Be proactive: by contacting agencies rather than expecting practitioners, managers and policy makers to attend national or regional conferences.
- Understand external factors, such as political sensitivities, financial and administrative mechanisms.

In conclusion, from many of the studies cited above, a number of factors influencing the use of research have been identified. Although factors related to the context in which research is to be implemented are more frequently reported than personal factors, it does not mean the same barriers will exist in every setting. It is also understandable that managers' support is one of the commonly reported impeding factors since it can influence, in turn, the time allocated to nurses, the distribution of workloads, access to research, opportunities for further training and education, financial rewards, autonomy, resistance to change and a host of other factors. However important contextual factors are, without a positive attitude and basic research training to access and to evaluate research, the utilisation of findings will be severely impeded. The starting point seems to be to create a culture in which learning about research is valued and opportunities to acquire knowledge and skills are present. This can be followed by devising strategies to implement research findings, where appropriate.

Strategies to enhance research utilisation

Practitioner research

A number of authors have questioned the existence of a research–practice or theory–practice gap in nursing practice and the way in which this issue is conceptualised. Larsen et al. (2002) claim that there is no research–practice gap, as nurses do not rely on research as a main source of knowledge for practice. They explain that clinical 'nurses are inspired and learn from the context, including each other, and they are active producers of knowledge, not simply recipients of knowledge'. Mulhall (2001) explains the limitations of 'conventional research in meeting the knowledge needs of practitioners as they also need the "know-how" knowledge in order to develop theory from practice'. Conventional research, according to her, produces only the 'know-that' knowledge and is therefore limited in its contribution to nursing practice. Mulhall (2001) supports Rolfe's (1998) view that practitioner-centred research is a useful strategy to complement research produced through more traditional academic routes.

Practitioner research (Reed and Proctor, 1995), practice development research (Clarke and Proctor, 1999) and practitioner-centred research (Rolfe, 1996, 1998; Bourner and O'Hara, 2003; McCormack, 2003) have all developed as ways to fill the research–practice gap by putting the emphasis on practice. Rolfe (1996) explains that the relationship between research and practice is an indirect one, and because of this much nursing research never gets translated into practice. Bourner and O'Hara (2003) propose that we change the formulation of the problem from 'how to raise the impact of research in professional practice' to 'how can professional practice be enhanced by research?'. The starting point for them, therefore, is practice not research.

The advantage of practitioner research is that the research process starts with practice and the research itself is carried out by practitioners with or without the collaboration of outside researchers. According to Clarke and Proctor (1999), this type of research is not separated from practice and therefore 'implementation is not a separate step to be achieved after the research has been completed', as is the case with the way in which research is traditionally carried out.

They point out that the practitioner researcher, by virtue of being an insider, has the knowledge, insight and opportunities to select relevant problems to research, be sensitive to the issues related to the process of collecting data, have a better understanding of the data and be more committed to the dissemination of the findings.

Some examples of practitioner research studies include 'a study of family networks and relationships in community midwifery' (Davies, 1995), 'patients' feelings about patients' (Skeil, 1995), 'reflections on evaluating a course of family therapy' (Stevenson, 1995) and 'the impact of child sexual abuse (Durham, 2002).

This research model, however, implies that practitioners should have enough research 'skills' to be proficient in research. According to Bourner and O'Hara (2003), practitioners would need more training in research. Many nurses who value the practice–research relationship may perceive that the researcher role they have to adopt could put too much pressure on their ever-expanding role.

While blending research with practice makes the study context more real, it raises ethical problems. There is 'potential for exploitation, through privileged access to vulnerable populations and insider information, which could be accessed without appropriate consent' (Durham, 2002). Both action research and practitioner research can, unintentionally, exert pressure on staff and patients to take part in the study. A member of staff who wants to opt out may fear victimisation, while patients may be concerned that refusal on their part may affect their care, since the researchers are also the carers. Disclosure of information by staff and patients may also be problematic (Durham, 2002). In 'conventional research', the researcher is often outside the network of professionals who deal with patients. Thus assurance of confidentiality can be more easily believed by participants than when their carers are also the researchers.

Another approach to bring research and practice together is action research (see also Chapter 10). It is popular with practitioners in a number of professions as it focuses on issues they want to explore and on changes they want to achieve. The contribution of action research towards closing the research–practice gap is in the way research and practice are entwined. The action research cycle of problem identification, data collection, implementation and evaluation of change (and starting again, if required) shows that research is not separated from practice.

Unlike practitioner-centred research, action research can involve practitioners working collaboratively with outside researchers to carry out the project. However, the success of this type of action research depends on how collaborative the project is and the degree of practitioner ownership. Rolfe (1996), believes that the best hope of closing the theory–practice gap is when practitioners and researchers work together and indeed are often the same people. To ensure that change does take place, Rolfe (1996) drawing on the work of Schön (1983), proposes a form of reflexive action research. Using this approach, 'the researcher-practitioner evaluates a situation, develops a theory to account for the situation, tests the theory by constructing and implementing a clinical intervention, evaluates the new situation, modifies the theory accordingly, and so on in a continuous cycle or spiral'.

An example of action research is Galvin et al.'s (1999) study, 'investigating and implementing change within the primary health care nursing team'.

Research utilisation through clinical guidelines

One of the ways in which to facilitate the instrumental use of research in practice is through clinical guidelines. Increasingly they are seen as an important tool to promote evidence-based practice. Clinical guidelines have been defined as 'systematically developed statements to assist practitioner and patient decisions about appropriate healthcare for specific clinical circumstances' (Field and Lohr, 1990). A number of terms such as 'protocols', 'procedures', and 'standards' have been used interchangeably to mean a set of instructions to guide clinical decisions. They provide procedures for practitioners to follow when faced with particular clinical problems.

There has been a significant increase in the number of guidelines in recent years. According to Hurwitz (1994), the annual rate at which the term 'guideline' or 'protocol' appeared in the titles and abstracts of medical articles from 1974 to 1993 was tenfold. Onion and Whalley (1998) noted that 'guidelines development' has become a business in which local and national groups produce competing and overlapping guidelines of varying quality.

The Royal College of Nursing (1995) explains that national clinical guidelines can provide a way for health professionals, patients and service users to work together to make decisions about appropriate care. According to Woolf et al. (1999), the potential benefits for patients are improved quality of clinical decisions and improved health outcomes. Potential limitations include the possibility that recommendations can be wrong and that the evidence on which some guidelines are based could have been wrongly interpreted (Woolf et al. 1999).

Developing guidelines

Clinical guidelines in the past were based mostly on the recommendations of a group of opinion leaders and these were termed 'consensus guidelines'. With the advent of evidence-based practice, more guidelines are being developed based on evidence from systematic reviews. These are referred to as evidence-based guidelines. Onion and Whalley (1998) identify two schools of thought on guidelines – those who think that guidelines should incorporate only the best evidence, and those who believe guidelines should be simple and practical, taking into account local resources, priorities, as well as local opinion and experience.

Guidelines are developed at local, regional and national levels. At local levels, resources and expertise are limited, while at national level it is possible to draw on the skills and expertise of a wider range of professionals. According to Eccles et al. (1996), local groups should identify valid regional and national guidelines and adapt them to local circumstances. However, there are few national guidelines although, within the context of evidence-based practice, more are being developed.

The development of guidelines can be a lengthy, complex process often involving multi-disciplinary groups and requiring considerable skills and resources – in particular, time. Eccles et al. (1996) described the process of the development of evidence-based guidelines for the primary care management of asthma in adults and for the stable angina. They discussed their experiences and the methodological issues they encountered to inform others who are involved in the process of guideline development and for those who wish to know more about the practicalities. The project comprised four groups: a 'project team' (to undertake the day-to-day running of the project), a 'project management team' (to provide technical advice), and two 'guideline development groups' (to produce guideline recommendations). The members of these groups were drawn from a range of backgrounds and disciplines, including general practitioners, practice nurses, physicians, health economists and patient representatives. A systematic review of the literature was carried out and recommendations from the evidence were discussed. There were areas for which no evidence existed or the evidence was poor. To resolve this one group looked at existing national consensus guidelines while the other made recommendations based on their experience.

The preliminary guidelines were each reviewed by nine reviewers. These consisted of 'methods experts', 'content area' experts (to review the interpretation, logic and clarity), and potential users (to appraise the clinical applicability and usefulness of the guidelines). The development of the guidelines was expected to take 12 months, but it took a further six months to complete (Eccles et al., 1996).

Validity of guidelines

The validity of guidelines is important as it can inspire confidence in practitioners to use them. This depends mainly on who develops the guidelines and the evidence on which they are based. Therefore the process of guideline development should be transparent and the methods used should be made explicit.

A number of strategies and methods that can be used together or singly include: focus groups, postal questionnaires, the Delphi technique, peer group consensus and literature review. There is no conclusive evidence that some of these methods to develop guidelines are more effective than others in changing practice (Grimshaw and Russell, 1994). The validity of guidelines developed without a literature review or after an unsystematic literature review can be questioned (Grimshaw and Russell, 1993). According to Grimshaw and Russell (1993), although guidelines developed locally are less likely to be scientifically valid through lack of technical skills in guideline development, clinical expertise and resources, they are more likely to change practice. This is supported by Worrall et al.'s (1997) study which showed that local guidelines produced significant improvements in practice when compared with national guidelines. Therein lies the contradiction. While the development of valid guidelines is most efficiently done at a regional and national level (Grimshaw et al., 1998), they are less likely to be used than local guidelines which tend to rely less on sound evidence. Stokes et al. (1998) point to the potential conflict between the need for validity and the relevance of guidelines to local circumstances.

The answer may be to adapt national guidelines to local use, but this could lead to bias as to which components of the original guideline are selected or rejected, thereby threatening the validity of the original guideline.

Disseminating guidelines

Once developed, guidelines have to be disseminated to those for whom they were intended. This process itself is poorly understood. A number of strategies have been used to disseminate guidelines. These include distributing hard copies of guidelines to practitioners and patients, computer-generated reminders in patients' notes and educational initiatives that focus specifically on the guidelines.

The evidence available on the relative effectiveness and efficiency of different disseminating strategies is still sparse (Grimshaw and Russell, 1994). This is echoed by Cheater and Closs (1997), who observed that although much attention is given to the development of guidelines, little is known about the relative effectiveness of different ways of communicating them to potential users, and ensuring that they are incorporated in practice. Worrall et al. (1997), who studied the effects of clinical practice guidelines on patient outcomes in primary care, found that computerised or automated reminder systems were more effective than physicians' recall. Thomas et al. (1999) concluded from their systematic review of clinical guidelines in nursing, midwifery and the therapies that apart from the provision of printed materials, the most commonly used method of dissemination was lectures or training sessions. Although they pointed out that research into the best means of dissemination and implementing clinical guidelines is in its infancy in nursing, they concluded from the findings of their review that active dissemination strategies, (e.g. educational interventions) may be more effective than passive dissemination (e.g. handouts) in bringing about change. It is also likely that a combination of dissemination strategies would be more effective than any single one, and that some may work better in some circumstances than in others.

Implementing guidelines

Davis and Taylor-Vaisey (1997) point out that the creation of guidelines without significant attention to their adoption is clearly a sterile exercise and that it wastes precious intellectual and human resources. Yet as Hunter (1998) remarked, the focus on implementation has so far taken second place behind the development of knowledge.

Although the dissemination and implementation of guidelines are discussed separately from the process of development, in practice the involvement of staff at the development stage is crucial to the likelihood of implementation. The dissemination and implementation strategies are interdependent. Davis and Taylor-Vaisey (1997) grade interventions to disseminate or implement guidelines as 'weak', 'moderately effective' and 'relatively strong'. Weak interventions comprise 'didactic traditional education' and the distribution of guidelines (in paper form). Moderately effective interventions include 'audit and feedback' as well as the involvement of peers and opinion leaders. Relatively strong interventions involve the use of reminder systems (in patients' notes), educational initiatives and multiple interventions.

Like all policies attempting to change professional practice, implementation of guidelines has proved difficult (Cluzeau et al., 1994). Cheater and Closs (1997) concluded that 'the implementation of strategies are likely to be most successful when they are: individualized; interactive; responsive to local problems; occur close to the time of clinical decision-making; and provided regularly'. Grimshaw and Russell (1994) believe that if guidelines are to achieve maximum benefit, more attention should be paid to the principles of change management, the need for leadership, the avoidance of unnecessary uncertainty, good communication, and, above all, time.

Outcomes of guidelines

One of the largest systematic reviews of published evaluations of clinical guidelines was carried out by Grimshaw and Russell (1993). Of the 59 studies which met their inclusion criteria for rigour, 55 showed significant improvements in the process of care, which was measured mainly by change in the practice of doctors, in particular their compliance with the recommendations of guidelines. Eleven of the studies reviewed also assessed the effects of guidelines on the outcome of care and nine of them showed significant improvements, in terms of fewer admissions, fewer complications, reduction in symptoms or more patient compliance with treatment or prevention. This rigorous review led Grimshaw and Russell (1993) to conclude that 'explicit guidelines do improve clinical practice'. The Nuffield Institute for Health (1994) reviewed 87 studies examining the effects of guidelines on the process of care (measured by adherence with recommendations) and concluded that there were significant improvements in 81 of them. Twelve out of 17 studies which assessed patient outcomes also reported significant improvements. The South Thames Evidence-based Practice (STEP) project, which involved the use of guidelines, was successful in showing 'measurable change in patient and staff outcomes, with some indications of organisational change and early signs of sustainability' (Ross et al., 2001).

The evidence on the effectiveness of guidelines is, however, by no means conclusive. Worrall et al. (1997) reviewed 13 studies (RCTs) which assessed the effectiveness of guidelines in improving patient outcomes in primary care. They found that only five out of 13 (38 per cent) studies showed significant improvements in outcomes. They also reported that in these studies 'improvement was noted for only a proportion of conditions studied, for only certain population subgroups, or for only a limited period'. Worrall et al. (1997) concluded that their review showed little evidence that guidelines were effective in improving patient outcomes in primary care and that 'even when the change was statistically significant, it was usually modest'. Another study that showed the difficulties with using guidelines was that carried out by Wye and McClenahan (2000), in which they evaluated the process and outcomes of 17 projects on the implementation of evidence in practice. Of these 17 projects, only three 'brought about a systematic change in clinical practice' and of these three, only two were reported to have improved patient care (Wye and McClenahan, 2000).

No reviews of studies evaluating the effects of guidelines on nursing practice or patient outcomes are available. Cheater and Closs (1997) reviewed studies on the dissemination and implementation of guidelines in nursing practice but found that none was readily available. They cautioned against extrapolating from studies on medical practice. Thomas et al. (1999), in their review of clinical guidelines in nursing and midwifery, also reported on their dissemination and implementation.

The complexity of change

According to Humphris (1997), it is important not to underestimate the complexity of the task of achieving changes in practice. The reasons for why change happens – or not – are not well understood. The usual distinction between traditionalists (those who resist change) and progressivists (those who are more receptive to the need for change) is too simplistic. Sometimes the same practitioners use some guidelines but not others. For example, Mansfield (1995), in a study of attitudes and behaviours towards clinical guidelines, found that 51 per cent of respondents only used half the guidelines they were aware of. Buchan (1993) believes that 'new knowledge' is not adopted as enthusiastically as 'new products'. According to her, doctors prescribe drugs for which they have received no formal education and eagerly adopt technical innovations such as laparoscopic surgery. These examples show that health care professions are selective in their change behaviour.

Drug manufacturers invest heavily in promoting their products while health care researchers lack the advantages of organised, aggressive, commercial marketing to sell their findings (Buchan, 1993). Being aware of guidelines and financial incentives (based on cost/benefit evaluations) are not enough to influence behavioural changes among health care professionals (Mittman et al., 1992). A number of models and conceptual frameworks for the implementation of research into practice have been offered (Mittman et al., 1992; Haines and Jones, 1994; Kitson et al., 1998; Moulding et al., 1999). Mittman et al.'s (1992) Social Influence Theory is based on a large body of theory and research in social psychology, sociology, health behaviour change and health services research. It suggests that 'decisions, actions and behaviour' are guided by 'habit and custom, by assumptions, beliefs and values held by peers and by prevailing practices and social norms that define appropriate behaviour' (Mittman et al., 1992). According to the Social Influence Theory, guidelines dissemination and implementation policies and interventions must take into account existing patterns of social interaction and influence, and must be carefully designed to meet the characteristics of target clinicians and practice settings. Social Influence Theory recognises that patterns of influence and interaction vary widely across specialities, practice settings and other situational variables (Mittman et al., 1992).

In Kitson et al.'s (1998) Multi-dimensional Framework for Implementing Research into Practice, successful implementation 'is a function of the interplay of three care elements – the level and nature of the evidence, the context or environment in which the research is to be placed, and the method or way in which the process is facilitated'. While Mittman et al. (1992) put more weight on the importance of patterns of social interaction and influences, Kitson et al. (1998) propose that each of the three core elements (evidence, context and facilitation) has equal standing. According to Kitson et al.'s (1998) framework, a combination of three dimensions – research, clinical experience and patient preferences – should be considered when assessing the nature and strength of the evidence. 'Context' is also subdivided into three core elements: an understanding of the prevailing culture, the nature of human relationships and the organisation's approach to routine monitoring of systems and services (Kitson et al., 1998). Finally, 'facilitation' is defined as 'the type of support required to help people change their attitudes, habits, skills, ways of thinking, and working' (Kitson et al., 1998).

Moulding et al.'s (1999) framework for effective management of change is based on the following theories: diffusion of innovation theory (Rogers, 1983); transtheoretical model of behaviour change (Prochaska and DiClemente, 1983); health education theory (Green et al., 1980); social influence theory (Mittman et al., 1992); and social ecology theory (Stokols, 1992).

They propose the following five steps for the successful dissemination and implementation of guidelines. These are:

Step 1:   assessment of practitioner's stage of readiness to change.
Step 2:   assessment of specific barriers to guideline use.
Step 3:   determination of appropriate level of intervention.
Step 4:   design of dissemination and implementation strategies.
Step 5:   evaluation of the implementation.

(Moulding et al., 1999)

What these and other conceptual frameworks for the implementation of guidelines or research findings in practice emphasise, is the complexity of behaviour change, the need to take into account a number of factors relating to the innovation, the practitioners and the environment in which they work. There is also a need to look at the broader political picture. As Rafferty et al. (1996) explain:

> Political as well as practical problems attend the 'translation' of theory into practice; understanding the ways in which nurses can influence the policy process and the possibilities for transformation are important preconditions for change.

Translating research into practice

Translating research into nursing practice has a history of over 30 years. Some of the best-known earlier projects in the USA include the Western Interstate Commission for Higher Education in Nursing (WICHEN) regional programme on nursing research development (Krueger et al., 1978); the Conduct and Utilization of Research in Nursing (CURN) project (Horsley et al., 1983); and the Nursing Child Assessment Satellite Training (NCAST) project (King et al., 1981). According to Titler (2004), findings from these studies showed that nursing practices could be changed. However, she explains, 'the contextual variables and the dose, type and frequency of the translation interventions were not clearly elucidated in these projects' (Titler, 2004).

In the UK, Hunt (1987) led a project involving nurse teachers and librarians from the schools of nursing on the management of mouth care and preoperative fasting. After evaluating and synthesising the literature on these topics, policies were drawn up following consultation with the relevant personnel, including central sterile supply department (CSSD) staff, anaesthetists, pharmacists, dental consultants and nursing staff. When staff found it difficult to translate the policy into practice, problem-solving and quality circles groups were set up. Hunt (1987) discussed a number of difficulties experienced during the project. These included the fact it took nearly two years for seven nurse teachers and a librarian to identify, evaluate and synthesise relevant information and produce a 'reference' package. Hunt (1987) explained that 'even at the end of two years' work the information collected on mouth care could not be regarded as up to date' and 'by the time the package was put together it was in need of updating'.

Titler (2004) points out that much of the effort in earlier 'translating research in practice' projects was spent on synthesis of evidence prior to implementing the evidence in practice and that many of the strategies used to promote the adoption of evidence-based practices were 'largely untested'. This problem is now partly addressed as the synthesis of evidence and the development of guidelines are increasingly being undertaken by national and international organisations. Some of these include the UK National Institute for Clinical Excellence (www.nice.org.uk), the Scottish Intercollegiate Guidelines Network (www.sign.ac.uk), the Royal College of Nursing (www.rcn.org.uk/guidelines.php), the Agency for Health Care Research and Quality (www.ahcpr.guidelines.php) and the Joanna Briggs Institute (www.joannabriggs.edu.au/about/home.php). There are, of course, many others which can be identified by a quick search on the worldwide web. For example, the Turning Research into Practice (TRIP) web-site (http://www.tripdatabase.com) is a useful database of publications and links to organisations involved in the development of guidelines and in evidence-based practice.

Recent projects focusing on the implementation and utilisation of research in clinical practice in the UK include: the Assisting Clinical Effectiveness in South Thames programme [ACE] (Miller et al., 1998); the Promoting Action on Clinical Effectiveness programme [PACE] (Dunning, 1998); and the South Thames Evidence-based Practice Project [STEP] (Redfern and Christian, 2003; Redfern et al., 2003).

From these and other similar projects, a number of factors which can lead to the successful utilisation of research practice have been identified. These are:

- The recognition that the linear model of change is simplistic. This model assumes that 'the process of change will proceed through a logical step-by-step progression from one stage to the next' (Redfern and Christian, 2003). There are many factors related to people, context and organisation which are unpredictable. Redfern and Christian (2003) found that the 'linear model of change can work in settings with high levels of certainty' but not in 'organisations characterised by uncertainty'.

- There should be an assessment of staff's needs and of what needs to be changed. Attitudes, motivation and skills are crucial to the success of change programmes.

- Projects should be underpinned by one or a combination of models or theories of change.

- Involving patients can help to improve outcomes (Dunning, 1998).

- Academic and practitioner partnerships can be helpful provided that partnerships have clear parameters, accountability pathways, transparent objectives and recognition of mutual benefits by all stakeholders (Ross et al., 2001).

- Opinion leaders/facilitators can provide the necessary leadership to motivate and empower those involved in the change process (McLaren et al., 2002; Tanner and Hale, 2002).

- Guidelines provide a useful vehicle for the implementation of evidence in practice.

- Projects should involve all relevant professionals.

For a thorough review of research implementation strategies see 'Getting Evidence into Practice' (NHS Centre for Reviews and Dissemination, 1999).

SUMMARY

Summary and conclusion

The research–practice gap continues to be a concern for health professionals and policy makers. The main barriers seem to be 'lack of time', 'lack of managers' support' and lack of authority to make changes. Others conceptualise the problem as the lack of research relevant to practice. A number of approaches such as practitioner-centred research, action research and the use of evidence-based guidelines have been proposed as a means to increase research utilisation in clinical practice. This chapter has also highlighted lessons which can be learnt from research utilisation projects.

What is clear is that change is a complex process which should take into account the change agent/s, the change or innovation to be implemented and the environment (including the support structure).

The success of evidence-based practice in nursing will ultimately depend on recognising all these factors at the local level and the influence of the broader socioeconomic and polical factors at the national level which impede or facilitate change.

References

Bourner T and O'Hara S (2003) Practitioner centred research. http://www.1mu.ac.uk/lss/staffsup/confreps/bourne-.htm. Accessed on 7 January 2003.

Bray J and Rees C (1995) The relevance of research. *Practice Nursing*, **6**, 7:33–4.

Buchan H (1993) Clinical guidelines: acceptance and promotion. *Quality in Health Care*, 2:213–14.

Caplan N (1982) Social research and public policy at the national level. In: D B P Kallen, G B Kosse, H C Wagenaar, J J J Kloprogge and M Vorbeck (eds), *Social Science Research and Public Policy-Making: A Reappraisal* (Netherlands: NFER).

Champion V L and Leach A (1989) Variables related to research utilization in nursing: an empirical investigation. *Journal of Advanced Nursing*, 14:705–10.

Cheater F M and Closs S J (1997) The effectiveness of methods of dissemination and implementation of clinical guidelines for nursing practice: a selective review. *Clinical Effectiveness in Nursing*, 1:4–15.

Clarke C and Procter S (1999) Practice development: ambiguity in research and practice. *Journal of Advanced Nursing*, **30**, 4:975–82.

Closs S J and Cheater F M (1994) Utilization of nursing research: culture, interest and support. *Journal of Advanced Nursing*, **19**:762–73.

Closs S J and Lewin B J P (1998) Perceived barriers to research utilization: a survey of four therapies. *British Journal of Therapy and Rehabilitation*, **5**, 3:151–5.

Cluzeau F, Littlejohns P and Grimshaw J M (1994) Editorial: Appraising clinical guidelines: towards a 'which' guide for purchasers. *Quality in Health Care*, **3**:121–2.

Davies J (1995) A study of family networks and relationships in community midwifery. In: J Reed and S Procter (eds), *Practitioner Research in Health Care* (London: Chapman & Hall).

Davis A D and Taylor-Vaisey A (1997) Translating guidelines into practice. *Canadian Medical Association*, **157**:408–16.

DeMey M T (1982) Action and knowledge from a cognitive point of view. In D B P Kallen, G B Kosse, H C Wagenaar, J J J Kloprogge and M Vorbeck (eds), *Social Science Research and Public Policy-Making: A Reappraisal* (Netherlands: NFER).

Drucker P F (1985) *Innovations and Entrepreneurship: Practice and Principles* (London: Heinemann).

Dunn V, Crichton N, Roe B, Seers K and Williams K (1998) Using research for practice: a UK experience of the BARRIERS Scale. *Journal of Advanced Nursing*, **27**:1203–10.

Dunning M (1998) Securing change: Lessons from the PACE programme. *Nursing Times*, **94**, 34:51–2.

Durham A (2002) Developing a sensitive practitioner research methodology for studying the impact of child sexual abuse. *British Journal of Social Work*, **32**:429–42.

Eccles M, Clapp Z, Grimshaw J, Adams P C, Higgins B, Purves I and Russell I (1996) Developing valid guidelines: methodological and procedural issues from the North of England Based Guideline Development Project. *Quality in Health Care*, **5**:44–50.

Edwards-Beckett J (1990) Nursing research utilization techniques. *Journal of Nursing Administration*, **20**, 11:25–30.

Ersser S and Tutton E (1991) *Primary Nursing in Perspective* (London: Scutari Press).

Estabrooks C A (1998) Will evidence-based nursing practice make practice perfect? *Canadian Journal of Nursing Research*, **30**, 1:15–36.

Estabrooks C A (1999) Mapping the research utilization field in nursing. *Canadian Journal of Nursing Research*, **31**, 1:53–72.

Estabrooks C A, O'Leary K A, Ricker K L and Humphrey C K (2003) The Internet and access to evidence: how are nurses positioned? *Journal of Advanced Nursing*, **42**, 1:73–81.

Estabrooks C A, Winther C and Derksen L (2004) Mapping the field: A bibliometric analysis of the research utilization literature in nursing. *Nursing Research*, **53**, 5:293–303.

Field M J and Lohr K N (1990) *Clinical Practice Guidelines: Direction of a New Program* (Washington, DC: National Academy Press).

Funk S G, Champagne M T, Wiese R A and Tornquist E M (1991) Barriers to using research findings in practice: the clinician's perspective. *Applied Nursing Research*, **4**, 2:90–5.

Galvin K, Andrews C, Jackson D, Cheesman S, Fudge T, Ferris R and Graham I (1999) Investigating and implementing change within the primary health care nursing team. *Journal of Advanced Nursing*, **30**, 1:238–47.

Green L, Kreuter M and Deeds S, et al. (1980) *Health Education Planning: A Diagnostic Approach* (Palo Alto, CA: Mayfield Press).

Grimshaw J M and Russell I T (1993) Effect of clinical guidelines on medical practice: a systematic review of rigorous evaluations. *The Lancet*, **342**:1317–22.

Grimshaw J M and Russell I T (1994) Achieving health gain through clinical guidelines II: Ensuring guidelines change medical practice. *Quality in Health Care*, **3**:45–52.

Grimshaw J M, Watson M S and Eccles M (1998) A false dichotomy. Commentary on 'Clinical guidelines: ways ahead'. *Journal of Evaluation in Clinical Practice*, **4**, 4:295–8.

Haines A and Jones R (1994) Implementing findings of research. *British Medical Journal*, **308**:1488–92.

Hicks C (1995) A factor analytic study of midwives' attitudes in research. *Midwifery*, **11**:11–17.

Hillan E M, McGuire M M and Cooper M (1998) Computers in midwifery practice: a view from the labour ward. *Journal of Advanced Nursing*, **27**:24–9.

Hodnett E D, Kaufman K, O'Brien-Pallas L, Chipman M, Watson-MacDonell J and Hunsburger W (1996) A strategy to promote research-based nursing care: effects on childbirth outcomes. *Research in Nursing and Health*, **19**:13–20.

Horsley J A, Crane J, Crabtree M K and Wood D J (1983) *Using Research to Improve Nursing Practice: A Guide* (New York: Grune & Stratton).

Hughes M and McNeish D (2000) *Linking Research and Practice* (Basildon: Barnado's Child Care Publications).

Humphris D (1997) Implementing research findings in practice. *Nursing Standard*, **11**, 33:49–56.

Humphris D, Hamilton S, O'Halloran P, Fisher S and Littlejohns P (1999) Do diabetes nurse specialists utilise research evidence? *Practical Diabetes International*, **16**, 2:47–50.

Humphris D, Littlejohns P, Victor C, O'Halloran P and Peacock J (2000) Implementing evidence-based practice: Factors that influence the use of research evidence by occupational therapists. *British Journal of Occupational Therapists*, **63**, 11:516–22.

Hundley V, Milne J, Leighton-Beck L, Graham W and Fitzmaurice A (2000) Raising research awareness among midwives and nurses: does it work? *Journal of Advanced Nursing*, **31**, 1:78–88.

Hunt J (1996) Editorial: Barriers to research utilization. *Journal of Advanced Nursing*, **23**, 3:423–5.

Hunt M (1987) The process of translating research findings into nursing practice. *Journal of Advanced Nursing*, **12**:101–10.

Hunter D (1998) Clinical guidelines, EBM and health policy. *Journal of Evaluation in Clinical Practice*, **4**, 4:305–7.

Hurwitz B (1994) Clinical guidelines: proliferation and medicolegal significance. *Quality in Health Care*, **3**:37–44.

Kane M and Parahoo K (1994) Lifting: why nurses follow bad practice. *Nursing Standard*, **8**, 25:34–8.

Kenrick M and Luker K A (1996) An exploration of the influence of managerial factors on research utilization in district nursing practice. *Journal of Advanced Nursing*, **23**:697–704.

King D, Barnard K E and Hoehn R (1981) Disseminating the results of nursing research. *Nursing Outlook*, **29**, 3:164–9.

Kitson A, Harvey G and McCormack B (1998) Enabling the implementation of evidence based practice: a conceptual framework. *Quality in Heath Care*, 7 149–58.

Krueger J, Nelson A and Wolanin M O (1978) *Nursing Research: Development, Collaboration and Utilization* (Germantown, ND: Aspen Systems).

Lacey E A (1994) Research utilisation in nursing practice – a pilot study. *Journal of Advanced Nursing*, **19**:987–95.

Larsen K, Adamsen L, Bjerregaard L and Madsen J K (2002) There is no gap 'per se' between theory and practice: research knowledge and clinical knowledge are developed in different contexts and follow their own logic. *Nursing Outlook*, **50**, 5:204–12.

Le May A, Mulhall A and Alexander C (1998a) Bridging the research–practice gap: exploring the research cultures of practitioners and managers. *Journal of Advanced Nursing*, **28**:428–37.

Le May A, Alexander C and Mulhall A, (1998b) Research-based practice: practitioners' and managers' view. *Managing Clinical Nursing*, **2**:87–92.

Luker K A (1984) Reading nursing: the burden of being different. *International Journal of Nursing Studies*, **21**, 1:1–7.

Mansfield C D (1995) Attitudes and behaviours towards clinical guidelines: the clinicians' perspectives. *Quality in Health Care*, **4**:250–5.

McCormack B (2003) Knowing and acting – A strategic practitioner-focused approach to nursing research and practice development. *Nursing Times Research*, **8**, 2:86–100.

McLaren S, Ross F, Redfern S and Christian S (2002) Focus: Leading opinion and managing change in complex organisations: findings from the South Thames Evidence-Based Practice Project. *Nursing Times Research*, **7**, 6:444–58.

Melia K M (1984) Student nurses' construction of occupational socialisation. *Sociology of Health and Illness*, **6**, 2:132–51.

Miller C, Scholes J and Freeman P (1998) *Evaluation of the 'Assisting Clinical Effectiveness' Programme* (Brighton: Centre for Nursing and Midwifery Research, University of Brighton).

Mittman B S, Tonesk X and Jacobson P D (1992) Implementing clinical practice guidelines: Social influence strategies and practitioner behavior change. *Quality Review Bulletin*, **18**:413–22.

Moulding N T, Silagy C A and Weller D P (1999) A framework for effective management of change in clinical practice: dissemination and implementation of clinical practice guidelines. *Quality in Health Care*, **8**:177–83.

Mulhall A (2001) Bridging the research–practice gap: breaking new ground in health care. *International Journal of Palliative Nursing*, **7**, 8:389–94.

NHS Centre for Reviews and Dissemination (1999) Getting evidence into practice. *Effective Health Care*, **5**, 1:1–16.

Nilsson Kajermo K N, Nordström G, Krusebrant A and Björvell H (2000) Perceptions of research utilization: comparisons between healthcare professionals, nursing students and a reference group of nurse clinicians. *Journal of Advanced Nursing*, **31**: 99–109.

Nolan M, Morgan L, Curran M, Clayton J, Gerrish K and Parker K (1998) Evidence-based care: can we overcome the barriers? *British Journal of Nursing*, **7**, 20:1273–8.

Nuffield Institute for Health (1994) Implementing clinical practice guidelines: can guidelines be used to improve clinical practice? *Effective Health Care*, **8**:1–12.

Onion C W R and Walley T (1998) Clinical guidelines: ways ahead. *Journal of Evaluation in Clinical Practice*, **4**, 4:287–93.

Parahoo K (2000) Barriers to, and facilitators of, research utilization among nurses in Northern Ireland. *Journal of Advanced Nursing*, **31**, 1:89–98.

Parahoo K and McCaughan E M (2001) Research utilization among medical and surgical nurses: a comparison of their self reports and perceptions of barriers and facilitators. *Journal of Nursing Management*, **9**:21–30.

Pettengill M M, Gillies D A and Clark C C (1994) Factors encouraging and discouraging the use of nursing research findings. *Image: Journal of Nursing Scholarship*, **26**, 2:143–8.

Prochaska J O and DiClemente C C (1983) Stages and processes of self-change of smoking: toward an integrative model of change. *Journal of Consultative Clinical Psychology*, **51**:390–5

Rafferty A M, Allcock N and Lathlean J (1996) The theory/practice 'gap': taking issue with the issue. *Journal of Advanced Nursing*, **23**:685–91.

Redfern S and Christian S (2003) Achieving change in health care practice. *Journal of Evaluation in Clinical Practice*, **9**, 2:225–38.

Redfern S, Christian S and Norman I (2003) Evaluating change in health care practice: lessons from three studies. *Journal of Evaluation in Clinical Practice*, **9**, 2:239–49.

Reed J and Procter S (eds) (1995) *Practitioner Research in Health Care* (London: Chapman & Hall).

Retsas A (2000) Barriers to using research evidence in nursing practice. *Journal of Advanced Nursing*, **31**, 3:599–606.

Rogers E (1983) *Diffusion of Innovations* (New York: The Free Press, Macmillan).

Rolfe G (1996) Going to extremes: action research, grounded practice and the theory–practice gap in nursing. *Journal of Advanced Nursing*, **24**:1315–20.

Rolfe G (1998) *Expanding Nursing Knowledge* (Oxford: Butterworth Heinemann).

Ross F, McLaren S, Redfern S and Warwick C (2001) Partnerships for changing practice: lessons from South Thames Evidence-Based Practice project (STEP). *Nursing Times Research*, **6**, 5:817–27.

Royal College of Nursing (1995) *Clinical Guidelines: What You Need to Know* (London: Royal College of Nursing).

Royle J and Blithe J (1998) Promoting research utilization in nursing: the role of the individual, organisation, and environment. *Evidence-Based Nursing*, **1**:71–2.

Royle J A, Blythe S, DiCenso A, Boblin-Cummongs Deber R and Hayward R (2000) Evaluation of a system for providing information resources to nurses. *Health Informatics Journal*, **6**:100–9.

Schön DA (1983) *The Reflective Practitioner* (London: Temple Smith).

Skeil D (1995) Patients' feelings about patients. In: J Reed and S Procter (eds), *Practitioner Research in Health Care* (London: Chapman & Hall).

Sleep J (1992) Research and the practice of midwifery. *Journal of Advanced Nursing*, **1**:1465–71.

Stetler C B and DiMaggio G (1991) Research utilization among clinical nurse specialists. *Clinical Nurse Specialist*, **5**, 3:151–5.

Stevenson C (1995) Reflections on evaluating a course of family therapy. In: J Reed and S Procter (eds), *Practitioner Research in Health Care* (London: Chapman & Hall).

Stokes T, Shukla R, Schober P and Baker R (1998) A model for the development of evidence-based clinical guidelines at local level – the Leicestershire Genital Chlamydia Guidelines Project. *Journal of Evaluation in Clinical Practice*, **4**, 4:325–38.

Stokols D (1992) Establishing and maintaining health environments: toward a social ecology of health promotion. *American Psychology*, **47**:6–22.

Tanner J and Hale C (2002) Research-active nurses' perceptions of the barriers to undertaking research in practice. *Nursing Times Research*, **7**, 5:363–77.

Thomas L H, McColl E, Cullum N, Rousseau N and Soutter J (1999) Clinical guidelines in nursing, midwifery and the therapies: a systematic review. *Journal of Advanced Nursing*, **30**, 1:40–50.

Thompson C, McCaughan D, Cullum N, Sheldon T A, Mulhall A and Thompson D R (2001) Research information in nurses' clinical decision-making: what is useful? *Journal of Advanced Nursing*, **36**, 3:376–88.

Thompson M A (1998) Closing the gap between nursing research and practice. *Evidence-Based Nursing*, **1**, 1:7–8.

Titler M G (2004) Methods in translation science. *Worldviews on Evidence-Based Nursing*, 1:38–48.

Titler M G, Kleiber C and Steelman V et al. (1994) Infusing research into practice to promote quality care. *Nursing Research*, **43**, 5:307–13.

Veeramah V (2004) Utilization of research findings by graduate nurses and midwives. *Journal of Advanced Nursing*, **47**, 2:183–91.

Walsh M (1997a) How nurses perceive barriers to research implementation. *Nursing Standard*, **11**, 29:34–9.

Walsh M (1997b) Perceptions of barriers to implementing research. *Nursing Standard*, 11, 19:34–7.

Weiss C (1979) The many meanings of research utilization. *Public Administration Review*, 39:426–31.

Woodgate R L and Degner L F (2004) Cancer symptom transition periods of children and families. *Journal of Advanced Nursing*, 46, 4:358–68.

Woolf S H, Grol R, Hutchinson A, Eccles M and Grimshaw J (1999) Clinical guidelines: Potential benefits, limitations, and harms of clinical guidelines. *British Medical Journal*, 318:527–30.

Worrall G, Chaulk P and Freake D (1997) The effects of clinical practice guidelines on patient outcomes in primary care: a systematic review. *Canadian Medical Association Journal*, 156, 12:1705–12.

Wye L and McClenahan J (2000) *Getting Better with Evidence: Experiences of Putting Evidence into Practice* (London: King's Fund Publishing).

Evidence-based Practice

OPENING THOUGHT

I once asked a worker at a crematorium, who had a curiously contented look on his face, what he found so satisfying about his work. He replied that what fascinated him was the way in which so much went in and so little came out. I thought of advising him to get a job in the NHS, it might have increased his job satisfaction, but decided against it.

Archie Cochrane

Introduction

The evidence-based movement which gathered momentum in the early 1990s has implications for the way health, social and other services are organised and delivered. In this chapter we will trace the factors which led to its emergence in the United Kingdom (UK). The meaning, objectives, benefits and limitations of evidence-based practice will be explored.

Finally, the criticisms of evidence-based practice and its implications for nursing practice will also be discussed.

Justifying practice

Suppose you are treating a wound using a particular dressing and your patient asks: 'Does it work?' 'How does it work?' 'Are there other treatments available?' 'Why did you decide that this is the best treatment for me?'

Would you also know what effects this intervention has on patients or what their views are on this treatment? When did you last read about the treatment of wound care? How often do you update your knowledge regarding your practice? Is there any research study or, better still, a systematic review of treatments for this particular type of wound care? Do you have the knowledge and skills to access and select a review? Are there guidelines on the treatment of wound care from your hospital or your professional organisation? How were these guidelines developed or adapted? Are they based on research? Do you follow these guidelines? Does your organisation have a written policy on wound care? Does your clinical environment have the facilities (on-line access to databases and training opportunities) to enable you to access and use relevant literature in your practice?

These are some of the questions which the evidence-based practice movement have sought to stimulate. No doubt many practitioners are aware of these issues and are well able to justify their practice on sound evidence. Many others, however, are unaware of what, and if, evidence exists on which to base their practice. They would find it hard to explain why they use particular interventions, other than that it has always been done in this way. Lang (1999) contends that not much is known about the thousands of decisions which nurses make every day and which have an impact on the people who are recipients of their practices.

The evidence-based practice movement places particular emphasis on the use of evidence, in particular research findings, in clinical decision making. It is a reaction to what was seen as an overreliance on experience, intuition and to the lack of knowledge of the effectiveness of interventions.

Background to evidence-based practice

The context which gave rise to the evidence-based practice movement in the UK includes the following:

- increasing cost of health care;
- glut of research;
- variation in health care;
- unnecessary interventions;
- changes to the management of heath services.

Increasing cost of health care

By far one of the most important reasons for the drive towards efficiency in health care is the increase in private and public spending on health worldwide. In the UK alone, the National Health Service (NHS) spending has increased from 3.9 per cent of the Gross Domestic Product (GDP) in 1949 to 5.5 per cent in 2000, with a projected increase to 6.3 per cent by 2004 (Emmerson et al., 2000). NHS spending for 2000–2001 was estimated at £54.2 billion (Department of Health, 2000).

Increasing costs can be attributed to increasing demands in health care. Although the NHS is treating more patients than before, waiting lists and waiting times have also increased (Emmerson et al., 2000). New technology has improved diagnostic and screening procedures with the result that more health problems are uncovered than would have been possible previously. The discovery or definition of new diseases such as the Acquired Immune Deficiency Syndrome (AIDS) and Chronic Fatigue Syndrome have added to the strain on already stretched resources. The increasing cost of drugs and the availability of new drugs also put pressure on health care expenditure.

It is believed that more efficient use of resources can help to keep down the cost of NHS spending. According to Hunter (1996), the release of resources through the adoption of evidence-based practice provides the most attractive way forward to cope with mounting demands and pressures on the NHS. This is reflected in the government's objective of achieving the greatest possible improvements in health by providing services that are effective in terms of results (National Health Service Executive, 1996). The heavy investment in evidence-based medicine and the high profile attached to it are expected to lead to the effectiveness of interventions and to massive savings in costs.

Glut of research

The UK government spends millions of pounds on research. In 1998 alone, £435 million was spend on Research and Development in the NHS (Millar, 1998). Ten years earlier, a House of Lords Report (1988) commented that most medical research in Britain had little relation to the needs of the NHS. Little is known about the effectiveness of most health interventions. According to Kirk (1996) only 15 per cent of modern clinical practice is of proven benefit. While this figure may be contentious, there is a general agreement that more should be done to evaluate the effectiveness of policy and practice in the health and other related sectors.

Although the number of research studies in nursing has increased in recent years there are insufficient synthesised research findings, in the form of systematic reviews, to provide practitioners with digestible and readily accessible material to use (Estabrooks, 1999). Allied health professionals such as occupational therapists have also reported that there is little research of relevance to the practising therapists and the clinical decisions they have to make (Taylor, 1997).

In medicine, on the other hand, the amount of research is such that it is almost impossible for doctors to keep up to date with publications. Over two million articles are published annually in the biomedical literature in over 2000 journals (Mulrow, 1995), and it is estimated that, in general, physicians would have to read 19 articles a day for each day of the year to keep up with developments in their own fields (Haynes, 1995). That was ten years ago; no doubt these figures have increased in the meantime. The main task facing the medical profession is to search, appraise and make sense of the findings of research on any particular intervention. The Cochrane Collaboration was set up to systematically review randomised controlled trials (RCTs). This network of collaborators in a number of countries was named after Archie Cochrane (1972), who was a strong advocate of the randomised controlled trial at a time when few

RCTs were carried out. Since then the number of RCTs has proliferated world-wide and it has therefore become necessary to create a database of studies evaluating the effectiveness of interventions.

Variation in practice

Variation in practice strikes at the heart of the principle of equity on which health services are built. The NHS was based on the principle that everyone irrespective of means, age, sex or occupation should have equal opportunity to benefit from the best and most up-to-date medical and allied services available (Timmins, 1995). Despite these lofty ideals, there are, in the UK, wide regional differences both in waiting lists and waiting times and in other indicators, such as death rates and the number of cases treated per hospital bed (Emmerson et al., 2000). Even within regions, there can be considerable differences between the best performing and the worst performing health authority and these differences are often seen as differences in efficiency (Emmerson et al., 2000). Post-code variations are well publicised; the term 'lottery' based on post-codes has been used, for example, to describe variations in cancer care (Kunkler, 1997).

Variation in health care organisation, delivery and use are almost impossible to eradicate as they depend on resources, personnel, attitudes, training and culture, amongst a number of factors. Whenever health services have been studied researchers have found substantial variations in the care which is delivered (Crombie and Davies, 1998). The less they know about what is effective in preventing or treating a disease or illness, the more likely it is that practitioners will provide a variety of interventions, mainly through trial and error.

The literature abounds with examples of variations in practice. In a study by Munson et al. (1999) on skin care practices in premature low birth weight infants, it was found that a quarter of units in 104 hospitals, in the United States, had no skin care protocols. Among units, there was considerable practice variation with respect to common nursing procedures such as bathing, adhesive application and wound care. In another study, Jaglal et al. (1997) examined trends in geographic variations in surgical treatment of femoral neck fractures. In 29,331 cases in hospitals across Canada they found that hemiarthroplasty (HA) was more likely to be performed on women, older patients and nursing home patients. There was a 38-fold variation for total hip arthroplasty and a nine-fold variation in use of HA among the different regions of Canada. Lavery (1995) surveyed skin care following radiotherapy in 48 radiotherapy units in the UK. The results showed that skin care practices were highly variable and included the use of talcum, steroids, simple creams, aloe vera and calamine. Even patients being treated in the same hospital know that treatment for the same conditions may differ according to consultants.

Peckham (1991), the first Director of Research and Development in the NHS in the UK, warned more than a decade ago that 'every clinician knows that there is indefensible diversity in the use of diagnostic methods and therapies and that there is unacceptable variation in the quality of treatment delivered by different clinical teams'.

Unnecessary practices

Those who promote evidence-based practice believe that a sure way of saving money is to wean out unnecessary practices. The literature is full of such examples. Physical restraint is extensively used despite virtually no evidence to support its use (Marks, 1992). There are different types and consequences of unnecessary practices. There are some for which there is no evidence of effectiveness, because they have not been evaluated. There are others which have been shown to be unnecessary, but are continued by practitioners who ignore the evidence. Webb and Hannaford (1996) point out that authoritative documents such as the *Handbook of Contraceptive Practice* still contain statements such as 'vaginal examinations, repeated at regular intervals, form the basis for good preventative care, even though the available evidence strongly suggests that this procedure should not be done in asymptomatic women'.

Unnecessary practices may be benign or harmful, but in both cases they are costly. Harmful effects cost more to remedy and also prolong the patient's discomfort and delay their return to normality. The evaluation of interventions is crucial if unnecessary interventions are to be stopped. A review of 5000 trials in prenatal medicine revealed that for about 50 per cent of practices there was no evaluation, for 20 per cent there was convincing evidence of ineffectiveness and for about 30 per cent there was evidence of effectiveness to support their use (Peckham, 1991).

Cochrane (1972) pointed out that doctors provide a mix of effective and ineffective therapies and that patients expect the doctor to help even when he or she has little to offer. He explained that there is a

> very widespread belief that for every symptom or group of symptoms there was a bottle of medicine, a pill, an operation, or some other therapy which would at least help. The doctor on his side was hardly to blame for aiding and abetting in the production of this myth.

There is almost a benign (but costly) complicity between the doctor and the patient, which Cochrane (1972) believed was due to the desire to help (on the part of doctors) and the desire to be helped (on the part of patients). The formation of the NHS in 1948 could have been perceived as providing a blank cheque to meet both the demands of patients and the wishes of doctors.

Changes to the management of health services

In April 1991 the reforms of the NHS in the UK introduced an internal market, separating the roles of purchaser and provider (Drummond, 1995). This was an attempt by the Conservative government to increase efficiency in the NHS, which was perceived as suffering from a chronic crisis of increasingly limited supply of medical resources but unlimited demand (McQuaide, 1996). These radical reforms were based on the assumption that clinicians, in particular doctors who managed the health service, were not trained to manage but to practise in their clinical fields. By relying on managers it was thought that the NHS would be run more efficiently than before. Another purpose of these changes was the introduction of the 'business ethos' in the NHS to enable purchasers to shop around for services based on the concept of 'value for money'. These purchasers would therefore be in a position to ask why some services were necessary or whether particular interventions were achieving the desired outcomes. In order to function appropriately, the internal market required detailed information on whether services were effective (Lloyd-Smith, 1997). Clinicians, on the other hand, regard such matters as their professional preserve. Marshall (1995) explains that 'when medical knowledge is based on evidence, neither the claim that it is the exclusive intellectual preserve of any one profession, nor claims for the prior authority of experts can be defended'.

Managers therefore saw the evidence-based practice movement as a useful vehicle to provide them with information on which to base their decisions. As such information would be in the public domain and in a form that could be understood by all, this fitted well with the objectives of the internal market. On the other hand, evidence-based practice was seen by a section of the medical profession as a threat to their clinical autonomy (this will be discussed later in this chapter).

Another factor which helped the evidence-based practice movement to thrive was the changing attitudes of consumers towards health and health care. There seems to be more willingness among some users to challenge the decisions and actions of health professionals. Successive UK governments have put emphasis on patients' rights to information and on their participation in decision making. These are possible if information is available freely and is easily accessible. Evidence-based practice can, potentially, satisfy customers in these respects.

The revolution in information technology, in particular the advent of the personal computer and on-line access to information in the early 1990s, was a perfect catalyst for the evidence-based movement. Information technology is now an integral part of evidence-based practice in that it facilitates the search for, and dissemination of, evidence. Clinicians are expected to click on the appropriate icons and access relevant, up-to-date information about their interventions instantly. It is difficult to imagine how the evidence-based practice movement would have gathered the momentum it has, if information were searched, appraised and disseminated by post or even by fax.

Together, the factors identified above contributed to, or facilitated, the emergence and progress of the evidence-based practice movement. In the next section, we will examine closely what evidence-based practice is and what it has to offer to practitioners and policy makers.

What is evidence-based practice?

The term 'evidence-based practice' is derived from definitions of evidence-based medicine. The Evidence Based Medicine Working Group (1992), based in Canada, describes evidence-based medicine as the process of de-emphasising

> intuition, unsystematic clinical experience, and pathophysiologic rationale as sufficient grounds for clinical decision making and stresses the examination of evidence from clinical research.

Later the McMaster University Evidence-Based Medicine Group (1996) offered this more comprehensive and workable definition:

> the collection, interpretation, and integration of valid, important and applicable patient-reported, clinician-observed, and research-derived evidence. The best available evidence, moderated by patient circumstances and preferences, is applied to improve the quality of clinical judgements and facilitate cost-effective health care.

The most quoted definition of evidence-based medicine comes from Sackett et al. (1996). It is described as:

> the conscientious, explicit and judicious use of current based evidence in making decisions about the care of individual patients. The practice of evidence based medicine means integrating individual clinical expertise with the best available external clinical evidence from systematic research.

Sackett et al. (1996) went on to add that evidence-based medicine involves the 'thoughtful identification and compassionate use of individual patients' predicaments, rights, and preferences in making clinical decisions about their care'.

A number of other professions have coined their own phrases such as 'evidence-based nursing', 'evidence-based occupational therapy', 'evidence-based public health', 'evidence-based policy' or 'evidence-based dentistry'. Others have offered their own versions of evidence-based practice (Gerrish and Clayton, 1998; Goode and Piedalue, 1999; and Ingersoll, 2000). While these definitions retain the use of the best available evidence, some do not rely on RCTs as their main source of evidence.

Evidence-based practice will be used in this chapter as a generic term to describe all decisions and actions which are based on the best available evidence taking into account clinical expertise and patients' wishes. Where appropriate, terms like 'evidence-based medicine' or 'evidence-based nursing' will be used to refer to the use of evidence in these professions. Evidence-based nursing will be discussed in a later section.

The evidence-based practice movement evolved out of developments at

McMaster University, in Ontario, Canada in the early 1990s. In the UK, it underpinned the Research and Development strategy (R&D) in 1991 (Department of Health NHS Executive, 1995). The aim of the R&D strategy was 'to create a knowledge-based health service in which clinical, managerial, and policy decisions are based on sound information about research findings and scientific developments'.

Main steps in evidence-based practice

The main steps of evidence-based practice involve the formulation of a clear question related to policy or practice, the search for relevant research studies, the appraisal of selected studies (based on their quality), the analysis and the synthesis of the findings of these studies, the dissemination of the results and the implementation of the evidence. At the heart of evidence-based practice lies the systematic review (see Chapter 7). However, evidence-based practice is more than systematic reviews; it involves the use of evidence, clinical expertise and patients' views to make clinical decisions.

The implementation of evidence can take place when a clinician looks for the evidence (often the result of a systematic review) and uses it to determine which treatment a particular patient will receive. Clinical guidelines (see previous chapter), based on research evidence, have also been developed to facilitate the use of evidence in practice.

Differences between evidence-based practice and research utilisation

Research is the systematic and rigorous collection and analysis of data to explain phenomena. It aims to contribute to the advancement of knowledge, often in the form of theories. Basic research is an example of research which may or may not have direct or immediate use in clinical practice. Applied research, as the term suggests, has direct application to the area being studied as, for example, when the benefits of two clinical interventions are compared. Therefore while research can answer questions directly related to clinical practice, its scope is broader than evidence-based practice. Researchers can make recommendations but these may or may not be implemented by clinicians.

The question that is often asked is why practitioners do not use research findings. The focus is on findings. These may or may not have direct application to one's practice. Evidence-based practice, on the other hand, starts with a clinical question (for example, which of the two types of treatment currently in use is more effective in treating a particular condition, in certain type of patients?). The focus is, therefore, on practice-relevant questions.

The practitioner looks for available evidence (in the form of a systematic review of studies already carried out) or sets in motion the process of producing the evidence (through primary research). The findings from the review or research study are then applied to practice. Therefore evidence-based practice starts with questioning practice and ends with using the evidence in practice. If the loop is not completed, evidence-based practice does not occur. Therefore evidence-based practice and research are interdependent.

Objectives of evidence-based practice

The main objective of evidence-based practice is to increase awareness of the effectiveness of decisions and actions of practitioners, educators and policy makers. In the health service it is designed to improve decision making and achieve clinical effectiveness by enabling clinicians to use the most effective interventions, thereby reducing waste and eliminating unnecessary practices.

With the dissemination of the best evidence to the widest audience imaginable with the use of information technology, it is expected that variations in the provision of services and in patients' outcomes will be reduced. The development and use of clinical guidelines based on evidence can also help to achieve this objective.

Finally, evidence-based practice also aims to reduce the reliance on expert knowledge and increase the transparency of decision making. With the evidence in the public domain lay persons can, potentially, look for and use the evidence to inform their discussions with health professionals.

Criticisms of evidence-based practice

Evidence-based practice has aroused a lot of different reactions, as reflected in the vast literature generated on the topic. Its advocates have been called 'arrogant', 'seductive' and 'controversial' (Polychronis et al., 1996b). It has its 'evangelists' and its 'enemies' (Hope, 1995). Although the evidence-based practice movement was initiated and led by doctors, the medical profession is itself divided on the importance, feasibility and implications of the movement for medicine and health care in general. The implications of evidence-based medicine in particular, and evidence-based practice in general, can be summed up at a number of levels: conceptual, political, economic and ethical.

Conceptual implications

At a conceptual level, by far the most contentious issue is what constitutes evidence. The evidence-based practice movement uses the following hierarchy of study designs for studies of effectiveness:

1. Experimental studies (e.g. RCT with concealed allocation).

2. Quasi-experimental studies (e.g. experimental study without randomisation).

3. Controlled observational studies.
   3a. Cohort studies
   3b. Case control studies

4. Observational studies without control groups.

5. Expert opinion based on pathophysiology, bench research or consensus.
   (Centre for Reviews and Disseminations, 2001)

The RCT is considered the 'gold standard' in producing evidence. In this hierarchy other designs or methods that do not include randomisation are perceived as producing lower forms of evidence.

Although the RCT is considered by many as a useful research design to evaluate the effectiveness of clinical interventions, in particular drugs and surgery, it is considered by others as having a number of limitations. RCTs are believed not to reflect the reality of clinical situations, in that participants are carefully selected in an attempt to control confounding variables and to have a sample who can complete the study. Thus exclusion criteria are set, and these are often used to exclude the very frail, those who cannot speak English and those with multiple conditions. The findings from these 'sanitised' samples are therefore not readily generalisable to all types of patients who seek help from health professionals.

Large-scale, multi-site RCTs are often required to establish the superiority of one treatment over another. However, RCTs are not appropriate for all types of interventions. Cochrane himself was sceptical about encouraging 'widespread RCTs in the care sector' because the objectives are more difficult to define and the technique (RCT) was less developed in that sector (Cochrane, 1972).

According to Clemence (1998), the interactive nature of much therapy and rehabilitation is not easily measured by RCTs. Even if the treatment is the same, the input of therapists would depend on their individual interactions with their clients. Some of the behavioural and therapeutic interventions used by nurses are complex and takes place over a period of time. They are not as clearly defined as some medical interventions such as drugs or surgery. Advocates of evidence-based practice acknowledge that RCTs are not appropriate for all types of interventions (Sackett et al., 1996). Yet the Research and Development programme reflects the preference for RCTs both in its commissioning of research and in its allocation of funding.

The National Health Service Executive (1996) made clear its preference for the use of RCTs to evaluate the effectiveness of interventions and recommended that only evidence from RCTs can be used in the contractual process. As nursing and the therapies are eclectic in their choice of methodologies, it leaves them in a confused position. There are mixed messages suggesting that it is fine to use other designs such as qualitative approaches, yet their evidence is, at the same time, also considered inferior. Evans (2003), on the other hand, proposes a hierarchy of evidence which 'acknowledges the valid contribution of evidence generated by a range of different types of research'. He emphasises the importance of assessing the quality of the evidence.

Turning a probability into a certainty

Policy makers, planners, managers need evidence to make and justify their decisions. When this evidence is available in numerical, quantitative forms, it makes decision making a 'black and white' issue. For example, if drug A is more effective than drug B and this is expressed in percentages of people cured then the use of 'A' is justified.

Emphasis is on 'statistically significant' results based on the probability of the results happening by chance or not. Clinicians faced with a statistically significant result may therefore use it as a certainty. Polychronis et al. (1996a) believe that advocates of evidence-based medicine 'glorify probabilism based on mathematical logic, synthesizing a certainty based on what is statistically probable, which – in the clinical setting – does not represent certainty at all'. The same views are expressed by Lewis (1996), who explains that overall

> there is still a tendency to regard statistics simply as mathematics: 'if you do your sums correctly, you get the right answer'. But of course this is not so. Applied statistics is like other applied sciences – full of assumptions and approximations. Because of this it requires critical judgement to apply and interpret it.

The danger of interpreting statistical data literally is illustrated in the well-publicised case of Sally Clark who was jailed for allegedly killing her babies. The statistical evidence produced by a well-known paediatrician is believed to have played a crucial part in the jury's decision. The statistic used in court stated that 'in a non-smoking, middle-class family like Sally's the chances of two cot deaths was one in 73 million' (Driscoll, 2003). As it happens, this statistic had been incorrectly calculated and the probabilities were simply irrelevant to the case. She was later released on appeal after her conviction was quashed and her name was cleared.

Evidence-based practice involves taking into account patients' views. It is not easy for health professionals, let alone patients, to interpret statistical probability. John Diamond (1998), the broadcaster and late husband of Nigella Lawson (the celebrity chef), explained (in his own inimitable style) their predicament when the couple faced the prospect of a foetal blood test:

> In a state of shock we went up to the foetal medicine department where a doctor talked to us about a foetal blood test with a one in 100 chance of

inducing a miscarriage balanced against the 1 in 250 chance that the cysts indicated something nasty.

As odds went they were reasonable ones and had I been standing in the bookies thinking about putting money on a healthy baby there would have been no problem. But under the circumstances the odds were meaningless. In these situations all odds are the same odds, or rather evens. Either the worst will happen or it won't: the baby will die or it won't. The odds always feel like 50:50.

Some years later when he was told by his surgeon about the odds of him being able to talk again after having part of his tongue removed as a result of cancer he reflected:

And as it was then so it was for me now. Either they'd cure me or they wouldn't. Everything was 50:50. When the official odds were 92 per cent they were really 50:50, and if the operation didn't work and the official odds dropped to 20 per cent or 10 per cent or worse, they'd still be 50:50. (Diamond, 1998)

Political implications

By making the process and results of systematic reviews transparent and accessible to professionals and laypersons, the evidence-based practice movement is believed to lead to the democratisation of clinical decision making (Marshall, 1995). Since the knowledge and opinion of experts is the lowest form of evidence in the hierarchy of evidence, any practitioner, armed with knowledge of the best available evidence, can (theoretically) challenge the authority of experts. Sackett (1995) believes that evidence-based practice appeals to mid-career doctors because it has the potential to 'replace authoritarian, one-way consultant rounds with two-way teaching (and, more important, learning) at the bedside'.

Open access to information about the best evidence can have implications for clinicians' autonomy. Managers can decide to challenge clinicians on the effectiveness of the interventions they carry out. There is the possibility that some control of clinical practice can shift from consultants to managers and bureaucrats. According to Hart (1997), Cochrane's ideas were appealing to managers because it fitted their ideology. The business ethos of managers often conflicts with the autonomy of practitioners. Doctors and the health professionals make decisions based on what they perceive as the best possible evidence. Managers, on the other hand, have to balance budgets, allocate resources and obtain maximum benefits from available, often limited, funding. To be able to challenge practitioners about their practice is a boost to managers' power and control. In particular, inefficient, unnecessary interventions as well as variations in practice can be questioned.

Economic implications

Sceptics point out that evidence-based practice is really about rationing health services (Hunter, 1996; Hart, 1997). Hunter (1996) sums up this position eloquently:

> Whatever researchers' own motivations, their work will be, and are already being, seized upon by policy makers intent on introducing cost-containment measures which can be defended on the grounds that health care resources will only be used on those interventions of proven efficacy. Decisions to limit or withdraw treatment will be justified and backed up by research evidence in order to reassure patients and silence critics.

In the 1970s and 1980s, efficiency and cost effectiveness were terms that were in fashion in the UK. With the advent of evidence-based practice in the early 1990s the two terms were separated. The emphasis was on clinical effectiveness although cost effectiveness was not entirely forgotten. The NHS spends millions of pounds on drug prescriptions. The National Institute for Clinical Effectiveness (NICE), set up to provide guidelines on the effectiveness of treatments, found itself accused of rationing when it decided, in October 1999, that NHS doctors should not prescribe the drug Relenza for all people with influenza. This caused uproar and upset Glaxo Wellcome, who at the time issued a veiled threat to quit the country and relocate elsewhere (Lynn, 1999).

Appraisal of the findings from 11 RCTs involving more than 3000 individuals from a number of countries concluded that while on average the duration of symptoms by all those who used the drug was reduced by 1–2 days, there was no statistically significant effect on overall mortality or hospitalisation rates (Barnett, 2001). Cost-effectiveness calculations were carried out taking into account the costs of additional consultations with general practitioners, cost of hospitalisation and cost of the drug itself. The guidelines subsequently issued by NICE stated that it did not recommend the use of Relenza for 'healthy adults with influenza'. Only those 'at risk' were to be prescribed the drug. This case shows that definition of clinical effectiveness for the same treatment can include a number of outcomes. While a drug or intervention can be effective for some of the outcomes (reduction of the duration of symptoms) and not for others (mortality rates), a decision needs to be taken whether overall the drug is effective or not. This is a subjective decision which can be influenced by the beliefs and agenda of the decision makers. This is illustrated by the conclusion by NICE that Relenza was not shown to be effective enough for it to be recommended for use by all patients. The drug company, Glaxo Wellcome, thought otherwise. Prescribing the drug would have meant £250 million for the drug company (Lynn, 1999), and considerable additional expenditure to the NHS. Drug companies have always resisted cost effectiveness as a criterion for allowing a drug on the NHS (Lynn, 1999) yet it was always likely that when large sums of money were involved, what counted as evidence could be perceived differently and hotly contested.

The panel who appraised the evidence about the effectiveness of Relenza also recommended that more research be carried out to fill the evidence-gap for this particular drug. They believed that such research would require 'several influenza seasons to complete' and that this 'might need to be set up on an international basis' (Barnett, 2001). Yet, a year later NICE lifted its ban on the prescription of Relenza.

Ethical implications

The main ethical implication for evidence-based practice is that it is population-based rather than individual-centred (Hope, 1995; Closs and Cheater, 1999). It is believed that evidence-based practice reflects the utilitarian philosophy of achieving the greatest good for the greatest number of people (Colyer and Kamath, 1999). In this scenario a blanket ban or the prescription of certain treatments for all patients with similar conditions are justified. And when purchasing of treatments is done by managers, it is difficult for practitioners to base their treatments on individuals. In 2000, another controversy surrounded the decision by NICE to restrict the use of the drug 'Interferon beta-1b' and 'glatiramer acetate' for patients with multiple sclerosis (MS) on the basis of lack of evidence of effectiveness. A number of nurses protested against the decision on the basis that they saw, in their practice, the benefits of the drug for their patients (Parish, 2000). They explained that MS patients were the best judges of the success of the treatment and that they (nurses) were acting as advocates for their patients.

Sackett et al.'s (1996) definition of evidence-based medicine recognises that it includes the 'thoughtful identification and compassionate use of individual patients' predicaments, rights, and preferences in making clinical decisions about their care'. Yet this example shows the difficulty of taking into account patients' preferences and wishes when guidelines dictates what should be prescribed or not.

Hope (1995) has concerns that evidence-based practice may be used to cut funding and to introduce systematic bias in purchasing those treatments for which there is good evidence of effectiveness. This would leave out treatments that have not been adequately researched and those which cannot be adequately studied by RCTs. Hope (1995) also believes that the evidence-based practice movement has tended to be doctor-centred rather than patient-centred.

The power of evidence can become so great that it can be used by politicians and policy makers to override the judgements of clinicians and the rights and wishes of patients. On the other hand, public access to information about the effectiveness of interventions can strengthen patients' hands in discussions with clinicians. This has to be weighed against the lobbying power of the drug companies whose aim is to maximise profits. According to Polychronis et al.

(1996a), it seems inevitable that the results of the evidence-based practice movement will be used selectively in an increasingly resource-limited service.

On the other hand, 'the ethics of ignorance' (Smith, 1992) relates to the use of treatments the benefits and risks of which clinicians remain ignorant of. Smith (1992) also points out that there may be 'a breach of contract in that the patients assume that the doctors know that the treatment they are using is beneficial'.

Evidence-based nursing

Evidence-based nursing has its roots in the evidence-based medicine movement. Most nursing authors have derived their definition or description of evidence-based nursing from Sackett et al.'s (1996) definition of evidence-based medicine. For example, The Royal College of Nursing (1996), while not using the term 'evidence-based nursing', describes evidence-based health care as:

> rooted in best available scientific evidence and takes into account patients' views of effectiveness and clinical expertise in order to promote clinically effective services. This is essential in ensuring that health care practitioners do the things that work and are acceptable to patients and do not do the things which do not work.

What is different in this definition when compared to Sackett et al.'s (1996) is that patients' views of effectiveness are given prominence.

Most nurses and allied health professionals would probably say that this is what they have been doing all the time. Nursing, in particular, claims that evidence-based practice began with Florence Nightingale, who collected statistical data to inform policy in the British military hospitals during the Crimean War (Lang, 1999). Briggs (1972), in the *Report on the Committee on Nursing* in the UK, called for nursing to be research-based and the phrase not only became one of the most quoted in nursing literature, but influenced the development of nursing research in the UK in the decades that followed.

While there is recognition by nurses that research evidence has a crucial role in decision making, there is little consensus as to what evidence-based practice in nursing means. Nurses do not fully understand the rules (Kitson, 1997). According to Estabrooks (1998), 'the term evidence-based practice has crept into nursing somewhat surreptitiously, and nursing has begun to use it without paying obvious attention to its origins or what it conveys to nurses, the public, politicians, and other health professionals'.

The reaction to the introduction of the current policy of evidence-based practice in nursing has been varied and often blunt. There are those who find it a rich opportunity to advance research utilisation in nursing (Cullum, 1998; Estabrooks, 1998) and for enhancing the reputation of nursing research and continuous quality improvement (French, 1999). Others describe it as a 'retrograde step' (Clarke, 1999), as a 'barren possibility' and 'an obstruction to the nursing process' (Mitchell, 1999), a regression back to practice based solely on the findings of quantitative research (Rolfe, 1999), and as having 'inherent contradictions and ethical dilemmas' (Colyer and Kamath, 1999). In between these two extremes, there are those who advise caution but not rejection of evidence-based practice (Kitson, 1997; Estabrooks, 1998).

Despite these differences among opinion leaders in nursing, evidence-based practice in the nursing profession seems 'to have gained wider popularity as demonstrated by the increasing number of nursing conferences with an evidence-based theme, journals that feature 'evidence-based, best practices in healthcare and professional nursing organisations that are developing or promoting clinical guidelines' (DiCenso et al., 2002). However, this popularity does not necessarily mean that nurses are practising evidence-based nursing.

In the next section we will examine some of the arguments for and against evidence-based practice in nursing.

A medical or nursing initiative?

Evidence-based medicine, from which offshoots such as evidence-based nursing, evidence-based policy or evidence-based dentistry are derived, is by definition and purpose a medical initiative. It is led by doctors and is best suited to medical practice. It is also a political initiative and is the base on which the NHS Research and Development agenda is built. To benefit from funding and other developments associated with evidence-based medicine, nursing and other allied health professions are expected to follow the lead of their medical colleagues. Salvage (1998) advises nurses not to naïvely rush to embrace evidence-based practice without considering the political implications of the NHS Research and Development agenda. These include curbing medical power and promoting research-based rationing of health care (Rafferty and Traynor, 1997). These goals may not be compatible with nurses' beliefs of how patient care can be improved.

Adopting the evidence-based medicine model for nursing can be seen as another attempt to impose the medical model on nursing. Once again nursing and the allied health professions are expected to walk in the shadow of medicine. Rafferty's (1996) review of government policy shows the limited extent to which internal reform within nursing can be achieved without government support. Both the refusal to ring-fence funds for nursing research and the lack of significant support to put into practice Briggs's (1972) recommendation for nursing to become a research-based profession are examples of the lack of government willingness to support nursing in its efforts to determine its own future on issues of research and what constitutes clinical effectiveness.

There is sometimes an underlying threat that if nurses do not 'join the bandwagon' of evidence-based practice, they will be left behind. Bonnell (1999) believes that if nurses do not embrace quantitative and experimental research (the preferred research methods in evidence-based practice) they will be marginalised and will relinquish their autonomy to managers. This is in sharp contrast to those who believe that evidence-based practice will lead to less clinical autonomy.

The nature of nursing knowledge

The needs of people cared for by nurses are varied and complex and require both technical and humanistic responses. Many nursing interventions are, in fact, interactions between nurses, patients and their families. Giving reassurance, allaying fears and anxiety, 'preparing' patients for surgery or counselling patients on how to stop smoking involve interactions in which the use of self is an important intervention. Mulhall (1998) explains that

> nursing is not merely concerned with the body, but is also in an 'intimate' and ongoing relationship with the person within the body. Thus nursing becomes concerned with 'untidy' things such as emotions and feelings, which traditional natural and social sciences have difficulty accommodating.

Much of what nurses do with patients is about the effects their presence, personalities and themselves have on patients. As well as expecting their symptoms to be relieved or their disease to be cured, patients want to be treated with respect and dignity. They value confidence, trust, privacy and want their rights respected. Such patients' outcomes are difficult to assess and are rarely used as measures of the effectiveness of nursing care. Closs and Cheater (1999) point out that 'there is abundant evidence demonstrating wide discrepancies between patients' and professionals' judgements about what constitutes desirable or successful outcomes'. Bradshaw (2000) asks if 'the notion of Evidence Based Practice which has its roots in positive science have sufficient relevance to the practise of nursing which embraces so many culturally, socially and spiritually constructed dimensions'?

Mulhall (1998) argues that because of the nature of nursing, nurses rely on many different ways of knowing and many different kinds of knowledge. To assess and respond to people's emotions, feelings or anxieties requires more than scales and questionnaires. It involves the use of self and all the senses that humans possess and it happens in ways that are often beyond human consciousness. Assessing a patient or a situation often involves not just hearing and seeing but also smelling, touching, as well as processing all this information while 'being there' with and for the patient. Professional expertise comprises intuition, personal and professional experience, tacit knowledge as well as external knowledge from research and other literature. Professionals often find it difficult to identify the sources of knowledge which led to particular decisions. This is because they build up their expertise from many different clinical situations as well as acquiring knowledge from a number of sources. Clarke (1999) believes that in nursing and the allied health professions, there is a tradition of taking an eclectic view of evidence, ranging from scientific and humanistic to personal experience. According to her, 'human beings require the benefits of science as well as the benefits of humanism and personal experience', and 'privileging one type of evidence is a narrow retrograde step' for nursing (Clarke, 1999).

The reliance on quantitative and experimental research to produce evidence for nursing and midwifery practice is also questioned (Hicks and Hennessy, 1997). Nursing research is pluralistic in its use of methodologies. In particular, qualitative research seems to be popular with nurses. Yet British medicine (the purveyor of evidence-based practice) does not understand qualitative methodologies (Bradshaw, 2000).

The way nursing and nursing knowledge are viewed by the medical profession in general, and the leaders of the evidence-based practice movement in particular, has implications for research in nursing. Medicine has a significant influence on the national Research and Development agenda and, by and large, those on research funding panels have, predominantly, a medical background. They tend to favour RCTs. Hicks and Hennessy (1997) explain that the emphasis on RCTs means that proposals employing this methodology are likely to be preferentially considered over and above any other when funding is being allocated. Bonnell (1999) warns that if nurses do not embrace RCTs they will be marginalised. The pressure on nursing research to produce the evidence for nursing practice by means of RCTs is maintained mainly through the 'carrot and stick' strategy. The message seems to be that funding is available for those who want to carry out RCTs (especially large, multi-site ones). Sometimes research designs other than RCTs are not considered rigorous enough and therefore receive less funding.

The inappropriateness of this approach for researching some of the main questions in medicine, nursing, midwifery or the allied health professions has been discussed extensively in the literature. Since RCTs are considered superior in providing evidence of the effectiveness of health interventions, the question which has remained unanswered is: if evidence produced by other research designs is inferior does it mean that those interventions not evaluated by RCTs are also of inferior quality?

Although the debates about the value of RCTs and qualitative research have sometimes been polarised, there is abundant recognition that nurses are prepared to use the most appropriate methods to study nursing phenomena. The increase in the number of publications in nursing journals of studies using a combination of methods attest to the willingness to be eclectic rather than dogmatic.

Medical treatments such as drugs, surgical interventions or the use of diagnostic and screening equipment, can to some extent be studied by means of RCTs. The more the number of confounding variables, the less easy it is to control or to account for them. With RCTs the less involvement professionals and researchers have with an intervention, the more likely the results will be attributed to the intervention itself than to other factors. Thus there are fewer variables to control if the treatment consists of patients taking a particular drug. On the other hand, a nursing intervention such as 'giving information to patients prior to discharge' cannot be as neatly packaged as can tablets or injections. The number of confounding variables involved in the 'information giving' session may be difficult to control or to account for, if an RCT is carried out.

The more control researchers exert over variables (which may work with or against the experimental intervention) the less the experiment resembles the real situations in which health professionals work. Closs and Cheater (1999) explain that 'depending on the aim of the research, less tightly controlled research designs produce findings of a different nature which may be equally valuable'. Thus quasi-experiment and single-case designs also have the potential to produce evidence for some nursing interventions. Mulhall (1998) points out that 'different questions require different designs and no single design has precedence over another, rather the design must fit the particular research question'. For example, comparing various ways in which cannula sites are cleansed and dressed to find out how they affect infection rates may be appropriate for an RCT (Mulhall, 1998). Rycroft-Malone et al. (2004) suggest a broader definition of evidence which includes research, professional knowledge/clinical experience, 'local' data and information, and patient experience and preferences.

RCTs, like other research approaches, have their strengths and limitations. What some have found objectionable is the pressure for practitioners to produce their evidence though RCTs and the downgrading of other forms of knowledge and evidence. Others see evidence-based practice with its emphasis on RCTs as an opportunity for nurses to use the experimental design to evaluate many of their practices. Although the prominence of quantitative approaches in the early years seemed to have been replaced by a preference for qualitative approaches, nursing research as a whole seems to be pluralistic in its use of methodologies. It is important, given the variety and complexity of nursing practice involving both technical and interactional activities, that researchers do not become entrenched in their preferred positions, refuse to listen to other viewpoints and impose their views on others. If evidence-based practice is perceived as an attempt to define for nurses what constitutes 'evidence' and 'effectiveness' of nursing practice, then its potential benefits to nursing will not be fully realised.

Implications of evidence-based practice for nursing

Nurses share some of the same problems as other health professionals. Variations in nursing practice are common and research utilisation is not happening on a significant scale. Nurses represent the largest group of health professionals throughout the world and spend considerably more time with patients than any other health professional group. As a profession, nursing must build its body of knowledge on solid grounds. This knowledge should be used to underpin the decisions which nurses take.

One – perhaps unintended – consequence of evidence-based practice is that it has highlighted the poor quality of a significant number of studies, and the lack of research in some clinical areas. Systematic reviews can be used as a tool to justify claims for funding underresearched areas.

Evidence-based practice has implications for the education and training of nurses. The skills to formulate clinical questions, search and appraise the literature, disseminate and implement evidence are crucial. This poses a challenge for curriculum planners and teachers and has implications for resources – in particular, for access to information technology. Nursing research is still at an early stage of its development and the challenge it faces worldwide is enormous. In the UK, nursing research came last out of 69 units of assessment in the 1996 Research Assessment Exercise (RAE) and last again in 2001. The RAE is a form of 'audit' which grades research performance over a number of years. Subsequent government funding for research is based on the rating awarded to individual disciplines.

Bradshaw (2000) concluded that Britain has a lack of the necessary scholarly traditions to fully embrace evidence-based practice. In practical terms there are insufficient nurses equipped to evaluate what evidence is available, let alone generate new evidence about the outcomes of practice. This is indeed a serious handicap which needs to be overcome through better education and training. But this does not mean that evidence-based practice can be ignored.

Before the advent of the evidence-based practice movement nurses, in some countries at least, began the long road towards making the profession research based. Given the nature of nursing and the knowledge required for nursing practice, it is unlikely that nurses would adopt the medical definition of evidence-based practice, with its heavy emphasis on systematic reviews and RCTs. The challenge for nursing is to take what it finds useful from it, while developing its own body of knowledge using a range of approaches. The strength of nursing research resides in its openness to different research and development methodologies. To impose a medical model of practice development on nursing will indeed be a retrograde step.

SUMMARY

Summary and conclusion

In this chapter we have traced the emergence of evidence-based practice as a movement whose objective is to revolutionise the basis on which clinical and other decisions are made. Its conceptual, political, ethical and economic implications have been discussed.

The reaction of nurses to evidence-based practice has ranged from cautious welcome to outright rejection. The nature of nursing and nursing knowledge does not seem to fit neatly into (what is perceived as) the medical model of evidence-based practice. Nursing research draws from a range of methodologies including, but not relying solely upon, the RCT.

What the evidence-based practice movement will achieve and how long it will last are questions that the future will answer. What is known, however, is that it has revolutionised the way evidence is perceived and its importance in clinical practice. The production, review, appraisal and dissemination of evidence has become a science in itself. It is likely that it will continue to develop as an important resource for health professionals in their daily work. Whether it reduces variation, ineffective practice and saves money on a significant scale remains to be seen. The future of the evidence-based practice movement will, no doubt, depend on evidence of its effectiveness in achieving the objectives set in the UK R&D strategy. Ironically, given the complexity of the NHS, it is hardly likely that the RCT will be the choice design for providing this evidence.

References

Barnett D (2001) Clinical effectiveness and cost effectiveness of zanamivir (Relenza): translating the evidence into clinical practice: a National Institute for Clinical Excellence view. *Philosophical Transactions of the Royal Society B*, **356**:1899–1903.

Bonnell C (1999) Evidence-based nursing: a stereotyped view of quantitative and experimental research could work against professional autonomy and authority. *Journal of Advanced Nursing*, **30**, 1:18–23.

Bradshaw P L (2000) Evidence-based practice in nursing – the current state of play in Britain. *Journal of Nursing Management*, **8**:313–16.

Briggs A (1972) *Report on the Committee on Nursing* (The Briggs Report), Cmnd 5115 (London: HMSO).

Centre for Reviews and Dissemination (2001) *Undertaking Systematic Reviews of Research on Effectiveness*, CRD Report no. 4, 2nd edn (York: University of York).

Clarke J B (1999) Evidence-based practice: a retrograde step? The importance of pluralisms in evidence generation for the practice of health care. *Journal of Advanced Nursing*, **8**:89–94.

Clemence M L (1998) Evidence-based physiotherapy: seeking the unattainable. *British Journal of Therapy and Rehabilitation*, **5**, 5:257–60.

Closs S J and Cheater F M (1999) Evidence for nursing practice: a clarification of the issues. *Journal of Advanced Nursing*, **30**, 1:10–17.

Cochrane A L (1972) *Effectiveness and Efficiency: Random Reflections on Health Services* (London: The Nuffield Provincial Hospitals Trust).

Colyer H and Kamath P (1999) Evidence-based practice: A philosophical and political analysis: some matters for consideration by professional practitioners. *Journal of Advanced Nursing*, **29**, 1:188–93.

Crombie I K and Davies H T O (1998) Beyond health outcomes: the advantages of measuring process. *Journal of Evaluation in Clinical Practice*, **4**, 1:31–8.

Cullum N (1998) Evidence-based practice. *Nurse Management*, **5**, 3:32–5.

Department of Health (2000) *The Government's Expenditure Plans 2000–01*. Cm 4603 (London: Stationery Office).

Department of Health NHS Executive (1995) *Research and Development: Towards an Evidence-based Health Service*, Information Pack (London: Department of Health).

Diamond J (1998) *C – Because Cowards Get Cancer Too* (London: Vermilion).

DiCenso A, Cullum N and Ciliska D (2002) Evidence-based nursing: 4 years down the road. *Evidence-Based Nursing*, **5**:4–5.

Driscoll M (2003) Learning to live again. *Sunday Times*, 2 February 2003, p. 19.

Drummond M (1995) The United Kingdom National Health Service Reforms: where are we now? *Australian Health Review*, **18**, 1:28–42.

Emmerson C, Frayne C and Goodman A (2000) *Pressures in UK Healthcare: Challenges for the NHS* (London: The Institute for Fiscal Studies).

Estabrooks C A (1998) Will evidence-based nursing practice make practice perfect? *Canadian Journal of Nursing Research*, **30**, 1:15–36.

Estabrooks C A (1999) Mapping the research utilization field in nursing. *Canadian Journal of Nursing Research*, **31**, 1:53–72.

Evans D (2003) Hierarchy of evidence: a framework for ranking evidence evaluating healthcare interventions. *Journal of Clinical Nursing*, **12**:77–84.

Evidence-based Medicine Working Group (1992) Evidence based medicine: a new approach to teaching the practice of medicine. *Journal of the American Medical Association*, **268**, 17:2420–5.

French P (1999) The development of evidence-based nursing. *Journal of Advanced Nursing*, **29**, 1:72–8.

Gerrish K and Clayton J (1998) Improving clinical effectiveness through an evidence-based approach: meeting the challenge for nursing in the United Kingdom. *Nursing Administration Quarterly*, **22**, 4:55–65.

Goode C J and Piedalue F (1999) Evidence-based clinical practice. *Journal of Nursing Administration*, **29**, 6:15–21.

Hart J T (1997) What evidence do we need for evidence based medicine? *Journal of Epidemiology and Community Health*, **51**:623–9.

Haynes B (1995) Letter to the editor. *The Lancet*, **346**:1171.

Hicks C and Hennessy D (1997) Mixed messages in nursing research: their contribution to the persisting hiatus between evidence and practice. *Journal of Advanced Nursing*, **25**:597–601.

Hope T (1995) Editorial: Evidence based medicine and ethics. *Journal of Medical Ethics*, **21**:259–60.

House of Lords Select Committee on Science and Technology (1988) *Priorities and Medical Research* (London: HMSO).

Hunter D J (1996) Rationing and evidence based medicine. *Journal of Evaluation in Clinical Practice*, **2**, 1:5–8.

Ingersoll G L (2000) Evidence-based nursing: what it is and what it isn't. *Nursing Outlook*, **48**, 4:151–2.

Jaglal S B, Sherry P G, Chua D and Schatzker J (1997) Temporal trends and geographic variations in surgical treatment of femoral neck fractures. *Journal of Trauma-Injury Infection and Critical Care*, **43**, 3:475–479.

Kirk S (1996) The NHS research and developmnt strategy. In: M R Baker and S Kirk (eds), *Research and Development for the NHS: Evidence, Evaluation and Effectiveness* (Oxford: Radcliffe Medical Press).

Kitson A (1997) Using evidence to demonstrate the value of nursing. *Nursing Standard*, **11**, 28:34–9.

Kunkler I H (1997) Variations in the management of cancer in the NHS: a legitimate cause for concern. *Journal of Evaluation in Clinical Practice*, **3**, 3:173–7.

Lang N M (1999) Discipline-based approaches to evidence-based practice: a view from nursing. *Journal on Quality Improvement*, **25**, 10:539–44.

Lavery B A (1995) Skin care during radiotherapy: a survey of UK practice. *Clinical Oncology*, 7, 3:184–7.

Lewis J A (1996) Editorial: Statistics and statisticians in the Regulation of Medicines. *Journal of the Royal Statistical Society*, **159**: 359–65.

Lloyd-Smith W (1997) Evidence-based practice and occupational therapy. *British Journal of Occupational Therapy*, **60**, 11:474–8.

Lynn M (1999) Drug wars. *Sunday Times*, 10 October 1999, p. 5.

Marks W (1992) Physical restraints in the practice of medicine. *Archives of Internal Medicine*, **152**, 11:2203–6.

Marshall T (1995) Letter to the Editor. *The Lancet*, **346**:1171–2.

McMaster University Evidence-Based Medicine Group (1996) Evidence based medicine: The new paradigm [on-line] http://www.hiru.mcmaster.ca/ebm.

McQuaide M (1996) The internal markets of the British National Health Service: prospects and problems. *American Journal of the Medical Sciences*, **311**, 3:122–9.

Millar B (1998) Failing the acid test. *Health Service Journal*, 26 March 1998, pp. 24–7.

Mitchell G J (1999) Evidence-based practice: critique and alternative view. *Nursing Science Quarterly*, **12**, 1:30–7.

Mulhall A (1998) Nursing, research, and the evidence. *Evidence-Based Nursing*, **1**, 1:4–6.

Mulrow C (1995) Rationale for systematic reviews. In: I Chalmers and D Altman D (eds), *Systematic Reviews* (London: B M J Publishing Group), pp. 1–8.

Munson K A, Bare D E, Hoath S and Visscher M O (1999) A survey of skin care practices for premature low birth infants. *Journal of Neonatal Nursing*, **18**, 3:25–31.

National Health Service Executive (1996) *Clinical Guidelines: Using Clinical Guidelines to Improve Patient Care within the NHS* (Leeds: National Health Service Executive).

Parish C (2000) MS drug guidelines ignore patients, nurses tell NICE. *Nursing Standard*, **14**, 50:5.

Peckham M (1991) Research and Development for the National Health Service. *The Lancet*, **338**:367–71.

Polychronis A, Miles A and Bentley P (1996a) Evidence-based medicine: reference? Dogma? Neologism? New orthodoxy? *Journal of Evaluation in Clinical Practice*, **2**, 1:1–3.

Polychronis A, Miles A and Bentley P (1996b) The protagonists of 'evidence-based medicine': arrogant, seductive and controversial. *Journal of Evaluation in Clinical Practice*, **2**, 1:9–12.

Rafferty A (1996) *The Politics of Nursing Knowledge* (London: Routledge).

Rafferty A and Traynor M (1997) Quality and quantity in research policy for nursing. *Nursing Times Research*, **2**, 1:16–27.

Rolfe G (1999) Insufficient evidence: the problems of evidence-based nursing. *Nurse Education Today*, 19:433–42.

Royal College of Nursing (1996) *The RCN Clinical Effectiveness Initiative: A Strategic Framework* (London: Royal College of Nursing).

Rycroft-Malone J, Seers K, Titchen A, Harvey G, Kitson A and McCormack B (2004) What counts as evidence in evidence-based practice? *Journal of Advanced Nursing*, **47**, 1:81–90.

Sackett D L (1995) Evidence-based medicine (letter). *The Lancet*, **346**:1171.

Sackett D L, Rosenberg W M C, Muir Gray J A, Haynes R B and Richardson W S (1996) Evidence based medicine: what it is and what it isn't. *British Medical Journal*, **312**:71–2.

Salvage J (1998) Evidence-based practice: a mixture of motives? *Nursing Times*, **94**, 23:61–2.

Smith R (1992) Editorial: The ethics of ignorance. *Journal of Medical Ethics*, **18**:117–18.

Taylor M C (1997) What is evidence-based practice? *British Journal of Occupational Therapy*, **60**, 11:470–4,

Timmins N (1995) *The Five Grants: A Biography of the Welfare State* (London: Harper)

Webb A M C and Hannaford P C (1996) Editorial: Opinions, evidence and good clinical practice. *The British Journal of Family Planning*, **22**:163–4.

Glossary

abstract   A brief summary usually found at the beginning of an article. It states briefly the aim of the study, the design (including the method/s, sample/s and sampling) and the main relevant findings.

accidental sample   It is a sample of convenience in which only those units which are available have a chance of being selected.

action research   Action research involves using research in order to plan, implement and evaluate change in practice.

alternate-form test   Alternate-form reliability test (also known as equivalence) is carried out by asking questions in different forms and comparing the data.

anonymity   In research the term is used to describe circumstances when respondents remain unknown to the researcher. It happens mainly when questionnaires are filled and posted by respondents without revealing their names.

attrition   The loss of participants to a study due to mortality, or to withdrawal for other reasons such as refusals, too ill to continue or moved away.

audit trail   This is the process used by qualitative researchers to track and record their crucial decisions and actions which could have influenced the collection of data and the interpretation of findings.

bias   Factors, other than those investigated, which may influence the findings of a study.

bracketing   It is the suspension of the researcher's preconceptions, prejudices and beliefs so that they do not interfere with or influence her description and interpretation of the respondent's experience.

case study   Case studies focus on specific populations (usually small) and events which are bounded by time and well defined. In-depth information can be collected by using a variety of methods.

central tendency   This term refers to 'average' or 'typical' scores, not extreme ones. The statistical measures of central tendency are the mode, median and mean.

clinical effectiveness   The most efficient and cost-effective way to assess, organise, deliver and evaluate care and treatment in order to achieve optimum benefit for clients.

cluster random sample A cluster or multi-stage random sample involves sampling the clusters before drawing samples from the selected clusters.

cluster randomisation The random allocation of clusters (e.g. hospitals or schools) instead of individuals, to the control or experimental groups.

coding The process of breaking up the data into segments to make sense of them.

comparative studies The purpose of a comparative study is to compare policies, practices, events and people.

conceptual/theoretical framework The use of concepts and/or theories to underpin a study.

confidentiality This refers to the assurance given by researchers that data collected from participants will not be revealed to others who are not connected with the study.

confounders These are variables which can work with or against the independent variable to produce an outcome in an experiment. It is difficult sometimes to separate the effects of each of these variables on the outcome.

construct validity This refers to the extent to which the questionnaire or scale reflects the construct which is being assessed or measured.

content validity The degree to which the questions or items in a questionnaire or observation schedule can adequately study or measure the phenomenon being researched.

control To account for the effect of unwanted variables, researchers introduce control in their experiments by making sure that another group (control group), similar in all respects (except for the intervention) to the experimental group, takes part in the experiment. Control is also exercised by the objective allocation of subjects to groups.

correlation The statistical association between two or more variables.

covert observation This is a form of participant observation in which researchers do not divulge that they are making observations for research purposes and when 'participants' are not aware they are being observed as part of a research study. Covert observation has serious ethical implications.

credibility The extent to which the findings of a study reflect the experience and perceptions of those who provided the data. They must also be credible to those who subsequently read the report.

criterion-related, concurrent and predictive validity A questionnaire's criterion-related validity can be assessed by comparing the data collected with data from other sources. When other such data are currently available, the concurrent validity of the questionnaire can thus be assessed. Predictive validity refers to data which may be available in the future and which may confirm the validity of the data from the present questionnaire.

data   The information collected by researchers during the course of a study.

database   A register of published materials, mostly in terms of articles, books, reports and audio-visuals.

deduction   Deduction is the process of knowledge acquisition by the formulation of a theory or hypothesis and the collection of data thereafter in order to support or reject it.

Delphi technique   This is a form of survey which consists of gathering the views of experts, normally individually, on a particular issue. It involves a number of rounds during which feedback is provided to respondents to allow them to reconsider their initial opinion, if necessary, for the purpose of reaching a consensus.

dependent and independent variables   Anything which varies can be called a variable. Variables can be dependent or independent. In the statement, 'lack of exercise causes constipation', the independent variable is 'lack of exercise' and the dependent one is 'constipation'. It is the relationship between variables which determines whether they are dependent or independent, not the variables themselves. In the statement, 'the degree of constipation determines one's level of well-being', constipation is the independent variable.

descriptive and correlational studies   In descriptive studies researchers describe phenomena about which little is normally known. From the data collected, patterns or trends may emerge and possible links between variables can be observed but the emphasis is on the description of phenomena. In correlational studies the primary aim is to examine or explore relationships between variables.

descriptive statistics   This type of statistics answers descriptive questions and does so by such measures as frequency, central tendency and dispersion.

determinism   It is the belief that phenomena have causes and effects and that experiments can find the answer to them.

discourse analysis   It is an approach based on the analysis of discourse (verbal, non-verbal and written communication). The purpose of this type of analysis is to uncover the values, meanings and intentions in interactions between people.

dispersion   To describe how scores vary, measures of dispersion such as standard deviation, variance, range and quartiles are used.

dissemination   The communication of research findings in a range of formats including published papers, conference presentations, reports and seminars.

ethnography   This is a research approach developed by anthropologists who go and live among the people they study. Ethnographers study human behaviour as it is influenced or mediated by the culture in which it takes place.

evaluative studies An evaluative study is normally carried out when a researcher wants to find out if, how and to what extent the objectives of particular activities, policies or practices have been or are being met.

evidence-based practice Practice based on the most valid and reliable research findings, the judgement and experience of practitioners and the views of clients.

explanatory trials This is an experimental design which is used to study the efficacy of interventions, under ideal circumstances, in order to gain a scientific understanding of interventions and their effects.

extraneous and confounding variables Extraneous variables are those which researchers are aware of at the start of the study but do not seek to study. They need to be controlled in order that they do not interfere with the experiment. Confounding variables are extraneous variables which researchers fail to or cannot control but which may work in the same or opposite direction with the independent variable. Sometimes the two terms are used interchangeably.

face validity Face validity is one form of content validity. It involves giving the questionnaire to anyone, not necessarily an expert on the subject, who can 'on the face of it' assess whether the questions or items reflect the phenomenon being studied.

factorial design This is a design (either survey or trial) in which the effect of one or more independent variables can be tested in the same study.

feminist research Research carried out by women, for women and on topics of relevance to women.

fittingness The degree to which the findings of qualitative studies 'fit' the reality of those who wish to use them.

focused group interview This can be described as interactions between one or more researchers and more than one respondent for the purpose of collecting data on a specific topic.

frequency This involves describing scores in absolute numbers, percentages and proportion.

grounded theory This term was coined by Glaser and Strauss (1967) to mean an inductive approach to research whereby hypotheses and theories emerge out of, or are 'grounded' in, data.

hypothesis A statement which normally specifies the relationship between variables.

hypothetico-deductive An approach whereby hypotheses and theories are put to the test by the deductive (see above) process during the course of research, especially experiments.

induction   This means that after a large number of observations have been made, it is possible to draw conclusions or theorise about particular phenomena.

inferential statistics   Inferential statistics describe correlational or casual links between variables.

informed consent   The process of agreeing to take part in a study based on access to all relevant and easily digestible information about what participation means, in particular, in terms of harms and benefits.

internal and external validity of experiments   Internal validity is the extent to which changes, if any, in the dependent variable can be said to have been caused by the independent variable alone. External validity is the extent to which the findings of an experiment can be applied or generalised to other similar populations or settings.

interpretivism   It is the belief that people continuously make sense of the world around them and different people may have different interpretations of the same phenomena. Interpretivism is a blanket term for a collection of approaches broadly called 'qualitative' that share an opposition to the logical positivists' notion (see positivism below) of studying humans as objects or particles.

interval scale   The numbers allocated to variables signify the order or hierarchy of these variables and they indicate the precise distance between them.

intervention/manipulation   The term intervention is used in an experiment to describe the independent variable whose effect the researcher is trying to assess or measure. Examples of interventions include medications, information programmes and therapies. By giving different medications (or the same medication in varying amounts) to different groups, the researcher is in fact manipulating the intervention, hence the term 'manipulation'.

intra- and inter-observer reliability   Intra-observer reliability is the consistency with which the same observer records the same behaviours in the same way on different occasions. Inter-observer reliability is the consistency with which two or more observers record the same behaviours in the same way on different occasions.

intuition   A form of knowing and behaving not apparently based on rational reasoning.

longitudinal and cross-sectional studies   A longitudinal study is one in which data are collected at intervals in order to capture any change which may take place over time. The same sample (cohort) is usually 'followed up' over a period of time. In cross-sectional studies, data are collected from different groups of people who are at different stages in their experience of the same phenomenon.

matched-pairs Matched-pairs allocation takes place when researchers try to pair a subject in the experiment with another in the control group, in terms of characteristics such as age, gender, illness condition, and so on. Usually researchers enter a subject in one of the two groups and allocate someone else with similar characteristics to the other group.

mean The mean is the arithmetical average of a set of values.

median The median is the mid-point value when the scores are arranged in ascending order.

meta-analysis This is a form of research on research. In its pure form it involves the statistical analysis of research findings in order to arrive at one final finding.

mode The mode is the most frequent value.

molar and molecular These are observation units or categories. Molar units are broad and sometimes abstract. Molecular units are more detailed and precise.

nominal group technique A structured meeting (led by a researcher or facilitator) designed to seek the views of a group of participants on a particular topic and to seek a consensus or agreement by asking them to rank or rate their responses.

nominal scale In a nominal scale the numbers allocated to variables have no value and are only used to label them.

non-respondents All those included in a survey who do not return the questionnaire or do not answer some questions on the questionnaire.

normal distribution In a normal distribution of scores most of the scores cluster around the mean and the extreme scores are few, and are (more or less) equally distributed above or below the mean.

null hypothesis This is the hypothesis which is tested in experimental research. It is stated in a format suggesting that no correlation (or link) exists between two or more variables. Data are collected in order to reject or confirm the hypothesis.

nursing research All research which pertains to the organisation, delivery, uses and outcomes of nursing care. It therefore includes research on clients, nurses, resources and nursing practice.

objectivity This term is used in research approaches in which researchers remain detached from respondents by not letting their subjective views influence the data they collect and analyse.

observer's effect Observer's effect, reactivity and the Hawthorne effect are terms used to describe changes in the participants' 'usual' or 'normal behaviour' as a reaction to being observed for research purposes.

operational definition   The process of communicating precisely the meaning of concepts and the ways in which they can be observed and recorded.

ordinal scale   In an ordinal scale, the numbers allocated to variables signify the order or hierarchy of these variables, but cannot specify the exact difference between them.

paradigm   A research paradigm can be described as the beliefs and values which particular research communities share about the type of phenomena which can or cannot be researched and the methodologies to be adopted.

Pearson product-moment correlation coefficient   A statistical test to measure the association between interval-ratio variables.

phenomenology   This is a philosophical theory about the way humans experience consciousness. The phenomenological approach focuses on individuals' interpretations of their lived experiences and the ways in which they express them.

placebo   A placebo is a substance of no pharmacological or therapeutic property which resembles, in all physical characteristics, the intervention used in the experimental group. Placebos are used in experiments to overcome the possible suggestive effect of new interventions.

population   The units (people, events, objects or institutions) from which data are collected.

positivism   A movement in the social sciences which evolved in the eighteenth century as a critique of the supernatural and metaphysical interpretations of phenomena. It is based on the belief that the methods of the natural sciences can be used to study human behaviour as well. It is the belief that only what can be observed by the human senses can be called facts. Logical positivism is one branch of positivism which makes use of mathematics in the interpretation of research findings.

postmodernism   This is an intellectual movement (towards the end of the 1950s) which rejects the notion of 'truth' and 'reality' as objective, and rationalism as the only way to think. Postmodernists believe that knowledge is co-created (by participants and researchers).

primary and secondary sources   Original publications are primary sources while publications which report, quote from or comment on original works are known as secondary sources.

probability and non-probability samples   With probability samples, every unit in the sample frame has a more than zero chance (known in advance) of being selected. Non-probability samples are made up of units whose chances of selection are not known.

prospective, retrospective and historical studies   A prospective study is one in which the researcher investigates a current phenomenon by seeking data which are to be collected in the future. A retrospective study relies on information from the past in order to understand a current problem. Both prospective and retrospective studies have a 'foot' in the present. A historical study does not need to have a link with the present. It seeks to understand phenomena embedded in the past.

purposive or judgemental sample   This involves making a judgement or relying on the judgement of others in selecting a sample. Researchers use their knowledge of potential participants to recruit them. The purpose of this type of sampling is to obtain as many perspectives of the phenomenon as possible.

qualitative interview   This is a broad term to denote a family of interviews with varying degrees of flexibility for the purpose of studying phenomena from the perspective of respondents.

quasi-experiment   Such an experiment does not meet all three components of a true experiment, but it must have an intervention. A quasi-experiment may or may not have a control group – and if it does, it does not have randomisation.

quota sample   When different groups of people take part in a study, the researcher allocates the number in each group beforehand and then uses non-probability sampling methods to select the units.

randomisation   The process of allocating subjects to experimental and control groups by an objective method.

randomised controlled trial (RCT)   These are true experiments which are normally carried out in clinical practice.

range   This is the lowest and highest value. Sometimes it is expressed as the difference between these two values.

ratio scale   A ratio scale is an interval scale with an absolute zero. The numbers on a ratio scale tell us not only the amount by which they differ but also by how many times.

reductionism   It means reducing complex phenomena to simple units that can be observed or recorded.

reflexivity   It is the continuous process of reflection by researchers of how their own values, perceptions, behaviour or presence and those of the respondents can affect the data they collect.

replication   This refers to the process of repeating the same study in the same or similar settings using the same method(s) with the same or equivalent sample(s).

research   It is the study of phenomena by rigorous and systematic collection and analysis of data. It is a private enterprise made public for the purpose of exposing it to the scrutiny of others, to allow for replication, verification or falsification, where possible.

research awareness   The term has three main components: the adoption of a questioning stance to one's practice, knowledge of existing research and the ability to use it.

research design   This is a plan of how, when and where data are to be collected and analysed.

research questions   Research involves asking questions. The term research question is used mainly to describe the broad question which is set at the start of a study. Some researchers may prefer to state aims, objectives or hypotheses instead.

research-based practice   It is a term to denote the use of research to inform and justify one's practice.

sample and population   A proportion or subset of the population is known as a sample. A population can be defined as the total number of units (such as individuals, organisations, events or artefacts) from which data can potentially be collected.

sample frame   A list of all the units of the target population from which random samples are normally drawn.

semi-quartile, lower-quartile and upper-quartile   The semi-quartile ranges are scores which fall below and above the median. The lower quartile is the midpoint between the lowest value and the median. The upper quartile is the midpoint between the highest value and the median.

semi-structured interview   In this type of interview respondents are all asked the questions from a predetermined list but there is flexibility in the phrasing and sequence of the questions.

simple random sample   Each unit in the sample frame has an equal chance of selection.

single-blind and double-blind trials   A single-blind trial is when either the subjects or the researcher is unaware which group is control or experimental. A design in which both subjects and researchers are unaware of which intervention each group is receiving is called a double-blind trial.

snowball sample   In this type of sampling, the first respondent refers someone they know to the study, who in turn refers someone they know until the researcher has an adequate sample.

split-half test   This test (of reliability) involves dividing or splitting the instrument (normally a scale) into two equal halves and finding out if their scores are similar.

standard deviation   The standard deviation is an average deviation of the scores from the mean.

stratified random sample A stratified random sample is drawn by separating the units in the sample frame into strata (layers), according to the variables the researcher believes are important for inclusion in the sample, before drawing simple random samples from each stratum.

structured interview In this type of interview, researchers ask all the questions as they are formulated on an interview schedule. They have some flexibility to rephrase the question but cannot alter the content or sequence of the questions.

structured observation A structured observation is one in which aspects of the phenomenon to be observed are decided in advance (predetermined) and a schedule or checklist is constructed (structured) and the same information is required of all observations (standardised).

survey A survey is a research design which aims to obtain descriptive and correlational data usually from large populations, usually by questionnaires, interviews and to a lesser extent, by observations.

systematic random sample A systematic random sample is drawn by choosing units on a list at intervals decided by the researcher in advance. Every unit on the list has an equal chance of selection.

systematic review This is one form of literature review in which all available research studies on a particular topic are identified, analysed and synthesised.

target population The target or study population is the population which meets the criteria for inclusion stipulated by the researcher.

test–retest Test–retest involves administering the questionnaire to the same respondents on two or more occasions and comparing their responses for the purpose of assessing the reliability of the questionnaire.

theory In its basic form a theory is an explanation of how and why a phenomenon occurs. Scientific theories are more precise in that they specify relationships between variables.

theory-generating research The aim of this type of theory is to generate hypotheses and/or theories. From the data collected researchers identify themes, patterns or relationships.

theory-testing research The aim of this type of research is to test particular hypotheses and/or theories. Researchers set hypotheses (often derived from theories) and collect data to confirm, modify or reject them.

time and event sampling These types of sampling are used mostly in studies which use observation. In time sampling, the sampling unit is time instead of people. Researchers may decide to sample the first 15 minutes of every hour of the day instead of observing the whole day. When 'events' are the focus of a study, the events become the units from which a sample is drawn.

true experiment In research terms a true experiment is characterised by three components: intervention (manipulation of), control and randomisation.

validity and reliability Validity refers to the degree or extent to which a questionnaire, interview or observation schedule and other methods of data collection studies or measures the phenomenon under investigation. Reliability refers to the consistency of a particular method in measuring or observing the same phenomena.

volunteer sample It is a sample of convenience over which the researcher has little control but instead is dependent on the sample volunteering to take part.

within-subject and between-subject designs When the same group of subjects receive the usual intervention and the experimental intervention alternately, the design is described as within-subject or cross-over. A between-subject design (or parallel groups) is one in which different subjects constitute the control and the experimental groups.

Index